APR 27 2011

NCLEX-PN®

Strategies, Practice, and Review

SIXTH EDITION

RELATED TITLES FOR NURSES

Test Preparation Flashcards

NCLEX-RN® Medications in a Box

Career

Change Your Career: Nursing as Your New Profession
First Year Nurse
How to Survive Clinical
Math for Nurses
Medical Terms for Nurses
Spanish for Nurses
Your Career in Nursing

Kaplan Voices: Nurses Series

Reflections on Doctors: Nurses' Stories about Physicians and Surgeons
Meditations on Hope: Nurses' Stories about Motivation and Inspiration
Final Moments: Nurses' Stories about Death and Dying
A Call to Nursing: Nurses' Stories about Challenge and Commitment
New Lives: Nurses' Stories about Caring for Babies
Lives in the Balances: Nurses' Stories from the ICU
Caring Beyond Borders: Nurses' Stories from Around the World

Memoir

Labor of Love: A Midwife's Memoir
Saving Lives: Why the Media's Portrayal of Nurses Puts Us All at Risk
Impaired: A Nurse's Story of Addiction and Recovery

SIXTH EDITION

NCLEX-PN

Strategies, Practice, and Review

Barbara J. Irwin, BSN, RN

Patricia A. Yock, BSN, RN, CRRN

Judith A. Burckhardt, PhD, RN

KAPLAN

PUBLISHING

New York

© 2011 by Kaplan, Inc.

Published by Kaplan Publishing, a division of Kaplan, Inc.
395 Hudson Street
New York, NY 10014

Printed in the United States of America

10 9 8 7 6 5 4 3 2 1

ISBN: 978-1-60714-828-9

Kaplan Publishing books are available at special quantity discounts to use for sales promotions, employee premiums, or educational purposes. For more information or to purchase books, please call the Simon & Schuster special sales department at 866-506-1949.

CONTENTS

FOR ANY TEST CHANGES OR LATE-BREAKING DEVELOPMENTS

kaptest.com/publishing

The material in this book is current at the time of publication. However, the National Council of State Boards of Nursing may have instituted changes in the test after this book was published. Be sure to carefully read the materials you receive when you register for the test. If there are any important late-breaking developments—or any changes or corrections to the Kaplan test preparation materials in this book—we will post that information online at *kaptest.com/publishing*.

FEEDBACK AND COMMENTS

kaplansurveys.com/books

We'd love to hear your comments and suggestions about this book. We invite you to fill out our online survey form at *kaplansurveys.com/books*. Your feedback is extremely helpful as we continue to develop high-quality resources to meet your needs.

ABOUT THE AUTHORS

BARBARA J. IRWIN, BSN, RN

Barbara Irwin is National Curriculum Director for Nursing Programs at Kaplan, Inc. She supervises development of the Kaplan courses for preparation for the NCLEX-RN® and NCLEX-PN exams for U.S. nursing students and international nurses, as well as integrated testing programs implemented by nursing schools. While tutoring students that had been unsuccessful on the NCLEX-RN exam, Irwin developed a series of innovative test-taking strategies that help students achieve success on this high-stakes test. She presents Strategy Seminars and Test-Taking Seminars for the NCLEX-RN to nursing school faculties and students nationwide. Irwin received her bachelor of science in nursing from the University of Oklahoma. Her professional background includes experience as a nursing educator and director of a home health agency.

PATRICIA A. YOCK, BSN, RN, CRRN

Patricia Yock is Director of the Practical Nursing Program at Front Range Community College, Boulder County Campus, Colorado, and continues as a consultant for Kaplan's Nursing Programs. She received a bachelor of science in nursing from Loyola University in Chicago. Her professional experience includes clinical nursing in varied settings from post-surgical care to comprehensive inpatient rehabilitation, and nursing education in diploma and practical nursing programs. Yock is certified in rehabilitation nursing and served as the nursing director for inpatient rehabilitation and transitional care units.

JUDITH A. BURCKHARDT, PHD, RN

Dr. Judith Burckhardt is Vice President of Strategic Development for the Kaplan University School of Nursing. She interacts with healthcare organizations and systems to develop strategic partnerships that advance the mission of the healthcare organization and the Kaplan University School of Nursing. After graduating from Loyola University in Chicago with a bachelor of science in nursing, she received a master's in education from Washington University and a doctorate in educational administration from the University of Nebraska, Lincoln. Her professional background includes many years of experience as an educator in diploma, A.D.N., and B.S.N. nursing programs. She has developed programs and materials to help prepare students for the NCLEX-RN and NCLEX-PN exams and has presented

NCLEX-RN exam preparation and career development seminars to students, nurses, and healthcare professionals in the United States and abroad. Burckhardt has also given item-writing workshops to nursing school faculties. She has written articles for nursing publications and has developed instructor-led continuing education programs for online delivery.

HOW TO USE THIS BOOK

STEP 1: Access Your Online Companion

Log on to *kaptest.com/booksonline* to access your online companion. You will be asked for a password derived from the text to access the online companion, so have your book available.

The online companion offers access to a 20-question sample of Kaplan's NCLEX-PN Question Bank. For more information and to order the full version of more than 1,000 questions, please visit *kaplannursing.com*. In addition to the Question Bank sample, you will be able to practice alternate format questions within a timed practice sample set and sign up for an Online Classroom Event. See "Sign up for an Online Classroom Event" for more details and to register.

STEP 2: Read Part 1

The chapters in Part 1 of this book contain a comprehensive, detailed strategy guide for each type of question on the NCLEX-PN exam. This information will teach you how to analyze each question and use your nursing knowledge to select the correct answer choice.

Chapter 12, Essentials for International Nurses, contains information on certification for graduates of foreign nursing schools, work visas, and programs that can help you prepare for the NCLEX-PN exam. This chapter also covers nursing practice in the United States, and includes practice questions with complete explanations designed to help you master NCLEX-PN exam-type questions on the important subject of nursing communication.

STEP 3: Take the Practice Test

Use the test in this book, complete with in-depth answer explanations, to prepare for the real NCLEX-PN exam. Take the test under timed conditions and then work through the explanations. Identify any areas of weakness, and use your remaining review time to address them, using the strategies outlined in this book. Note your strengths as well—these will help you on the test, and can give you a sense of confidence.

STEP 4: Register for the Exam

When you are prepared to take the NCLEX-PN exam, use the contact information and licensure requirements provided in Appendix D, State Licensing Requirements, in Part 3 to initiate the registration process. All of the steps you'll need to follow are contained in Chapter 10, The Licensure Process.

SIGN UP FOR AN ONLINE CLASSROOM EVENT

Kaplan's NCLEX-PN online classroom sessions are interactive, instructor-led NCLEX-PN prep lessons that you can participate in from anywhere you can access the Internet.

The online sessions are held in a state-of-the-art virtual classroom—actual lessons in real time, just like a physical classroom experience. Interact with your teacher and other class-mates using audio, instant chat, whiteboard, polling, and screen-sharing functionality. And just like courses at Kaplan centers, a NCLEX-PN online classroom session is led by an experienced Kaplan instructor.

To register for your NCLEX-PN online classroom session:

1. Go to *kaptest.com/booksonline* and sign up for the online companion. See "How to Use This Book" for more information on how to sign up.

2. Once you've signed up for the online companion, then sign in to your student home page and go to Your Course Syllabus.

3. In the All Sessions drop down menu, click on "Online Class Registration."

4. Click on "Access Your Online Classroom Event." A separate window will appear with registration instructions.

For upcoming NCLEX-PN online classroom events, please check your online companion for dates and times.

Please note: Registration begins one month before the session date. Be sure to sign up early, since spaces are reserved on a first-come, first-served basis.

PART 1

PREPARING FOR THE NCLEX-PN® EXAM

CHAPTER 1

OVERVIEW OF THE NCLEX-PN® EXAM

The NCLEX-PN® exam, is among other things, an endurance test, like a marathon. If you don't prepare properly, or approach it with confidence and rigor, you'll quickly lose your composure. Here is a sample, test-like question:

> A man had a permanent pacemaker implanted one year ago. He returns to the outpatient clinic because he thinks the pacemaker battery is malfunctioning. It is MOST important for the LPN/LVN to assess which of the following?
>
> 1. Abdominal pain, nausea, and vomiting
> 2. Wheezing on exertion, cyanosis, and orthopnea
> 3. Peripheral edema, shortness of breath, and dizziness
> 4. Chest pain radiating to the right arm, headache, and diaphoresis

As you can see, the style and content of the NCLEX-PN® exam is unique. It's not like any other exam you've ever taken, even in nursing school!

The content in this book was prepared by the experts on Kaplan's Nursing team, the world's largest provider of test prep courses for the NCLEX-PN® exam. By using Kaplan's proven methods and strategies, you will be able to take control of the exam, just as you have taken control of your nursing education and other preparations for your career in this incredibly challenging and rewarding field. The first step is to learn everything you can about the exam.

WHAT IS THE NCLEX-PN® EXAM?

NCLEX-PN® stands for *National Council Licensure Examination-Practical Nurse*. The *NCLEX-PN®* examination is administered by The National Council of State Boards of Nursing (NCSBN), whose members include the boards of nursing in each of the 50 states in the United States, the District of Columbia, and four U.S. territories: American Samoa, Guam, the Northern Mariana Islands, and the Virgin Islands. These boards have a mandate to protect the public from unsafe and ineffective nursing care, and each board has been given responsibility to regulate the practice of nursing in its respective state. In fact, the NCLEX-PN® exam is often referred to as "the Boards" or "State Boards."

The NCLEX-PN® exam has only one purpose: to determine if it is safe for you to begin practice as an entry-level practical/vocational nurse.

Why Must You Take the NCLEX-PN® Exam?

The NCLEX-PN® exam is prepared by the NCSBN. Each state requires that you pass this exam to obtain a license to practice as a practical/vocational nurse. The designation *licensed practical/vocational nurse* or *LPN/LVN* indicates that you have proven to your state board of nursing that you can deliver safe and effective nursing care. The NCLEX-PN® exam is a test of minimum competency and is based on the knowledge and behaviors that are needed for the entry-level practice of practical/vocational nursing. This exam tests not only your knowledge, but also your ability to make competent nursing decisions.

What Is Entry-Level Practice of Practical/Vocational Nursing?

In order to define *entry-level* practice of practical/vocational nursing, the National Council conducts a job-analysis study every three years to determine what entry-level nurses do on the job. The kinds of questions they investigate include: In which clinical settings does the beginning practical/vocational nurse work? What types of care do beginning practical/vocational nurses provide to their clients? What are their primary duties and responsibilities? Based on the results of this study, National Council adjusts the content and level of difficulty of the test to accurately reflect what is happening in the workplace.

What the NCLEX-PN® Exam Is *NOT*

It is not a test of achievement or intelligence. It is not designed for nurses who have years of experience. The questions do not involve high-tech clinical nursing or equipment. It is not predictive of your eventual success in the career of nursing. You will not be tested on all the content that you were taught in practical/vocational nursing school.

What Is a CAT?

CAT stands for *Computer Adaptive Test*. Each test is assembled interactively based on the accuracy of the candidate's response to the questions. This ensures that the questions you are answering are not "too hard" or "too easy" for your skill level. Your first question will be relatively easy; that is, below the level of minimum competency. If you answer that question correctly, the computer selects a slightly more difficult question. If you answer the first question incorrectly, the computer selects a slightly easier question (Figure 1). By continuing to do this as you answer questions, the computer is able to calculate your level of competence.

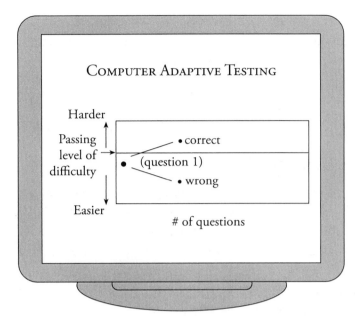

Figure 1

In a CAT, the questions are adapted to your ability level. The computer selects questions that represent all areas of nursing, as defined by the NCLEX-PN® test plan and by the level of item difficulty. Each question is self-contained, so that all of the information you need to answer a question is presented on the computer screen.

Taking the Exam

There is no time limit for each individual question. You have a maximum of five hours to complete the exam, but that includes the beginning tutorial, an optional 10-minute break after the first two hours of testing, and an optional break after an additional 90 minutes of testing. Everyone answers a minimum of 85 questions to a maximum of 205 questions. Regardless of the number of questions you answer, you are given 25 questions that are experimental. These questions, which are indistinguishable from the other questions on the test, are being tested for future use in NCLEX-PN® exams, and your answers do not count for or against you.

Your test ends when one of the following occurs:

- You have demonstrated minimum competency and answered the minimum number of questions (85) (Figure 2).
- You have demonstrated a lack of minimum competency and answered the minimum number of questions (85) (Figure 3).
- You have answered the maximum number of questions (205).
- You have used the maximum time allowed (five hours).

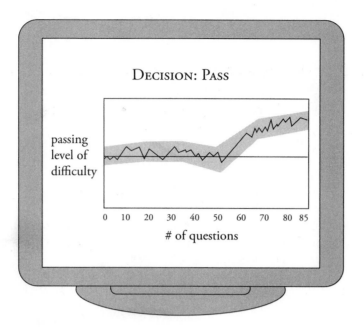

Figure 2

Try not to be concerned with the length of your test. In fact, you should plan on testing for five hours and seeing 205 questions. You are still in the game as long as the computer continues to give you test questions, so focus on answering them to the best of your ability.

Remember, every question counts. There is no warm-up time, so it is important for you to be ready to answer questions correctly from the very beginning. Concentration is also key. You need to give your best to each question because you do not know which will put you over the top.

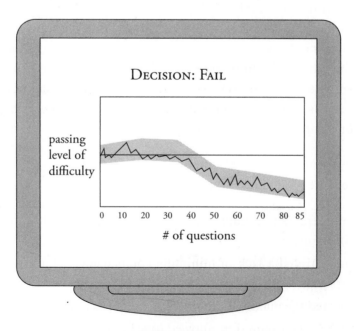

Figure 3

CONTENT OF THE NCLEX-PN® EXAM

The NCLEX-PN® exam is not divided into separate content areas. It tests integrated nursing content. Many nursing programs are based on the medical model. Students take separate medical, surgical, pediatric, psychiatric, and obstetric classes. On the NCLEX-PN® exam, all content is integrated.

Look at the following question.

> A woman with type 1 diabetes is returned to the recovery room one hour after an uneventful delivery of a 9 lb., 8 oz., baby boy. The nurse would expect the woman's blood sugar to do which of the following?
>
> 1. Change from 220 to 180 mg/dL.
> 2. Change from 110 to 80 mg/dL.
> 3. Change from 90 to 120 mg/dL.
> 4. Change from 100 to 140 mg/dL.

Is this an obstetrical question or a medical/surgical question? In order to select the correct answer, (2), you must consider the pathophysiology of diabetes along with the principles of labor and delivery. This is an example of an integrated question.

The NCLEX-PN® Exam Blueprint

The NCLEX-PN® exam is organized according to the framework "Meeting Client Needs." There are four major categories of client needs and six subcategories. This information is distributed by NCSBN, the developer of the NCLEX-PN® exam.

Client Need #1: Safe and Effective Care Environment

The first subcategory for this client need is **Coordinated Care**, which accounts for **13–19** percent of the questions on the exam. Nursing actions that are covered in this subcategory include:

- Advance directives
- Advocacy
- Client care assignments
- Client rights
- Collaboration with interdisciplinary team
- Concepts of management and supervision
- Confidentiality/information security
- Continuity of care

- Establishing priorities
- Ethical practice
- Information technology
- Informed consent
- Legal responsibilities
- Performance improvement (quality improvement)
- Referral process
- Resource management

Here is an example of a typical question from the Coordinated Care subcategory:

> The LPN/LVN knows that an assignment to which of the following clients would be appropriate?
>
> 1. A 56-year-old woman with emphysema scheduled to be discharged later today
> 2. A 41-year-old woman in traction with a fractured femur
> 3. A 34-year-old woman with low back pain scheduled for a myelogram in the afternoon
> 4. A newly diagnosed 43-year-old woman with type 1 diabetes mellitus

The correct answer is (2). This client is in stable condition and can be cared for by an LPN/LVN.

Here is another example of a Coordinated Care question:

> After receiving report from the RN, which of the following clients should the LPN/LVN see *FIRST*?
>
> 1. A 31-year-old woman refusing sucralfate (Carafate) before breakfast
> 2. A 40-year-old man with left-sided weakness asking for assistance to the commode
> 3. A 52-year-old woman complaining of chills who is scheduled for a cholecystectomy
> 4. A 65-year-old man with a nasogastric tube who had a bowel resection yesterday

The correct answer is (3). This is the least stable client.

The second subcategory for this client need is **Safety and Infection Control**, which accounts for **11–17** percent of the questions on the exam. Nursing actions that are covered in this subcategory include:

- Accident/error/injury prevention
- Emergency response plan
- Ergonomic principles
- Handling hazardous and infectious materials
- Home safety
- Internal and external disaster plans
- Medical and surgical asepsis
- Reporting of incident/event/irregular occurrence/variance
- Restraints and safety devices
- Safe use of equipment
- Security plan
- Standard precautions/transmission-based precautions/surgical asepsis

Here is an example of a question from the Safety and Infection Control subcategory:

> The physician orders amoxycillin 150 mg PO in oral suspension every 8 hours for a 3-year-old boy. The LPN/LVN enters the client's room to administer the medication and discovers that the boy does not have an identification bracelet. Which of the following should the LPN/LVN do?
>
> 1. Ask the parents at the child's bedside to state their child's name.
> 2. Ask the child to say his first and last name.
> 3. Have a coworker identify the child before giving the medication.
> 4. Hold the medication until an identification bracelet can be obtained.

The correct answer is (1). This action will allow the nurse to correctly identify the child and enable the nurse to give the medication on time.

Client Need #2: Health Promotion and Maintenance

This client need accounts for **7–13** percent of the questions on the exam. Nursing actions that are covered in this category include:

- Aging process
- Ante/intra/postpartum and newborn care
- Data collection techniques
- Developmental stages and transitions
- Health promotion/disease prevention
- High risk behaviors
- Lifestyle choices
- Self-care

It is important to understand that not everyone described in the questions will be sick, hospitalized, or in a long-term care facility. Some clients may be in a clinic or home-care setting. Some clients may not be sick at all. Wellness is an important concept on the NCLEX-PN® exam. It is necessary for a safe and effective practical/vocational nurse to know how to promote health and prevent disease.

The following is an example of a typical question from the Health Promotion and Maintenance category:

> The LPN/LVN in the outpatient clinic notes that the blood pressure for an 88-year-old client is 190/100. The LPN/LVN should take which of the following actions?
>
> 1. Report the blood pressure reading to the RN.
> 2. Wait 20 minutes and retake the blood pressure.
> 3. Use a different cuff and retake the blood pressure.
> 4. Position the client supine with feet elevated.

The correct answer is (1). The LPN/LVN is responsible for data collection and should report findings that are abnormal to the supervising RN. Immediate action should be taken, so (2) is incorrect. It is unnecessary to recheck the blood pressure using other equipment (3) or to position the client supine with feet elevated (4).

Client Need #3: Psychosocial Integrity

This client need accounts for **7–13** percent of the questions on the exam. Nursing actions that are covered in this category include:

- Abuse/neglect
- Behavioral management
- Chemical and other dependencies
- Coping mechanisms
- Crisis intervention
- Cultural awareness
- End-of-life concepts
- Grief and loss
- Mental health concepts
- Religious and spiritual influences on health
- Sensory/perceptual alterations
- Stress management
- Support systems

- Therapeutic communications
- Therapeutic environment

This is an example of a typical question from the Psychosocial Integrity category:

> A 50-year-old male client comes to the nurses' station and asks the LPN/LVN if he can go to the cafeteria to get something to eat. When told that his privileges do not include visiting the cafeteria, the client becomes verbally abusive. Which of the following approaches by the LPN/LVN would be *MOST* effective?
>
> 1. Tell the client to lower his voice, because he is disturbing the other clients.
> 2. Ask the client what he wants from the cafeteria and have it delivered to his room.
> 3. Calmly but firmly escort the client back to his room.
> 4. Assign a nursing assistant to accompany the client to the cafeteria.

The correct answer is (3). The nurse should not reinforce abusive behavior. Clients need consistent and clearly defined expectations and limits.

Client Need #4: Physiological Integrity

The first subcategory for this client need is **Basic Care and Comfort**, which accounts for **9–15** percent of the questions on the exam. Nursing actions that are covered in this subcategory include:

- Assistive devices
- Elimination
- Mobility/immobility
- Non-pharmacological comfort interventions
- Nutrition and oral hydration
- Personal hygiene
- Rest and sleep

The following question is representative of the Basic Care and Comfort subcategory:

> A cast is applied to a 9-month-old girl for the treatment of talipes equinovarus. Which of the following instructions is *MOST* essential for the LPN/LVN to give to the child's mother regarding her care?
>
> 1. Offer appropriate toys for her age.
> 2. Make frequent clinic visits for cast adjustment.
> 3. Provide an analgesic as needed.
> 4. Do circulatory checks of the casted extremity.

The correct answer is (4). A possible complication that can occur after cast application is impaired circulation. All of these answer choices might be included in family teaching, but checking the child's circulation is the highest priority.

The second subcategory for this client need is **Pharmacological Therapies** and accounts for **11–17** percent of the questions on the exam. Nursing actions that are covered in this subcategory include:

- Adverse effects/contraindications/side effects/interactions
- Dosage calculations
- Expected effects/outcomes
- Medication administration
- Pharmacological pain management

Try this question from the Pharmacological Therapies subcategory:

> The LPN/LVN notes the client is allergic to an ordered medication. Which of the following is the correct action by the LPN/LVN?
>
> 1. Administer the medication as the physician ordered it.
> 2. Administer the medication and closely observe the client.
> 3. Call the pharmacist to verify potential allergic responses.
> 4. Call the physician and report the medication allergy.

The correct answer is (4). The LPN/LVN must notify the physician regarding the client's allergy to revise the medication order.

The third subcategory for this client need is **Reduction of Risk Potential**, which accounts for **9–15** percent of the questions on the exam. Nursing actions that are covered in this subcategory include:

- Changes/abnormalities in vital signs
- Diagnostic tests
- Laboratory values
- Potential for alterations in body systems
- Potential for complications of diagnostic tests/treatments
- Potential for complications from surgical procedures and health alterations
- Therapeutic procedures

This is a an example of a question from the Reduction of Risk Potential subcategory:

> A 7-year-old girl with type 1 insulin-dependent diabetes mellitus (IDDM) has been home sick for several days and is brought to the Emergency Department by her parents. If the child is experiencing ketoacidosis, the LPN/LVN would expect to see which of the following lab results?
>
> 1. Serum glucose 140 mg/dL
> 2. Serum creatine 5.2 mg/dL
> 3. Blood pH 7.28
> 4. Hematocrit 38%

The correct answer is (3). Normal blood pH is 7.35–7.45. This indicates diabetic ketoacidosis.

The fourth subcategory for this client need is **Physiological Adaptation**, which accounts for **9–15** percent of the questions on the exam. Nursing actions that are covered in this subcategory include:

- Alterations in body systems
- Basic pathophysiology
- Fluid and electrolyte imbalances
- Medical emergencies
- Radiation therapy
- Unexpected response to therapies

The following is an example of a Physiological Adaptation question:

> The LPN/LVN delivers external cardiac compressions to a client while performing cardiopulmonary resuscitation (CPR). Which of the following actions by the LPN/LVN is *BEST*?
>
> 1. Maintain a position close to the client's side with the nurse's knees apart.
> 2. Maintain vertical pressure on the client's chest through the heel of the nurse's hand.
> 3. Recheck the nurse's hand position after every 10 chest compressions.
> 4. Check for a return of the client's pulse after every 8 breaths by the nurse.

The correct answer is (2). The nurse's elbows should be locked, arms straight, with shoulders directly over hands. Incorrect pressure or improperly placed hands could cause injury to the client.

The Nursing Process

Several processes are integrated throughout the NCLEX-PN® exam. The most important of these is *the nursing process.*

For the practical/vocational nurse the nursing process involves *data collection, planning, implementation,* and *evaluation* of nursing care. You will help the registered nurse, or other qualified health professional, formulate a plan of nursing care for clients in a variety of settings. As a graduate practical/vocational nurse, you are very familiar with each step of the nursing process and how to assist in writing a care plan using this process. Knowledge of the nursing process is essential to the performance of safe and effective care. It is also essential to answering questions correctly on the NCLEX-PN® exam.

Now we are going to review the steps of the nursing process and show you how each step is incorporated into test questions. The nursing process is a way of thinking. Using it will help you select correct answers.

Data collection. Data collection is the process of establishing and verifying a database of information about the client. This permits you to collaborate in the identification of actual and/or potential health problems. The practical/vocational nurse obtains subjective data (information given to you by the client that can't be observed or measured by others), and objective data (information that is observable and measurable by others). This data is collected by interviewing and observing the client and/or significant others, reviewing the health history, performing a physical assessment, gathering lab results, and interacting with the registered nurse and members of the healthcare team.

An example of a data collection test question is:

> The LPN/LVN obtains a health history from a client admitted with acute glomerulonephritis that is associated with beta-hemolytic *Streptococcus.* The LPN/LVN expects which of the following to be significant in the health history?
>
> 1. The client had a sore throat 3 weeks earlier.
> 2. There is a family history of glomerulonephritis.
> 3. The client had a renal calculus 2 years earlier.
> 4. The client had an accident involving renal trauma several years ago.

The correct answer is (1). Glomerulonephritis is an immunologic disorder that is caused by beta-hemolytic Streptococcus. *It occurs 21 days after a respiratory or skin infection.*

Planning. During the planning phase of the nursing process, the nursing care plan is formulated collaboratively with the registered nurse. Steps in planning include:

- Assigning priorities to nursing diagnosis
- Specifying goals
- Identifying interventions
- Specifying expected outcomes
- Documenting the nursing care plan

Goals are anticipated responses and client behaviors that result from nursing care. Nursing goals are client-centered and measurable, and they have an established time frame. *Expected outcomes* are the interim steps needed to reach a goal and the resolution of a nursing diagnosis. There will be multiple expected outcomes for each goal. Expected outcomes guide the practical/vocational nurse in planning interventions.

This is an example of a planning question:

A client is admitted to the medical/surgical unit complaining of nausea, vomiting, and severe right upper quadrant pain. His temperature is 101.3° F (38.5° C) and an abdominal X-ray reveals an enlarged gallbladder. He is scheduled for surgery. Which of the following actions should the LPN/LVN take *FIRST*?

1. Assess the client's need for dietary teaching.
2. Evaluate the client's fluid and electrolyte status.
3. Examine the client's health history for allergies to antibiotics.
4. Determine whether the client has signed consent for surgery.

The correct answer is (2). Hypokalemia and hypomagnesemia commonly occur after repeated vomiting.

Implementation. Implementation is the term for the actions that you take in the care of your clients. Implementation includes:

- Assisting in the performance of activities of daily living (ADLs)
- Implementing the educational plan for the client and family
- Giving care to clients

It is important for you to remember that nursing interventions may be:

- *Independent* actions that do not require supervision by others. These nursing interventions are usually not within the scope of practice for practical/vocational nurses. However, the LPN/LVN can follow established care plans, standards of care, and established protocols.
- *Dependent* actions based on the written orders of a physician.
- *Interdependent* actions shared with the registered nurse or other members of the health team.

The NCLEX-PN® exam includes questions that involve all three types of nursing interventions.

Here is an example of an implementation question:

A client is being treated in the burn unit for second- and third-degree burns over 45% of his body. The physician's orders include the application of silver sulfadiazine (Silvadene cream). The best way for the LPN/LVN to apply this medication is to use which of the following?

1. Sterile 4 × 4 dressings soaked in saline
2. Sterile tongue depressor
3. Sterile gloved hand
4. Sterile cotton-tipped applicator

The correct answer is (3). A sterile, gloved hand will cause the least amount of trauma to tissues and will decrease the chances of breaking blisters.

Evaluation. Evaluation measures the client's response to nursing interventions and indicates the client's progress toward achieving the goals established in the care plan. You compare the observed results to expected outcomes in collaboration with the registered nurse.

This is an evaluation question:

When caring for a client with anorexia nervosa, which of the following observations indicates to the LPN/LVN that the client's condition is improving?

1. The client eats all the food on her meal tray.
2. The client asks friends to bring her special foods.
3. The client weighs herself daily.
4. The client's weight has increased.

The correct response is (4). The client's weight is the most objective outcome measure in the evaluation of this client's problem.

Integrated Processes

Several other important processes are integrated throughout the NCLEX-PN® exam. They are:

Caring. As you take the NCLEX-PN® exam, remember that the test is about caring for people, not working with high-tech equipment or analyzing lab results.

Communication and Documentation. For this exam, you are required to understand and utilize therapeutic communication skills with all professional contacts, including clients, their families, and other members of the healthcare team. Charting or documenting your care and the client's response is both a legal requirement and an essential method of communication in nursing. On this exam you may be asked to identify appropriate documentation of a client behavior or nursing action.

Teaching/Learning Principles. Nursing frequently involves sharing information with clients and families so optimal functioning can be achieved. You may see questions concerning teaching a client about his diet and/or medications.

You might see some questions on the NCLEX-PN® exam that contain graphics (pictures). These questions may include the picture of a client in traction or a pregnant woman's abdomen. These questions do count, so take them seriously. We have included several questions with graphics in the practice test found in this book and others can be found online at *kaptest.com/booksonline.*

Knowledge Is Power

The more knowledgeable you are about the NCLEX-PN® exam, the more effective your study will be. As you prepare for the exam, keep the content of the test in mind. Thinking like the test maker will enhance your chance of success on the exam.

Are you still thinking about the question involving the pacemaker battery on page 3? What do you think the correct answer is?

> A man had a permanent pacemaker implanted one year ago. He returns to the outpatient clinic because he thinks the pacemaker battery is malfunctioning. It is *MOST* important for the LPN/LVN to assess for which of the following?
>
> 1. Abdominal pain, nausea, and vomiting
> 2. Wheezing on exertion, cyanosis, and orthopnea
> 3. Peripheral edema, shortness of breath, and dizziness
> 4. Chest pain radiating to the right arm, headache, and diaphoresis

The correct answer is (3). These are symptoms of decreased cardiac output. These symptoms occur with pacemaker battery failure. Other symptoms include changes in pulse rate, irregular pulse, and palpitations.

Gastrointestinal symptoms (1) are not found with pacemaker malfunction. The items listed in (2) are not symptoms of pacemaker failure. And although chest pain may occur with decreased output (4), chest pain that radiates to the right arm is suggestive of angina. Headache and diaphoresis are not seen with pacemaker failure.

CHAPTER 2

GENERAL TEST STRATEGIES

As a nursing student, you are used to taking multiple-choice tests. In fact, you've taken so many tests by the time you graduate from nursing school, you probably believe that there won't be any more surprises on any nursing test, inlcuding the NCLEX-PN® exam.

But if you've ever talked to graduate practical/vocational nurses about their experiences taking the NCLEX-PN® exam, they probably told you that the test wasn't like *any* nursing test they had ever taken. How can that be? How can the NCLEX-PN® exam seem like a practical/vocational nursing school test but be so different? The reason is that the NCLEX-PN® exam is a standardized test that analyzes a different set of behaviors from those tested in nursing school.

STANDARDIZED EXAMS

Many of you have some experience with standardized exams. You may have been required to take the SAT or ACT to get into nursing school. Remember taking that exam? Was your experience positive or negative?

All standardized exams share the same characteristics:

- Tests are written by content specialists and test-construction experts.
- The content of the exam is researched and planned.
- The questions are designed according to test construction methodology (all answer choices are about the same length, the verb tenses all agree, etc.).
- All the questions are tested before use on the actual exam.

The NCLEX-PN® exam is similar to other standardized exams in some ways yet different in others:

- The NCLEX-PN® exam is written by nurse specialists who are experts in a content area of nursing.
- All content is selected to allow the beginning practical/vocational nurse to prove minimum competency on all areas of the test plan.

- Minimum-competency questions are most frequently asked at the application level, not the recognition or recall level. All the responses to a question are similar in length and subject matter, and are grammatically correct.
- All test items have been extensively tested by NCSBN. The questions are valid; all correct responses are documented in two different sources.

What does this mean for you?

- NCSBN has defined what is minimum-competency, entry-level nursing.
- Questions and answers will be written in such a way that you cannot, in most cases, predict or recognize the correct answer.
- NCSBN is knowledgeable about strategies regarding length of answers, grammar, and so on. It makes sure that you can't use these strategies in order to select correct answers. English majors have no advantage!
- The answer choices have been extensively tested. The people who write the test questions make the incorrect answer choices look attractive to the unwary test taker.

WHAT BEHAVIORS DOES THE NCLEX-PN® EXAM TEST?

The NCLEX-PN® exam does *not* just test your nursing knowledge: It assumes that you have a body of knowledge and you understand the material because you have graduated from nursing school. So what does the NCLEX-PN® exam test? The NCLEX-PN® exam primarily tests your nursing decisions. It tests your ability to think critically and solve problems.

Critical Thinking

What does the term *critical thinking* mean? Critical thinking is problem solving that involves thinking creatively. It requires that the practical/vocational nurse:

- Observe.
- Decide what is important.
- Look for patterns and relationships.
- Identify normal and abnormal.
- Identify the problem.
- Transfer knowledge from one situation to another.
- Apply knowledge.
- Evaluate according to criteria established.

You successfully solve problems every day in the clinical area. You are probably comfortable with this concept when actually caring for clients. Although you've had lots of practice critically thinking in the clinical area, you may have had less practice critically thinking your way through test questions. Why is that?

During nursing school, you take exams developed by nursing instructors to test a specific body of content. Many of these questions are at the knowledge level. This involves recognition and recall of ideas or material that you read in your nursing textbooks and discussed in class. This is the most basic level of testing. Figure 1 illustrates the different levels of questions on nursing exams.

The following is an example of a knowledge-based question you might have seen in nursing school.

Which of the following is a complication that occurs during the first 24 hours after a percutaneous liver biopsy?

(1) Nausea and vomiting

(2) Constipation

(3) Hemorrhage

(4) Pain at the biopsy site

The question restated is, "What is a common complication of a liver biopsy?" You may or may not remember the answer. So, as you look at the answer choices, you hope to see an item that looks familiar. You do see something that looks familiar: "Hemorrhage." You select the correct answer based on recall or recognition. The NCLEX-PN® exam rarely asks passing questions at the recall/recognition level.

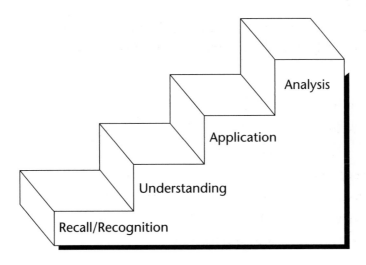

Figure 1: Levels of Questions in Nursing Tests

In nursing school, you are also given test questions written at the comprehension level. These questions require you to understand the meaning of the material. Let's look at this same question written at the comprehension level.

> **The LPN/LVN understands that hemorrhage is a complication of a liver biopsy due to which of the following reasons?**
>
> (1)   There are several large blood vessels near the liver.
> (2)   The liver cells are bathed with a mixture of venous and arterial blood.
> (3)   The test is performed on clients with elevated enzymes.
> (4)   The procedure requires a large piece of tissue to be removed.

The question restated is, "Why does hemorrhage occur after a liver biopsy?" In order to answer this question, the nurse must understand that the liver is a highly vascular organ. The portal vein and the hepatic artery join in the liver to form the sinusoids that bathe the liver in a mixture of venous and arterial blood.

The NCLEX-PN® exam asks few minimum-competency questions at the comprehension level. It assumes you know and understand the facts you learned in practical/vocational nursing school.

Minimum-competency NCLEX-PN® exam questions are written at the application and/or analysis level. Remember, the NCLEX-PN® exam tests your ability to make safe judgments about client care. Your ability to solve problems is not tested with questions at the recall/recognition or comprehension level.

Let's look at this same question written at the application level.

> **Which of the following symptoms observed by the LPN/LVN during the first 24 hours after a percutaneous liver biopsy would indicate a complication from the procedure?**
>
> 1.   Anorexia, nausea, and vomiting
> 2.   Abdominal distention and discomfort
> 3.   Pulse 112, blood pressure 100/60, respirations 20
> 4.   Pain at the biopsy site

Can you select an answer based on recall or recognition? No. Let's analyze the question and answer choices.

The question is: What is a complication of a liver biopsy? In order to begin to analyze this question, you must *know* that hemorrhage is the major complication. However, it's not listed as an answer. Can you find hemorrhage in one of the answer choices?

ANSWERS:

(1) Anorexia, nausea, and vomiting. Does this indicate that the client is hemorrhaging? No, these are not symptoms of hemorrhage.

(2) Abdominal distention and discomfort. Does this indicate that the client is hemorrhaging? Perhaps. Abdominal distention could indicate internal bleeding.

(3) Pulse 112, blood pressure 100/60, respiration 20. Does this indicate that the client is hemorrhaging? Yes. An increased pulse, a decreased blood pressure, and increased respirations indicate shock. Shock is a result of hemorrhage.

(4) Pain at the biopsy site. Does this indicate the client is hemorrhaging? No. Pain at the biopsy site is expected due to the procedure.

Ask yourself, "Which is the best indicator of hemorrhage?" Abdominal distention or a change in vital signs? Abdominal distention can be caused by liver disease. The correct answer is (3).

This question tests you at the application level. You were not able to answer the question by recalling or recognizing the word *hemorrhage*. You had to take information you learned (hemorrhage is the major complication of a liver biopsy) and select the answer that best indicates hemorrhage. Application involves taking the facts that you know and using them to make a nursing judgment. You must be able to answer questions at the application level in order to prove your competence on the NCLEX-PN® exam.

Let's look at a question that is written at the analysis level.

> The LPN/LVN is caring for a 56-year-old man receiving haloperidol (Haldol) 2 mg PO bid. The LPN/LVN assists the client to choose which of the following menus?
>
> 1. 3 oz. roast beef, baked potato, salad with dressing, dill pickle, baked apple pie, and milk
> 2. 3 oz. baked chicken, green beans, steamed rice, one slice of bread, banana, and milk
> 3. Cheeseburger on a bun, french fries with catsup, chocolate-chip cookie, apple, and milk
> 4. 3 oz. baked fish, slice of bread, broccoli, ice cream, and pineapple drink taken 30 to 60 minutes after the meal

Many students panic when they read this question because they can't immediately recall any diet restriction required by a client taking Haldol. Because students can't recall the information, they assume that they didn't learn enough information. Analysis questions are often written so that a familiar piece of information is put in an unfamiliar setting. Let's think about this question.

What type of diet do you choose for a client receiving Haldol? In order to begin analyzing this question, you must first recall that Haldol is an antipsychotic medication used to treat psychotic disorders. There are *no* diet restrictions for clients taking Haldol. Because there are no diet restrictions, you must problem-solve to determine what this question is *really* asking. Based on the answer choices, it is obviously a diet question. What kind of diet should you choose for this client? Because you have been given no other information, there is only one type of diet that can be considered: a regular balanced diet. This is an example of taking the familiar (a regular balanced diet) and putting it into the unfamiliar (a client receiving Haldol). In this question, the critical thinking is deciding what this question is *really* asking.

QUESTION: "What is the most balanced regular diet?"

ANSWERS:

(1) 3 oz. roast beef, baked potato, salad with dressing, dill pickle, baked apple pie, and milk. Is this a balanced diet? Yes, it certainly has possibilities.

(2) 3 oz. baked chicken, green beans, steamed rice, one slice of bread, banana, and milk. Is this a balanced diet? Yes, this is also a good answer because it contains foods from each of the food groups.

(3) Cheeseburger on a bun, french fries with catsup, chocolate-chip cookie, apple, and milk. Is this a balanced diet? No. This diet is high in fat and does not contain all of the food groups. Eliminate this answer.

(4) 3 oz. baked fish, slice of bread, broccoli, ice cream, and pineapple drink taken 30 to 60 minutes after the meal. Does this sound like a balanced diet? The choice of foods isn't bad, but why would the intake of fluids be delayed? This sounds like a menu to prevent dumping syndrome. Eliminate this answer.

Which is the better answer choice: (1) or (2)? Dill pickles are high in sodium, so the correct answer is (2).

Choosing the menu that best represents a balanced diet is not a difficult question to answer. The challenge lies in determining that a balanced diet is the topic of the question. Note that answer choices (1) and (2) are very similar. Because the NCLEX-PN® exam is testing your discretion, you will be making decisions between answer choices that are very close in meaning. Don't expect obvious answer choices.

These questions highlight the difference between the knowledge/comprehension-based questions that you may have seen in nursing school, and the application/analysis-based questions that you will see on the NCLEX-PN® exam.

STRATEGIES THAT DON'T WORK ON THE NCLEX-PN® EXAM

Whether you realize it or not, you developed a set of strategies in nursing school to answer teacher-generated test questions that are written at the knowledge/comprehension level. These strategies include:

- "Cramming" in hundreds of facts about disease processes and nursing care
- Recognizing and recalling facts rather than understanding the pathophysiology and the needs of a client with an illness
- Knowing who wrote the question and what is important to that instructor
- Predicting answers based on what you remember or who wrote the test question
- Selecting the response that is a different length compared to the other choices
- Selecting the answer choice that is grammatically correct
- When in doubt, choosing answer choice (C)

These strategies will not work on the NCLEX-PN® exam. Remember, the NCLEX-PN® exam is testing your ability to make safe, competent decisions.

BECOMING A BETTER TEST TAKER

The first step to becoming a better test taker is to assess and identify the following:

- The kind of test taker you are
- The kind of learner you are

Successful NCLEX-PN® Exam Test Takers
- Have a good understanding of nursing content.
- Have the ability to tackle each test question with a lot of confidence because they assume that they can figure out the right answer.
- Don't give up if they are unsure of the answer. They are not afraid to think about the question, and the possible choices, in order to select the correct answer.
- Possess the know-how to correctly identify the question.
- Stay focused on the question.

Unsuccessful NCLEX-PN® Exam Test Takers
- Assume that they either know or don't know the answer to the question.
- Memorize facts to answer questions by recall or recognition.
- Read the question, read the answers, re-read the question, and pick an answer.
- Choose answer choices based on a hunch or a feeling instead of thinking carefully.

- Answer questions based on personal experience rather than nursing theory.
- Give up too soon, because they aren't willing to think hard about questions and answers.
- Don't stay focused on the question.

If you are a successful test taker, congratulations! This book will reinforce your test-taking skills. If you have many of the characteristics of an unsuccessful test taker, don't despair! You can change. If you follow the strategies in this book, you will become a successful test taker.

What Kind of Learner Are You?

It is important for you to identify whether you think predominantly in images or words. Why? This will assist you in developing a study plan that is specific for your learning style. Read the following statement:

A nurse walks into a room and finds the client lying on the floor.

As you read those words, did you hear yourself reading the words? Or did you see a nurse walking into a room, and see the client lying on the floor? If you heard yourself reading the sentence, you think in words. If you formed a mental image (saw a picture), you think in images.

Students who think in images sometimes have a difficult time answering nursing test questions. These students say things like:

"I have to study harder than the other students."
"I have to look up the same information over and over again."
"Once I see the procedure (or client), I don't have any difficulty understanding or remembering the content."
"I have trouble understanding procedures from reading the book. I have to see the procedure to understand it."
"I have trouble answering test questions about clients or procedures I've never seen."

Why is that? For some people, imagery is necessary to understand ideas and concepts. If this is true for you, you need to visualize information that you are learning. As you prepare for the NCLEX-PN® exam, try to form mental images of terminology, procedures, and diseases. For example, if you're reviewing information about traction but you have never seen traction, it would be ideal for you to see a client in traction. If that isn't possible, find a picture of traction and rig up a traction setup with whatever material you have available. As you read about traction, use the photo or model to visualize care of the client. If you can visualize the theory that you are trying to learn, it will make recall and understanding of concepts much easier for you.

It is also important that you visualize test questions. As you read the question and possible answer choices, picture yourself going through each suggested action. This will increase your chances of selecting correct answer choices.

Let's look at a test question that requires imagery.

> An adolescent is seen in the emergency room for a fracture of the left femur sustained in a sledding accident. The fracture is reduced and a cast is applied. The client is taught how to use crutches for ambulating without bearing weight on the left leg. The LPN/LVN would expect the client to learn which of the following crutch-walking gaits?
>
> 1. Two-point gait
> 2. Three-point gait
> 3. Four-point gait
> 4. Swing-through gait

Don't panic if you can't remember crutch-walking gaits. Instead, visualize!

Step 1. "See" a person (or yourself) walking normally. First the right leg and left arm are extended, and then the left leg and right arm are extended.

Step 2. Put crutches in your hands. Now walk. Each foot and each crutch is a point.

Step 3. "See" a person (or yourself) with a full cast on the left leg, with the foot never touching the ground.

Step 4. Visualize the answers.

(1) Two-point gait. One leg and one crutch would be touching the ground at the same time. Sounds like normal walking. Eliminate this choice because the client is non-weight-bearing.

(2) Three-point gait. Both crutches and one foot are on the ground. This would be appropriate for a non-weight-bearing client.

(3) Four-point gait. This would require both legs and crutches to touch the ground. However, in this question the client is non-weight-bearing. Eliminate this option.

(4) Swing-through gait. This gait means advancing both crutches, then both legs, and requires weight-bearing. The gait is not as stable as the other gaits. Eliminate this option: the client in this question is non-weight-bearing.

The correct answer is (2).

Even if you are unsure of crutch walking gaits, imagining and thinking through the answer choices will enable you to select the correct answer.

CHAPTER 3

COMPUTER-ADAPTIVE TEST STRATEGIES

The NCLEX-PN® exam is composed primarily of multiple-choice, four-option, text-based questions written at the application/analysis level of difficulty. These questions may include charts, tables, or graphic images.

Your NCLEX-PN® exam may also contain questions in a format other than traditional four-option, text-based, multiple-choice questions. These other types of questions, called *alternate questions*, are part of the test pool of questions for the NCLEX-PN® exam. These alternate question types include:

- Multiple-response questions that require you to select all answer choices that apply from among five or six answer options
- "Hot spot" questions that require you to identify a "hot spot" or specific area on a graphic image by clicking on the correct area with the mouse
- Fill-in-the-blank questions that require you to type in a number that you calculate into a blank space provided after the question
- Drag-and-drop/ordered-response questions that ask you to place answers in a specific order

There are also three types of alternate questions that are variations on the traditional four-option multiple-choice question. These include:

- Chart/exhibit questions that require you to click an Exhibit button to display charts and/or exhibits that provide information needed to answer the question. Once you have done so, you then select the correct choice from four multiple-choice answer options.
- Audio questions that present you with an audio clip that you listen to on headphones. After listening to the clip, you then select the correct choice from among four multiple-choice answer options.
- Graphics questions that present you with graphics instead of text as the four multiple-choice answer options.

These questions either are counted toward your NCLEX-PN® exam results or they are experimental questions for future exams that are not counted.

This book contains strategies that help you correctly answer both alternate questions and traditional four-option, text-based, multiple-choice questions.

ALTERNATE TEST QUESTIONS

Let's take a look at the individual alternate question types and the strategies that help you correctly answer these questions.

Select All That Apply—Click on all appropriate answer choices

Take a look at the following question:

> The LPN/LVN cares for a client diagnosed with a left-sided cerebrovascular accident (CVA) with dysphagia. Which of the following actions by the LPN/LVN reflects appropriate care for the client? **Select all that apply.**
>
> ☐ 1. The LPN/LVN assesses the client's ability to swallow.
> ☐ 2. The LPN/LVN offers the client apple juice.
> ☐ 3. The LPN/LVN positions the client at a 45-degree angle.
> ☐ 4. The LPN/LVN offers the client scrambled eggs.
> ☐ 5. The LPN/LVN instructs the client to place food on the right side of the mouth.
> ☐ 6. The LPN/LVN turns off the television.

You will know that the question is a "Select all that apply" alternate question because after the question stem and before the answer choices you are instructed to **"Select all that apply."** You will note that there are more than four possible answer choices; usually five or six are provided. Also, there is a box in front of each answer choice rather than the radio button you see with multiple-choice, four-option, text-based questions.

To answer this type of question, determine which of the answer choices provided are correct. It is important to remember that in order for the question to be scored as correct you must select *all* of the correct responses that apply, not just the *best* response. You will not receive any partial credit if you do not. Left-click on the box in front of each answer choice that you think is correct. A small check mark appears in the box indicating that you selected that answer. If you change your mind about a particular answer choice, just click on the box again: the check mark disappears and the answer choice is no longer selected.

How should you approach this type of question? What doesn't work is to compare and contrast the individual answer choices. For a "Select all that apply" question, any number of answer choices may be correct. Instead, consider each answer choice a True/False question. Reword this question to ask, "What is appropriate care for a client with a left-sided CVA who has dysphagia?" Dysphagia means the client is having difficulty swallowing; if the CVA is in the left hemisphere, the client's right side is affected.

Let's look at the answers. The strategy is to change each answer choice into a statement, and then determine whether the statement is true or false.

(1) "I should assess the client's ability to swallow." Is this true for a client with dysphagia? Yes. This is a correct response because the nurse needs to make sure that the client can swallow food before giving him anything to eat. Select this answer choice.

(2) "I should offer the client apple juice." Is this an appropriate fluid for a client with dysphagia? Yes. Although the client may have some difficulty taking oral fluids, it is important to offer them slowly. Select this answer choice.

(3) "I should position the client at a 45-degree angle." Is this the correct position for a client with dysphagia? No. The client should be sitting upright in a chair or the bed. Eliminate this answer choice.

(4) "I should offer the client scrambled eggs." Is this an appropriate food for a client with dysphagia? Yes. Soft or semi-soft foods are more easily tolerated than a regular diet. Select this answer choice.

(5) "I should instruct the client to place food on the right side of his mouth." Is this what should be done? If the client has a left-sided CVA, that means the right side of the client's body is affected. The food should be placed on the unaffected side. This is the left side of the mouth for this client. Eliminate this answer.

(6) "I should turn off the television." What are they getting at with this statement? Many clients after a CVA are easily distracted. If the client has dysphagia, you don't want him to aspirate because he is distracted by the television. It is best to turn off the TV during meals. Select this answer choice.

So, which answers should be checked as correct? For this question, choices (1), (2), (4), and (6) are correct. Left-click on the box in front of each of these answer choices to select them. When you have selected all the responses you believe to be correct, click on the NEXT (N) button in the bottom left of the screen or press the Enter key on the keyboard to lock in your answer and go on to the next question. Remember, once you click on the NEXT (N) button or press the Enter key, you have entered your answer to the question and you cannot return to the question.

> The LPN/LVN cares for a client diagnosed with a left-sided cerebrovascular accident (CVA) with dysphagia. Which of the following actions by the LPN/LVN reflects appropriate care for the client? **Select all that apply.**
>
> ☑ 1. The LPN/LVN assesses the client's ability to swallow.
> ☑ 2. The LPN/LVN offers the client apple juice.
> ☐ 3. The LPN/LVN positions the client at a 45-degree angle.
> ☑ 4. The LPN/LVN offers the client scrambled eggs.
> ☐ 5. The LPN/LVN instructs the client to place food on the right side of the mouth.
> ☑ 6. The LPN/LVN turns off the television.

Hot Spot—Select the correct area and click the mouse

This type of alternate question asks you to identify a location on a graphic or table. It is important to understand that this is not a test of your fine motor skills but is designed to evaluate your knowledge of nursing content, anatomy, physiology, and pathophysiology.

Let's take a look at a question that involves a hot spot.

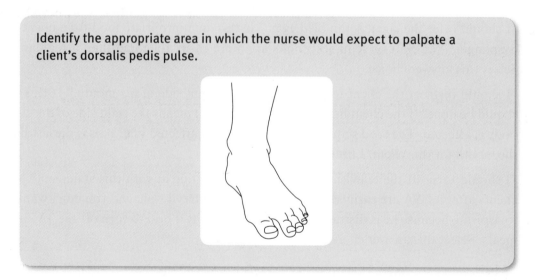

> Identify the appropriate area in which the nurse would expect to palpate a client's dorsalis pedis pulse.

The question asks you to identify where you would palpate one of the two commonly assessed peripheral pulses found in the foot. The strategy you should use is to locate anatomical landmarks. You need to know that the dorsalis pedis pulse is located on the top (dorsum) of the client's foot. It is found between the first and second metatarsal bones (between the great and first toes) over the dorsalis pedis artery.

Using the computer's mouse, move the cursor to the location you think is correct. Then, left-click the mouse. Check to make sure that you have selected the location you wanted. Then enter your answer by clicking on the NEXT (N) button or pressing the Enter key. If you click between the second and third toes, for example, the location would be inaccurate for the dorsalis pedis pulse and the question would be counted wrong. Just do your best and use the anatomical landmarks to get your bearings and select the location.

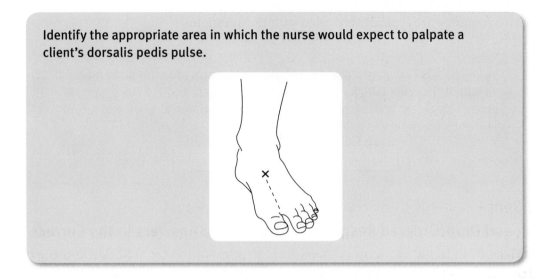

Identify the appropriate area in which the nurse would expect to palpate a client's dorsalis pedis pulse.

Fill in the Blank—Enter the answer

This type of alternate question asks you to fill in the blank with a number based on a calculation.

The following is a sample of a fill-in-the-blank question that is a calculation.

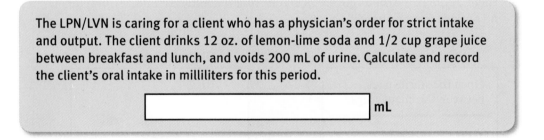

The LPN/LVN is caring for a client who has a physician's order for strict intake and output. The client drinks 12 oz. of lemon-lime soda and 1/2 cup grape juice between breakfast and lunch, and voids 200 mL of urine. Calculate and record the client's oral intake in milliliters for this period.

mL

To answer this question, calculate the client's intake from the information provided. **Note: Pay close attention to the unit of measure you need for your final answer.** In this situation you are asked for the client's intake in milliliters, not cups or ounces.

You can use the drop-down calculator provided on the computer to do the math. The button that displays the calculator is on the bottom of the right side of the computer screen. Use your mouse to click on the numbers or functions you want. Remember, the slash (/) is used for division.

First, convert cups into ounces. One cup of fluid = 8 oz. Then convert ounces into milliliters. One ounce = 30 milliliters. The client's intake is:

12 oz. lemon-lime soda = 360 mL

1/2 cup grape juice = 4 oz. = 120 mL

Use the computer mouse to move the cursor inside the text box. Left-click on the cursor. Type in the correct intake using the number keys on the keyboard. The correct answer is 480. Do not put "mL" or any unit of measure after the number. Only the number goes into the box. Rules for rounding are typically provided with the question.

> The LPN/LVN is caring for a client who has a physician's order for strict intake and output. The client drinks 12 oz. of lemon-lime soda and 1/2 cup grape juice between breakfast and lunch, and voids 200 mL of urine. Calculate and record the client's oral intake in milliliters for this period.
>
> | 480 | mL |

Drag and Drop/Ordered Response—Arrange the Answers in the Correct Order

This is one of the newer alternate question types introduced by the NCSBN. These questions ask you to place answers in a specific order.

Take a look at the following question.

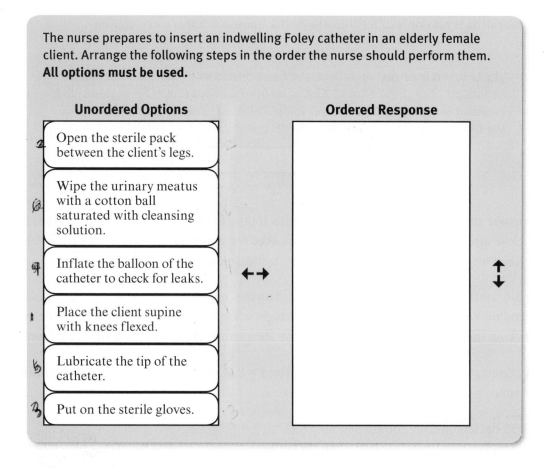

The nurse prepares to insert an indwelling Foley catheter in an elderly female client. Arrange the following steps in the order the nurse should perform them. **All options must be used.**

Unordered Options

- Open the sterile pack between the client's legs.
- Wipe the urinary meatus with a cotton ball saturated with cleansing solution.
- Inflate the balloon of the catheter to check for leaks.
- Place the client supine with knees flexed.
- Lubricate the tip of the catheter.
- Put on the sterile gloves.

Ordered Response

The strategy to use to answer this kind of question is to picture yourself performing the procedure. First, prepare the client. Next, prepare the equipment in the correct order using sterile technique. Open the sterile pack between the client's legs. Next, put on the sterile gloves. Inflate the balloon of the catheter to check for leaks. Lubricate the tip of the catheter. Once the equipment is ready, prepare the client for the insertion of the catheter. The last step from those provided is to wipe the urinary meatus with a cotton ball saturated with cleansing solution.

To place the options in the correct order, click on an option and drag it to the box on the right. You can also move an answer from the left column to the right column by highlighting the option and clicking the arrow key that points to the column on the right. You may also rearrange the order of the options in the right column using the arrow keys pointing up and down.

Here's the answer to this question.

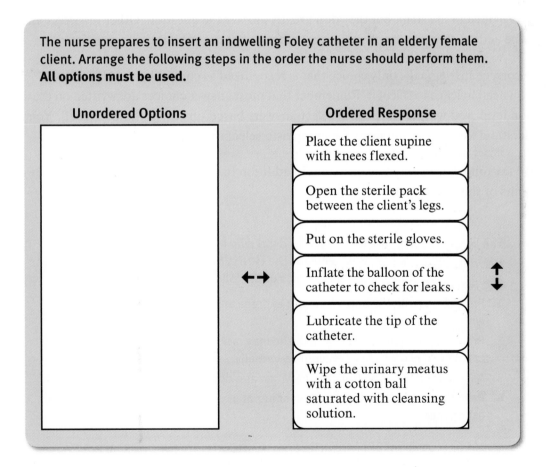

MULTIPLE-CHOICE TEST QUESTIONS

Multiple-choice questions with four answer options may take the form of a traditional text-based question, or may be in the form of an alternate question that includes an exhibit/chart, is based on an audio clip, or contains graphics in place of some of the text. No matter the form, to effectively apply the strategies discussed in this book, you need to understand the components of an NCLEX-PN® multiple-choice question. They are as follows::

- The *stem* of the question. The stem includes the situation that describes the client, his or her problems or healthcare needs, and other relevant information. It also includes a question or an incomplete statement. This is the question that you must answer.
- Three incorrect answers, referred to here as *distracters.*
- The correct answer.

The three distracters will probably sound logical to you. They may even be based on information provided in the stem, but they don't really answer the question. Other incorrect answers may be actions that are common nursing practice but not ideal nursing practice.

The correct answer is the only choice that is recognized as correct by the NCLEX-PN® exam, so you need to learn to select it. Remember that most answer choices are written on the application level: you will not be able to select answers based on recognition or recall. You must understand the *whys* of nursing care in order to select the correct response.

Read the following exam-style question. In addition to selecting an answer, identify the components of this question.

The LPN/LVN plans care for a 4-year-old girl who has been sexually abused by her father. Play therapy is scheduled. The LPN/LVN knows that the **PRIMARY** goal of play therapy for a 4-year-old is which of the following?

1. Provide her with the opportunity to express anger and hostility by playing with dolls.
2. Promote communication because she may lack the emotional and intellectual capacity to express her perceptions verbally.
3. Assess whether she is functioning at an age-appropriate developmental level.
4. Reveal through direct observation of her at play what type of abuse has been experienced.

The Components

- The stem:
  - 4-year-old girl
  - Sexually abused by her father

- Play therapy is scheduled
- What is the primary goal of play therapy for a 4-year-old?

- The answer choices:

(1) Opportunity to express anger and hostility. Play therapy will allow children to express anger and hostility if that's what they want to communicate. Some students select this answer because they focus on the treatment of sexual abuse mentioned in the situation. This is a distracter.

(2) Promote communication. Play is the universal language of children. The purpose of play therapy is to give children the opportunity to communicate using their own "language." This is the correct answer.

(3) Assess her developmental level. The nurse might be able to assess whether a child is functioning at an age-appropriate level, but this is not the primary purpose of play therapy. This is a distracter.

(4) Find out what type of abuse she has experienced. The child might communicate the type of abuse she has experienced if that is what she chooses to communicate. The nurse should focus on the purpose of play therapy, not the type of abuse. This is a distracter.

Let's try another question.

> A client is being treated for heart failure with diuretic therapy. Which of the following assessments **BEST** indicates to the LPN/LVN that the client's condition is improving?
>
> 1. The client's weight has remained stable since admission.
> 2. The client's systolic blood pressure has decreased.
> 3. There are fewer crackles heard when auscultating the client's lungs.
> 4. The client's urinary output is 1,500 mL per day.

The Components

- The stem:
  - Heart failure
  - Treatment is diuretic therapy
  - How do you know the client's condition is improving?

- The answer choices:

(1) Weight has remained stable. Client's weight should decrease because he is taking a diuretic. Weight addresses issues involved with diuretic therapy. However, it is not the best indication of improvement in a client with heart failure. This is a distracter.

(2) The systolic blood pressure has decreased. Decreased blood pressure may be the result of diuretic therapy, but the reduction could also be due to other causes (change of position, calm rather than an excited state, etc.). This is not the best indication of an improvement in a client with heart failure. This is a distracter.

(3) There are fewer crackles. A client with heart failure has crackles due to pulmonary edema. Diuretics are given to promote excretion of sodium and water through the kidneys. Decreased crackles would indicate that the pulmonary edema is improving. This is the correct answer.

(4) Output of 1,500 mL in 24 hours. This is within normal limits. Although a normal output addresses diuretic therapy, it is not the best indication of improvement of heart failure. This is a distracter.

CRITICAL THINKING STRATEGIES

- The NCLEX-PN® exam is not a test about recognizing facts.
- You must be able to correctly identify what the question is asking.
- Do not focus on background information that is not needed to answer the question.
- The NCLEX-PN® exam focuses on thinking through a problem or situation.

Now that you are more knowledgeable about the components of a multiple-choice test question, let's talk about specific strategies that you can use to problem-solve your way to correct answers on the NCLEX-PN® exam.

Remember, the NCLEX-PN® exam tests your ability to think critically. Critical thinking for the practical/vocational nurse involves:

- Observation
- Deciding what is important
- Looking for patterns and relationships
- Identifying the problem
- Transferring knowledge from one situation to another
- Applying knowledge
- Discriminating between possible choices and/or courses of action
- Evaluating according to criteria established

Are you feeling overwhelmed as you read these words? Don't be! We are going teach you a step-by-step method to choose the appropriate path.

There are some strategies that you must follow on *every* NCLEX-PN® exam test question. You must *always* figure out what the question is asking, and you must *always* eliminate answer choices.

Choosing the right answer often involves choosing the best of several answers that have correct information. This may entail your correct analysis and interpretation of what the question is really asking. So let's talk about how to figure out what the question is asking.

REWORD THE QUESTION

The first step to correctly answering NCLEX-PN® exam questions is to find out what each question is *really* asking.

Step 1. Read each question carefully from the first word to the last word. Do not skim over the words or read them too quickly.

Step 2. Look for hints in the wording of the question stem. The adjectives *most, first, best, primary,* and *initial* indicate that you must establish priorities. The phrase *further teaching is necessary* indicates that the answer will contain incorrect information. The phrase *client understands the teaching* indicates that the answer will be correct information.

Step 3. Reword the question stem in your own words so that it can be answered with a *yes* or a *no,* or with a specific bit of information. Begin your questions with *what, when,* or *why.* We will refer to this reworded version as THE REWORDED QUESTION in the examples that follow.

Step 4. If you can't complete step 3, read the answer choices for clues.

Let's practice rewording a question.

> A preschooler with a fractured femur is admitted to the pediatric unit. When asked how the injury occurred, the child's parents state that she fell off the sofa. On examination, the LPN/LVN finds old and new lesions on the child's buttocks. Which of the following statements **MOST** appropriately reflects how the LPN/LVN should document these findings?
>
> 1.
> 2.
> 3.
> 4.

We omitted the answer choices to make you focus on the question stem this time. The answer choices will be provided and discussed later in this chapter.

Step 1. Read the question stem carefully.

Step 2. Pay attention to the adjectives. *Most appropriately* tells you that you need to select the best answer.

Step 3. Reword the question stem in your own words. In this case, it is, "What is the best charting for this situation?"

Step 4. Because you were able to reword the question, the fourth step is unnecessary. You didn't need to read the answer choices for clues.

We have all missed questions on a test because we didn't read accurately. The following question illustrates this point.

> A construction worker is admitted to the hospital for treatment of active tuberculosis (TB). The LPN/LVN reinforces a teaching plan for the client about TB. Which of the following statements by the client indicates to the LPN/LVN that further teaching is necessary?
>
> 1.
> 2.
> 3.
> 4.

Again, just the question stem is given to encourage you to focus on rewording the question. We will discuss the answer choices for this question later in this chapter.

Step 1. Read the question stem carefully.

Step 2. Look for hints. Pay particular attention to the statement "further teaching is necessary." You are looking for negative information.

Step 3. Reword the question stem in your own words. In this case, it is, "What is incorrect information about TB?"

Step 4. Because you were able to reword the question, the fourth step is unnecessary. You didn't need to read the answer choices for clues to determine what the question is asking.

Try rewording this test question.

A woman admitted to the hospital in premature labor has been treated successfully. The client is to be sent home on an oral regimen of terbutaline (Brethine). Which of the following statements by the client indicates to the LPN/LVN that the client understands the discharge teaching about the medication?

1.
2.
3.
4.

Again, just the question stem is given to encourage you to focus on rewording the question. We will discuss the answer choices for this question later in this chapter.

Step 1. Read the question stem carefully.

Step 2. Look for hints. Pay attention to the words *client understands*. You are looking for true information.

Step 3. Reword the question stem. This question is asking, "What is true about Brethine?"

Step 4. Because you were able to reword this question, the fourth step is unnecessary. You didn't need to obtain clues about what the question is asking from the answer choices.

ELIMINATE INCORRECT ANSWER CHOICES

Now that you've mastered rewording the question, let's examine how to select the correct answer.

Remember the characteristics of unsuccessful test takers? One of their major problems is that they do not thoughtfully consider each answer choice. They react to questions using feelings and hunches. Unsuccessful test takers look for a specific answer choice. The following strategy will enable you to consider each answer choice in a thoughtful way.

Step 1. Do not look at any of the answer choices except answer choice (1).

Step 2. Read answer choice (1). Then repeat THE REWORDED QUESTION after reading the answer choice. Ask yourself, "Does this answer THE REWORDED QUESTION?" If you know the answer choice is wrong, eliminate it. If you aren't sure, leave the answer choice in for consideration.

Step 3. Repeat the above process with each remaining answer choice.

Step 4. Note which answer choices remain.

Step 5. Reread the question to make sure you have correctly identified THE REWORDED QUESTION.

Step 6. Ask yourself, "Which answer choice best answers the question?" That is your answer.

Let's practice the elimination strategy using the same questions.

A preschooler with a fractured femur is admitted to the pediatric unit. When asked how the injury occurred, the child's parents state that she fell off the sofa. On examination, the LPN/LVN finds old and new lesions on the child's buttocks. Which of the following statements most appropriately reflects how the LPN/LVN should document these findings?

1. "Six lesions noted on buttocks at various stages of healing."
2. "Multiple lesions on buttocks due to child abuse."
3. "Lesions on buttocks due to unknown causes."
4. "Several lesions on buttocks caused by cigarettes."

THE REWORDED QUESTION: "What is good charting?"

Step 1. Do not look at any of the answer choices except for answer choice (1). Thoughtfully consider each answer choice individually.

Step 2. Read answer choice (1). Does it answer the question, "What is good charting for this situation?"

(1) "Six lesions noted on buttocks at various stages of healing." Is this good charting? Maybe. Leave it in for consideration.

Step 3. Repeat the process with each remaining answer choice.

(2) "Multiple lesions on buttocks due to child abuse." Is this good charting? No, because the nurse is making a judgment about the cause of the lesion.

(3) "Lesions on buttocks due to unknown causes." Is this good charting? Maybe. Leave it in for consideration.

(4) "Several lesions on buttocks caused by cigarettes." Is this good charting? No. The question does not include information about how the burns occurred.

Step 4. Answer choices (1) and (3) remain.

Step 5. Reread the question. This question asks you to identify good charting.

Step 6. Which is the best charting? "Six lesions noted on buttocks at various stages of healing," or "Lesions due to unknown causes"? Good charting is accurate, objective, concise, and complete. It must reflect the client's current status. The correct answer is (1).

Some students will select answer (3), thinking, "How can I be sure about the stages of healing?" But the purpose of this question is to test your ability to select good charting. Select the answer choice that shows you are a safe and effective nurse. Remember, questions on the NCLEX-PN® exam are not designed to trick you. Stay focused on the question.

Let's select the correct answer for the second question.

> A construction worker is admitted to the hospital for treatment of active tuberculosis (TB). The LPN/LVN reinforces a teaching plan for the client about TB. Which of the following statements by the client indicates to the LPN/LVN that further teaching is necessary?
>
> 1. "I will have to take medication for 6 months."
> 2. "I should cover my nose and mouth when coughing or sneezing."
> 3. "I will remain in isolation for at least 6 weeks."
> 4. "I will always have a positive skin test for TB."

THE REWORDED QUESTION: What is incorrect information about TB?

Step 1. Do not look at any of the answer choices except answer choice (1).

Step 2. Read answer choice (1). Does it answer THE REWORDED QUESTION, "What is incorrect (or wrong) information about TB?"

(1) "I will have to take medication for 6 months." Is this wrong information? No, it is a true statement. The client will need to take a medication, such as isonicotinyl hydrazine (INH), for 6 months or longer. Eliminate this choice.

Step 3. Repeat the process with each remaining answer choice.

(2) "I should cover my nose and mouth when coughing or sneezing." Is this wrong information about TB? No, this is a true statement. TB is transmitted by droplet contamination. Eliminate it.

(3) "I will remain in isolation for at least 6 weeks." Is this wrong information about TB? Maybe. Leave it in for consideration.

(4) "I will always have a positive skin test for TB." Is this a wrong statement about TB? No, this is true. A positive skin test indicates that the client has developed antibodies to the tuberculosis bacillus. Eliminate this choice.

Step 4. Only answer choice (3) remains.

Step 5. Reread the question. The question is, "What is wrong information about TB?"

Step 6. The correct answer is (3). You "know" this is the correct answer because you've eliminated the other three answer choices. The client does not need to be isolated for 6 weeks. The client's activities will be restricted for about 2–3 weeks after medication therapy is initiated.

A couple of things to remember when using this strategy:

- Eliminate only what you know is wrong. However, once you eliminate an answer choice, do not retrieve it for consideration. You may be tempted to do this if you do not feel comfortable with the one answer choice that is left. Resist the impulse!
- Stay focused on THE REWORDED QUESTION. How many of you have missed a question that asked for negative information because you selected the answer choice that contained correct information?

Here's another question.

> A woman admitted to the hospital in premature labor has been treated successfully. The client is to be sent home on an oral regimen of terbutaline (Brethine). Which of the following statements by the client indicates to the LPN/LVN that the client understands the discharge teaching about the medication?
>
> 1. "As long as I take my medication, I can be sure I will not deliver prematurely."
> 2. "It is important that I count the fetal movements for one hour, twice a day."
> 3. "I may feel a rapid heartbeat and some muscle tremors while on this medication."
> 4. "Bedrest is necessary in order for the medication to work properly."

THE REWORDED QUESTION: What is true about Brethine?

Step 1. Do not look at any of the answer choices except answer choice (1).

Step 2. Read answer choice (1). Does it answer the question, "What is true about Brethine?"

(1) "As long as I take my medication, I can be sure I will not deliver prematurely." Is this true about Brethine? No. Brethine will inhibit uterine contractions, but there is no guarantee that there won't be a premature delivery. Eliminate it.

Step 3. Repeat the process with each remaining answer choice.

(2) "It is important that I count the fetal movements for one hour, twice a day." Is this true about Brethine? Maybe. Clients are told to be aware of fetal movement. Keep it as a possibility.

(3) "I may feel a rapid heartbeat and some muscle tremors while on this medication." Is this true of Brethine? Yes. Brethine is a smooth-muscle relaxant. Side effects include increased maternal heart rate, palpitations, and muscle tremors. Leave this choice in for consideration.

(4) "Bedrest is necessary in order for the medication to work properly." Is this true about Brethine? No. Brethine will work whether the client is on bedrest or not. Eliminate it.

Step 4. Note that only answer choices (2) and (3) remain.

Step 5. Reread the question to make sure you are answering the right question. The question is, "What is true about Brethine?"

Step 6. Which choice best answers the question, (2) or (3)? If you are focused on the question, you will select (3). Some students focus on the background information (pregnancy). This question has nothing to do with pregnancy. If you chose (2), you fell for a distracter.

Remember: Focus on the question, and not the background information. If you can answer the question—"What is true about Brethine?"—without considering the background information (pregnancy), do it. Many students answer a question incorrectly because they don't focus on THE REWORDED QUESTION. Don't fall for the distracters.

At this point you're probably thinking, "Will I have enough time to finish the test using these strategies?" or "How will I ever remember how to answer questions using these steps?" Yes, you will have time to finish the test. Unsuccessful test takers spend time agonizing over test questions. By using these strategies, you will be using your time productively. You will remember the steps because you are going to practice, practice, practice with test questions. You will not be able to absorb this strategy by osmosis; the process must be practiced repeatedly.

DON'T PREDICT ANSWERS

On the NCLEX-PN® exam, you are asked to select the best answer from the four choices that you are given. Many times, the "ideal" answer choice is not there. Don't sit and moan because the answer that you think should be there isn't provided. Remember:

- Identify THE REWORDED QUESTION.
- Select the best answer *from the choices given.*

Look at this question.

> The LPN/LVN describes the procedure for collecting a clean-catch urine specimen for culture and sensitivity to a male client. Which of the following explanations by the LPN/LVN would be **MOST** accurate?
>
> 1. "The urinary meatus is cleansed with an iodine solution and then a urinary drainage catheter is inserted to obtain urine."
> 2. "You will be asked to empty your bladder one-half hour before the test; you will then be asked to void into a container."
> 3. "Before voiding, the urinary meatus is cleansed with an iodine solution and urine is voided into a sterile container; the container must not touch the penis."
> 4. "You must void a few drops of urine, then stop; then void the remaining urine into a clean container, which should be immediately covered."

Step 1. Read the question stem.

Step 2. Focus on the adjectives. "*Most accurate*" tells you that more than one answer may seem correct.

Step 3. Reword the question stem. What is true about a clean-catch urine specimen for culture and sensitivity?

Step 4. Read each answer choice and ask yourself, "Is this true about a clean-catch urine specimen for culture and sensitivity?"

(1) This choice describes how to obtain a catheterized urine specimen. Urine isn't usually collected by catheterization due to the increased risk of infection. This answer does not answer the question about a clean-catch urine specimen. Eliminate.

(2) This describes a double-voided specimen. This action is usually done when testing urine for glucose and ketones. It is not relevant to a clean-catch urine specimen. Eliminate.

(3) This is true of a clean-catch urine specimen for culture and sensitivity. The urinary meatus is cleansed, a sterile container is used, and the penis must not touch the container. Leave this answer in for consideration.

(4) This does describe a clean-catch urine specimen. The client does void a few drops of urine, stops, and then continues voiding into the container. There is only one problem. For a culture and sensitivity, the container must be sterile. Eliminate.

The correct answer is (3). Many students will select answer choice (4) because they see the expected words: "Void a few drops, stop, continue voiding." Be careful. This question is a good example of why scanning for expected words could get you into trouble. You may see expected words in an answer choice that is not correct.

Okay. You've practiced how to identify the topic of the question and how to eliminate answer choices. You know that predicting answers does not work on the NCLEX-PN® exam. You are well on your way to correctly answering NCLEX-PN® exam test questions. Unfortunately, this is just the starting point. Let's talk about specific paths and how you can correctly decide which paths to use on the NCLEX-PN® exam. Remember, the correct answer is at the end of the path!

RECOGNIZE EXPECTED OUTCOMES

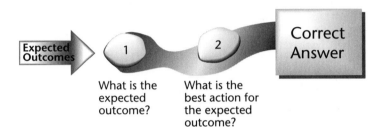

You spent much of your time in practical/vocational nursing school learning about what might go wrong with clients and their care. This makes sense; after all, nurses need to deal with problems and illnesses. Many test questions that your practical/vocational nursing school faculty wrote focused on what was wrong with clients and their care. In order to prove minimum competence, the beginning practical/vocational nurse must demonstrate the ability to make appropriate nursing judgments. Competent nursing judgments include recognizing both expected and unexpected behaviors, so it is important for you to recognize expected outcomes on the NCLEX-PN® exam. Expected outcomes are the behaviors and changes you think are going to occur as a result of nursing care. These outcomes allow the nurse to evaluate whether goals have been met.

Look at the following question.

> The LPN/LVN checks the morning's serum electrolyte results for a client. The nurse notes that the client's Na+ (sodium) is 142 mEq/L, K+ (potassium) is 4.4 mEq/L, and Cl− (chloride) is 102 mEq/L. Which of the following should the nurse do *FIRST*?
>
> 1. Encourage the client to drink additional fluids.
> 2. Notify the physician of the client's electrolyte results.
> 3. Record the electrolyte results in the client's chart.
> 4. Withhold the client's morning potassium supplement.

If this question were included on one of your fundamentals tests, you would assume that a problem was being described. You would choose an answer that involved "fixing" the problem. Let's look at this question.

THE REWORDED QUESTION: What should you do with a client with these electrolyte results?

Step 1. Recognize normal. Interpret the serum electrolyte results. All are within normal limits.

Step 2. Decide how you should use this information. Because the values are all normal, let's reword the question again using this information.

Now THE REWORDED QUESTION is: What should you do for a client with normal serum electrolytes?

ANSWERS:

(1) Encourage the client to drink additional fluids. Although good fluid intake is usually recommended, this is not a priority because the serum electrolytes are within normal limits. Eliminate.

(2) Notify the physician of the client's electrolyte results. This is unnecessary because the serum electrolytes are normal. Most physicians request notification only for abnormal test results. Eliminate.

(3) Record the electrolyte results in the client's chart. This action should be done because the electrolyte results are normal.

(4) Withhold the client's morning potassium supplement. The client's K+ is within normal limits, which suggests that the potassium supplement has helped maintain this serum level. There is no indication with the information you have been given that this would be necessary or prudent. Eliminate.

The correct answer is (3). The electrolytes are within normal limits. Some students select answer choice (1) because they think there's something they missed, or it must be a trick question. The "trick" is deciding whether the information that you are given is normal or abnormal, and then answering the question accordingly.

Try this question.

A client is brought to the emergency room complaining of pressure in her chest. Her blood pressure is 150/90, pulse 88, respirations 20. The LPN/LVN administers nitroglycerine 0.4 mg sublingually as ordered. After 5 minutes the client's blood pressure is 100/60, pulse 96, respirations 20. Which of the following should the LPN/LVN do next?

1. Notify the physician that the client has become hypotensive.
2. Place the client in semi-Fowler's position, and administer O_2 at 4 L.
3. Administer a second dose of nitroglycerine.
4. Document the results, and continue to monitor the client.

THE REWORDED QUESTION: What should you do for this client?

To answer this question you need to know what these vital signs indicate.

Step 1. Recognize normal. Nitroglycerine is a potent vasodilator with anti-anginal, anti-ischemic, and antihypertensive actions. It increases blood flow through the coronary arteries. Side effects include orthostatic hypotension, tachycardia, dizziness, and palpitations. A decreased blood pressure, increased pulse, and stable respirations after administration of a potent vasodilator is normal and expected.

Step 2. Decide how you should use this information. The question should be reworded as, "What should you do for a client who has responded as expected to a dose of nitroglycerin?"

ANSWERS:

(1) Notify the physician that the client has become hypotensive. The blood pressure has decreased due to vasodilation. Decreased blood pressure is expected. Eliminate.

(2) Place the client in semi-Fowler's position and administer O_2 at 4 L. Respirations are stable and there is no indication of respiratory distress. Eliminate.

(3) Administer a second dose of nitroglycerine. The nurse should assess the client for chest pain first, and administer a second dose of the medication only if the client continues to complain of chest pain. Eliminate.

(4) Document the results and continue to monitor the client. This is the correct choice because you recognized the client's response as normal, thus eliminating the other three answer choices.

The correct answer is (4). You would expect a client's blood pressure to decrease after administration of nitroglycerine. The key to this question is understanding how the medication works, and correctly identifying the expected outcome.

READ ANSWER CHOICES TO OBTAIN CLUES

Because the NCLEX-PN® exam tests your critical thinking, the topic of the questions may be unstated. You may see a question that concerns a disease process or procedure with which you are unfamiliar. Most test takers who are "clueless" about a question will read the question and answer choices over and over again. They do this because they hope that:

- They will remember seeing the topic in their notes or on a textbook page.
- The light will dawn and they will remember something about the topic.
- They believe there is some clue in the question that will point them toward the correct answer.

What usually happens? Absolutely nothing! The student then randomly selects an answer choice. When you randomly select an answer, you have 1 chance in 4 of getting it right. You can better those odds, and here's how: when you encounter a question that deals with unfamiliar nursing content, look for clues in the answer choices instead of in the question stem.

If you find yourself "clueless" after you carefully read a question, follow these steps:

Step 1. Resist the impulse to read and reread the question. Read the question only once. Identify the topic of the question. It is often unstated.

Step 2. Read the answer choices, not to select the correct answer, but to figure out, "What is the topic of the question," or "What should I be thinking?" You are looking for clues from the answer choices.

Step 3. After reading the answer choices, reword the question using the clues that you have obtained.

Step 4. Then use the strategies previously discussed to answer the question you have formulated.

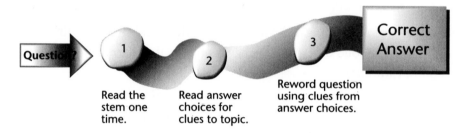

Question? 1 Read the stem one time. 2 Read answer choices for clues to topic. 3 Reword question using clues from answer choices. Correct Answer

Let's try this strategy with a question.

> A client contacts his home care LPN/LVN with complaints of nausea and abdominal pain. He has type I diabetes. The LPN/LVN should advise the client to do which of the following?
>
> 1. "Hold your regular dose of insulin."
> 2. "Check your blood glucose level every 3–4 hours."
> 3. "Increase your consumption of foods containing simple sugars."
> 4. "Increase your activity level."

Step 1. Read the stem of the question. Can you identify the topic of the question? No, you can't. The LPN/LVN is telling the client to do something, but about what topic? The topic is unstated in the question.

Step 2. Read the answer choices to obtain clues about the topic of the question. Each answer choice deals with ways to maintain a normal blood sugar.

Step 3. Reword the question. "What does the LPN/LVN tell the client about 'sick day rules'?"

ANSWERS:

(1) Hold his regular dose of insulin. This is an implementation that would increase the blood glucose level. The LPN/LVN should collect data first. Eliminate.

(2) Check his blood glucose level every 3–4 hours. This is data collection. Before you can advise the client, you must identify whether the client is hypoglycemic or hyperglycemic. Keep this answer for consideration.

(3) Increase his consumption of foods containing simple sugars. This is an implementation and would increase the client's blood glucose level. The LPN/LVN should collect data first. Eliminate.

(4) Increase his activity level. This is an implementation that would decrease the client's blood glucose level. The LPN/LVN should collect data first. Eliminate.

The nurse should always collect data before implementing nursing care. The correct answer is (2).

No matter how much you prepare for the NCLEX-PN® exam, there may be topics you see on your test with which you are unfamiliar. Reading the answer choices for clues will increase your chances of selecting a correct answer. Remember, you do have a body of knowledge. You just have to calm down and access this knowledge.

Read this question.

> A client is being treated for Addison's disease. The physician orders cortisone 25 mg PO daily. The LPN/LVN should explain to the client that adjustment of the dosage may be required in which of the following situations?
>
> 1. Dosage is increased when the blood glucose level increases.
> 2. Dosage is decreased when dietary intake is increased.
> 3. Dosage is decreased when infection stimulates endogenous steroid secretion.
> 4. Dosage is increased relative to an increase in the level of stress.

Not sure what Addison's disease is? Not sure how to adjust the dose of cortisone?

Step 1. Read the question once. Resist the impulse to reread the question.

Step 2. Read the answer choices. What should you be thinking? The question concerns cortisone. If the client is receiving cortisone, Addison's disease must be something that requires cortisone, a hormone from the adrenal glands. You notice that dosages are both increased and decreased.

Step 3. Use these clues to find the answer to THE REWORDED QUESTION, "What is true about adjusting cortisone dosage?"

(1) Dosage is increased when the blood glucose level increases. Is this true about cortisone? No. This sounds like insulin. Eliminate.

(2) Dosage is decreased when dietary intake is increased. Is this true about cortisone? No. Cortisone requirements are not related to diet. Eliminate.

(3) Dosage is decreased when infection stimulates endogenous steroid secretion. Endogenous means "within the client." If the client is receiving cortisone for Addison's disease, he must have adrenal insufficiency. Therefore, infection can't stimulate steroid secretion. Eliminate.

Step 4. The correct answer is (4) because it is the only choice remaining. Even if you are not confident that cortisone is increased during periods of stress, you can conclude that this is the correct answer because the other choices have been eliminated.

If you're not sure about the topic of the question, read the answer choices for clues.

Let's look at another path.

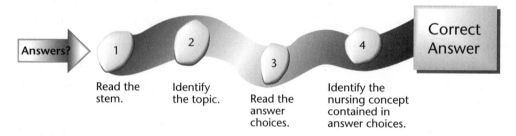

In some questions, the NCLEX-PN® exam asks you to figure out the topic of the question. In other questions, you are required to use critical thinking skills to figure out what the answer choices *really* mean. The NCLEX-PN® exam can take a concept with which you are very familiar, and make it difficult to recognize. The following question illustrates this point.

> A client with a history of heart failure visits the clinic. He states, "I have not been feeling like my old self for about 2 weeks." It would be **MOST** important for the LPN/LVN to ask which of the following questions?
>
> 1. "Do your ankles swell at the end of the day?"
> 2. "Where do you sleep at night?"
> 3. "How do you feel after you eat dinner?"
> 4. "Do you have chest pain when you inhale?"

It is not difficult to identify the topic of this question, "What is a priority for a client with heart failure?" Many students get tripped up on this question by not thinking through the answers as carefully as they should. In some questions, you have to figure out the topic of the question. In this question, you have to figure out what the answer choices mean.

Step 1. Read the stem of the question.

Step 2. Reword the question in your own words.

Step 3. Read the answer choices.

Step 4. Think: "What nursing concept should I identify in the answer choices?"

THE REWORDED QUESTION: What is a priority for a client with heart failure?

ANSWERS:

(1) "Do your ankles swell at the end of the day?" Why would you ask a client this question? Because edema is a symptom of right-sided heart failure. Is right-sided failure your priority? No, left-sided failure takes priority because it affects the lungs. Eliminate this answer.

(2) "Where do you sleep at night?" Why would you ask a client this question? If he is sleeping in his bed, his breathing is not compromised. If he has to sleep in his recliner, he is having orthopnea. Orthopnea is a symptom of left-sided failure, and this would be a priority. Keep this answer for consideration.

(3) "How do you feel after you eat dinner?" Why would you ask a client this question? Bloating after meals is a symptom of right-sided failure. This is not as important as breathing problems. Eliminate this answer.

(4) "Do you have chest pain when you inhale?" Why would you ask a client this question? It does indicate a breathing problem. The student who reacts rather than thinks may select this answer. Pain on inspiration may indicate irritation of the parietal pleura of the lung, which is not associated with heart failure. Eliminate this answer.

The correct answer is (2). In order to select this answer, you must recognize that "Where do you sleep at night?" represents orthopnea. The NCLEX-PN® exam can take important concepts such as this, and "hide" the concept in some fairly simple behaviors.

Let's try another question where you have to figure out, "What do the answer choices really mean?"

> **The LPN/LVN is caring for a client immediately after a paracentesis. It is *MOST* important for the LPN/LVN to ask which of the following questions?**
>
> 1. "Do your clothes still feel tight?"
> 2. "Do you need to void?"
> 3. "Are you feeling dizzy?"
> 4. "Do you have any pain?"

Step 1. Read the stem of the question.

Step 2. Reword the question in your own words.

Step 3. Read the answer choices.

Step 4. Think: "What nursing concept should I identify in the answer choices?"

THE REWORDED QUESTION: What is the highest priority for a client after a paracentesis?

ANSWERS:

(1) "Do your clothes still feel tight?" Why would you ask a client this question? Clothes should fit looser because the abdominal girth has decreased after fluid has been removed with a paracentesis. This is an expected outcome. Eliminate.

(2) "Do you need to void?" Why would you ask a client this question? It is imperative to empty the bladder prior to the procedure, not after the procedure. There is no compelling reason to ask the client this question. Eliminate.

(3) "Are you feeling dizzy?" What makes a client dizzy? One of the causes is a decrease in cerebral perfusion due to a fall in blood pressure. Could this client have a decreased blood pressure? Yes. Hypotension and hypovolemic shock are complications of a paracentesis due to removal of a large volume of fluid. Keep this answer for consideration.

(4) "Do you have any pain?" You ask this question to assess pain level. This client may have discomfort where the paracentesis was performed, but this is an expected outcome. Eliminate.

The correct answer is (3).

These questions illustrate why knowing nursing content is not enough to answer application/analysis-level questions. You must be able to effectively use the information you learned in practical/vocational nursing school to answer NCLEX-PN® exam-style test questions. Review the lessons that you learned in this chapter:

- Reword the question.
- Eliminate answer choices you know to be incorrect.
- Don't predict answers.
- Recognize expected outcomes.
- Read answer choices to obtain clues.

CHAPTER 4

THE NCLEX-PN® EXAM VERSUS REAL-WORLD NURSING

Some of you are nursing assistants or CNAs completing your practical/vocational nursing studies, while others are EMTs. Some of you worked during school as student techs. All of you, however, spent time in clinical during your practical/vocational nursing education. All of this adds up to a lot of experience. Experience will help you get a job, but answering questions based on your experience can be dangerous on the NCLEX-PN® exam.

Look at the following question.

> On admission to the hospital, an elderly client appears disheveled and is restless and confused. During the client's second day on the unit, an LPN/LVN approaches the client to administer medication. The LPN/LVN is unable to identify the client because his armband is missing. Which of the following actions by the nurse is the *BEST*?
>
> 1. Have the client's roommate identify him.
> 2. Ask the client to state his full name.
> 3. Ask another LPN/LVN to identify the client.
> 4. Look in the chart at the picture of the client.

Let's see how someone using his or her real-world experience would approach this question:

(1) "The roommate is never involved in identification of a client."

(2) "A confused client cannot be relied on for an accurate identification."

(3) "Sounds reasonable. I have seen this done in some circumstances."

(4) "A picture? What picture? I've never seen a picture of a client in a chart!"

Possible conclusions drawn by this person would include: *"OK, I've seen one LPN/LVN ask another for information so (3) must be the answer,"* or *"Well, maybe the client isn't all that confused, so I'll select (2)."*

According to nursing textbooks, asking another healthcare professional is not the correct way to identify a client. Many acute-care settings now include a photo of the client in the chart for just this type of situation. The correct answer to this question is (4). Many students reject this answer because there are rarely pictures of clients in the charts. Real-world experience doesn't count, though; in this case, the client does have a picture in his chart.

The NCLEX-PN® exam is a standardized exam administered by the NCSBN. Because the NCLEX-PN® exam is a national exam, students should be aware that in some parts of the country, practical/vocational nursing is practiced slightly differently. However, to ensure that the test is reflective of national trends, questions and answers are all carefully documented. The test makers ensure that the correct answers are documented in at least two standard nursing textbooks or one textbook and one nursing journal.

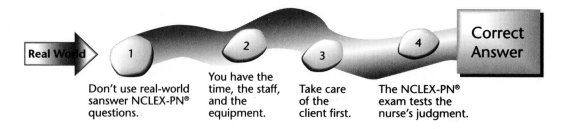

Real World → 1 — Don't use real-world sanswer NCLEX-PN® questions. 2 — You have the time, the staff, and the equipment. 3 — Take care of the client first. 4 — The NCLEX-PN® exam tests the nurse's judgment. → Correct Answer

When you are unsure of an answer choice, don't ask yourself, "What do they do on my floor?" but "What does the medical/surgical textbook writer Brunner say?" or "What do Potter and Perry say to do?" This test does not necessarily reflect what happens in the "real world," but is based on textbook nursing.

Remember the following when taking the NCLEX-PN® exam:

- You have all of the time and resources you need to provide appropriate care to your client. (Checking for bowel sounds for 5 minutes in all four quadrants, no problem!)
- You have all of the equipment you need. (Remember the bath thermometer you learned to use in the nursing lab? For the NCLEX-PN® exam, you will have one available to test the temperature of bath water.)
- There are no staffing problems on the NCLEX-PN® exam. You are caring only for the client described in the question, and that person is your only concern.
- All care given to clients is "by the book." No shortcuts are used.

Answer the following question.

> The LPN/LVN prepares an agitated and confused elderly client for surgery. The physician has ordered morphine sulfate 5 mg IM and lorazepam (Ativan) 0.5 mg IM as preoperative medications. The LPN/LVN administers these medications at the appropriate time. The LPN/LVN should take which of the following precautions after the preoperative medication is administered?
>
> 1. Ask the security guard to stay with the client.
> 2. Assign a nursing assistant to stay at the client's bedside.
> 3. Leave the client in his room alone with the side rails up.
> 4. Place the client in a vest restraint and dim the room lights.

Let's look at this using real-world logic.

(1) Ask the security guard to stay with the client. Yes, in the real world, security is called when clients are agitated.

(2) Assign a nursing assistant to stay with the client. Sounds good, but what if you don't have enough staffing to assign a nursing assistant to sit with the client?

(3) Leave the client in his room alone with the bedside rails up. Yes, that is done in the real world for most medicated preoperative clients, but this client is agitated and confused. This is not the best answer.

(4) Place the client in a vest restraint and dim the lights. Yes, this is done in the real world.

According to real-world logic, the correct answer must be (1) or (4). However, textbook theoretical nursing practice states that this client should not be left alone while in an agitated state. A member of the healthcare staff should remain with the client. Therefore, the correct answer is (2).

Use your real-world experience to help you visualize the client described in the test question, but select your answers based on what is found in nursing textbooks.

Your nursing faculty has been very conscientious about instructing you in the most up-to-date nursing practice. According to the National Council, the primary source for documenting correct answers is in nursing textbooks, and the most up-to-date practice might not always agree with the textbooks. When in doubt, always select the textbook answer!

The next question illustrates this point.

> A woman is admitted to the hospital and delivers a healthy 7 lb., 2 oz., girl. The mother decides to bottle-feed her infant. Which of the following statements by the mother after a teaching session indicates to the LPN/LVN that the client needs further instruction?
>
> 1. "I'll pump my breasts and use warm packs to relieve breast pain."
> 2. "I'll use a tight bra and ice packs to relieve engorgement discomfort."
> 3. "I'll take the medication prescribed by the doctor for pain."
> 4. "I'll take the pills ordered by my doctor to help stop the production of milk."

Let's look at these answers more closely.

(1) Pumping the breasts will stimulate milk production. This is clearly wrong.

(2) Wearing a tight bra and using ice packs are appropriate interventions for a non-breast-feeding mother.

(3) Taking a medication (mild analgesic) is an appropriate intervention for a non-breastfeeding mother.

(4) Medication to prevent lactation is not frequently prescribed because of potentially dangerous side effects. However, a medication may be prescribed to prevent lactation. This would be considered an appropriate intervention.

The correct answer is (1).

FIRST TAKE CARE OF THE CLIENT, THEN THE EQUIPMENT

The NCLEX-PN® exam tests your ability to use critical thinking skills to make nursing judgments. It is very important that you remember to:

- Take care of the client first.
- Take care of the equipment second.

Look at the following question.

> A client sustains a fractured left femur in a car accident. She is placed in balanced-suspension skeletal traction using a Thomas splint and a Pearson attachment. The client tells the LPN/LVN that she has "terrible" pain in her left thigh. Which of the following should the LPN/LVN do *FIRST?*
>
> 1. Determine that all the weights and ropes from the traction apparatus are in line and hanging free.
> 2. Ask the client for more information about the location and characteristics of her pain.
> 3. Check the Thomas splint and Pearson attachment to make sure they are properly positioned.
> 4. Explain to the client that the pain she is experiencing in the affected leg is a common occurrence.

Let's review the answers:

(1) All weights should be hanging free in balanced-suspension skeletal traction. This answer choice has you checking the equipment, not the client. Your first concern should be the client, not the traction.

(2) The LPN/LVN should focus on assessing the client and her problem before assessing the function of the equipment. All complaints of pain should be thoroughly investigated by the LPN/LVN.

(3) This answer choice has you checking the equipment, not the client. Your first concern should be the client, not the traction.

(4) Any complaints of pain are considered abnormal and should be thoroughly investigated by the LPN/LVN.

The correct answer is (2).

LABORATORY VALUES

Answering questions about lab values is another example of how the real world does not work on the NCLEX-PN® exam. In practical/vocational nursing school, you learned lab values for specific tests and you may not have remembered them after the test. While you were in the clinical setting, the emphasis was on interpretation of lab values. Because most lab slips contained a listing of normal values, you were able to compare the client's results to the normal levels. Questions on the NCLEX-PN® exam will not provide you with a listing of normal lab values.

To answer questions on the NCLEX-PN® exam, you must:

- Know normal lab test results.
- Correctly interpret normal or abnormal lab test results.

Compare the following two questions.

> A client is admitted to the hospital with flu-like symptoms. When taking the history, the LPN/LVN learns that the client has been taking digoxin (Lanoxin) 0.125 mg PO daily and furosemide (Lasix) 40 mg PO daily for 3 years. Last month her physician changed the prescription for digoxin to 0.25 mg qd. The LPN/LVN would expect the physician to order which of the following laboratory tests?
>
> 1. Serum electrolytes and digoxin level
> 2. White blood cell count and hemoglobin and hematocrit
> 3. Cardiac enzymes and an arterial blood gas
> 4. Blood cultures and urinalysis

Most of you are probably familiar with the concepts presented in this question. The physician has increased the client's dose of digoxin. Lasix is a potassium-wasting diuretic. The client will likely develop digitalis toxicity if she has a low potassium level. Serum electrolytes and digoxin level (1) is the correct answer.

Now look at this question.

> The LPN/LVN implements care for a teenager admitted with complaints of fever, vomiting, and diarrhea. The LPN/LVN sees the following nursing diagnosis on the client's care plan: "fluid volume deficit." Which of the following changes in laboratory values would demonstrate an improvement in the client's condition?
>
> 1. Urine specific gravity, 1.015; hematocrit, 37%
> 2. Urine specific gravity, 1.020; hematocrit, 45%
> 3. Urine specific gravity, 1.032; hematocrit, 52%
> 4. Urine specific gravity, 1.025; hematocrit, 35%

In order to correctly answer this question, you must know:

- The normal levels of hematocrit (male 42–50%, female 40–48%) and the specific gravity of urine (1.010–1.030)
- How the hematocrit and specific gravity levels are affected by a fluid volume deficit

Fluid volume deficit occurs when water and electrolytes are lost in the same proportion as they exist in the body. When a client is dehydrated, both the specific gravity of urine and the hematocrit become elevated. The correct answer is (2).

Answer this question:

> A client is hospitalized with a diagnosis of atrial fibrillation. Heparin 5,000 units is ordered every 12 hours to be given subcutaneously. The physician orders daily partial thromboplastin times (PTTs). The result of the client's most recent PTT is 55 seconds. Which of the following actions should be taken by the LPN/LVN?
>
> 1. Document the results and administer the heparin.
> 2. Withhold the heparin.
> 3. Notify the physician.
> 4. Have the test repeated.

In order to answer this question you need to know:

- The normal range for a PTT is 20–45 seconds.
- The therapeutic range for a client receiving heparin, an anticoagulant, is 1.5–2 times the control or normal level.

Evaluate the answer choices:

(1) Document the results and give the heparin. The client's most recent PTT is 55 seconds. This is not 1.5–2 times the control or normal so the medication should be given.

(2) Withhold the heparin. The PTT level is not yet within what is considered an effective therapeutic level. This client needs the anticoagulant.

(3) Notify the physician. There is no reason to notify the physician. The client has not reached the therapeutic level of heparin.

(4) Have the test repeated. There is no reason to have the test repeated. The client has not achieved the therapeutic level.

The correct answer is (1).

MEDICATION ADMINISTRATION

An important function in providing safe and effective care to clients is the administration of medications. Because this is one of the responsibilities of a beginning LPN/LVN, questions about medications are often an important part of the NCLEX-PN® exam. The LPN/LVN who is minimally competent is knowledgeable about medications and uses the "six rights" when administering medication.

In nursing school, most questions about medication followed the same pattern. You were told the client's diagnosis, the name of the medication, and then were asked a question. Even if you didn't know the information about the medication, sometimes you were able to select the correct answer by knowing the diagnosis.

The NCLEX-PN® exam does not give you any clues from the context of the question. The questions on this exam include the name of the medication, almost always identifying it by both trade and generic names. Most of the time, you will not be given the reason the client is receiving the medication.

Let's look at some medication questions.

> The physician orders furosemide (Lasix) and spironolactone (Aldactone) for a client. Prior to administering the medication, the LPN/LVN determines that the client's potassium is 3.2 mEq/L. In addition to notifying the supervising RN, the LPN/LVN should anticipate taking which of the following actions?
>
> 1. Do not administer the Lasix or Aldactone.
> 2. Administer the Aldactone only.
> 3. Administer the Lasix only.
> 4. Administer the Lasix and Aldactone.

This is a typical exam-style medication question. The question concerns the side effects and nursing implications of Lasix and Aldactone.

(1) The potassium level is below normal (3.5–5.0 mEq/L). Lasix is a potassium-wasting diuretic. Aldactone is a potassium-sparing diuretic. There is no reason to hold the Aldactone because the client has a low potassium level. Eliminate this answer.

(2) The Aldactone should be administered.

(3) Do not administer the Lasix because it is a potassium-wasting diuretic. The client's potassium level is already low. Eliminate.

(4) Do not administer the Lasix. Eliminate.

The correct answer is (2).

Let's try this next question.

> A client returns to the clinic 2 weeks after being started on allopurinol (Zyloprim) 200 mg PO daily. The LPN/LVN reviews information about this medication with the client. Which of the following statements by the client indicates that the teaching was effective?
>
> 1. "I should take my medication on an empty stomach."
> 2. "I should take my medication with orange juice."
> 3. "I should increase my intake of protein."
> 4. "I should drink at least 8 glasses of water every day."

To answer this question you need to know information about Zyloprim, an antigout agent that reduces uric acid.

(1) Zyloprim is best tolerated with or immediately after meals to reduce gastrointestinal (GI) irritation. Eliminate.

(2) Orange juice makes the urine acidic. Zyloprim is more soluble in alkaline urine. Eliminate.

(3) It is not necessary to increase the intake of protein when taking Zyloprim. Eliminate.

(4) Zyloprim can cause renal calculi. The client should drink 3,000 mL/day to reduce the risk of kidney stone formation.

The correct answer is (4). You must know the side effects and nursing implications of medications for the NCLEX-PN® exam.

NOTIFY THE PHYSICIAN

Another behavior that commonly occurs in the real world is calling the physician. In nursing school you were encouraged to notify your instructor of changes in your client's condition. Be very careful how you handle this on the NCLEX-PN® exam. More often than not, the answer choice that states "call the physician," "contact the social worker," or "refer to the chaplain" is the WRONG answer. Usually there is something you need to do first before you make that call. The NCLEX-PN® exam does not want to know what the physician is going to do. The NCLEX-PN® exam wants to know what you, the LPN/LVN, will do in a given situation.

Answer this question.

> The LPN/LVN notes that there is no urine in the client's urinary drainage bag 3 hours after the bag was last emptied. Which of the following actions should the LPN/LVN take *FIRST*?
>
> 1. Check for kinks in the tubing.
> 2. Insert a new indwelling catheter.
> 3. Irrigate the urinary catheter.
> 4. Notify the client's physician.

THE REWORDED QUESTION: What should you do *first* for this client? Have this client's kidneys stopped producing urine? Is there an obstruction in the urinary drainage system?

(1) If there is no urine in the urine drainage bag, could there be an obstruction in the drainage system? Checking for kinks in the drainage tubing has virtually no risks and could provide a simple explanation for your observations.

(2) Inserting a new indwelling catheter may address a "possible" obstruction in the tubing, but provides a new opportunity for the client to contract a nosocomial urinary tract infection. Are you sure you want to do this first?

(3) Irrigating the urinary catheter in hopes of dislodging a "possible" obstruction again opens the client up to contract a nosocomial urinary tract infection. Are you sure you want to do this first?

(4) If you notify the client's physician of "no urinary output in 3 hours" as your first action, will you be able to answer potential questions from the physician regarding the client and the lack of urinary output? Are you avoiding your responsibility and transferring your responsibility to the physician? Is there something YOU should do first?

The correct answer is (1).

Before you choose the answer choice that involves "call the physician," look at the other answer choices very carefully. Make sure that there isn't an answer that contains data collection or an action you should take before making the phone call. The test makers want to know what you would do in a situation, not what the doctor would do!

Here is one more real-world question.

> Upon returning from lunch, the LPN/LVN is approached in the elevator by a hospital employee from another unit. The employee states that her close friend is a client on the nurse's unit. The employee asks how her friend is doing and if all of her tests were normal. The LPN/LVN should do which of the following?
>
> 1. Answer the employee's questions softly so other people on the elevator will not hear.
> 2. Refuse to discuss her friend's medical condition. Suggest that she visit her friend.
> 3. Give the employee the name of the client's physician to call for this information.
> 4. Tell the employee about the results of the client's tests because they were within normal limits.

THE REWORDED QUESTION: What should an LPN/LVN do when asked about a client by a hospital employee?

(1) Discussing client information in a public place is a breach of confidentiality. Eliminate.

(2) This does not violate the client's right to privacy and confidentiality. Keep in consideration.

(3) Providing any information about a client to someone not directly involved in the client's care is a breach of privacy. Eliminate.

(4) It is a breach in the client's right to privacy to share any information with others without the client's permission. Eliminate.

The correct answer is (2).

Expect to see real-world situations on your NCLEX-PN® exam, but make sure that you do not choose real-world answers! These strategies should help you use your previous nursing experience without encountering any pitfalls.

CHAPTER 5

STRATEGIES FOR PRIORITY QUESTIONS

One of the biggest challenges facing you as a candidate for practical/vocational nursing licensure is to correctly answer priority questions. You will recognize these questions because they will ask you what is the "best," "most important," "first," or "initial" response by the nurse.

Take a look at this sample question.

> An hour after admission to the nursery, the LPN/LVN observes a newborn baby having spontaneous jerky movements of the limbs. The infant's mother had gestational diabetes mellitus (GDM) during pregnancy. Which of the following actions should the LPN/LVN take *FIRST*?
>
> 1. Give dextrose water.
> 2. Call the physician immediately.
> 3. Determine the blood glucose level.
> 4. Observe closely for other symptoms.

As you read this question you are probably thinking, "All of these look right!" or "How can I decide what I will do first?" The panic sets in as you try to decide what the best answer is when they all seem "correct."

As a licensed practical/vocational nurse, you will be caring for clients who have multiple problems and needs. You must be able to establish priorities by deciding which needs take precedence over other needs. You probably recognized the baby's jerky movements as an indication of hypoglycemia. Don't forget that an important part of the data collection process is *validating* what you observe. You must complete data collection before you plan and implement nursing care. The correct answer is (3).

The following situation might sound familiar: You are called to a client's room by a family member and find the client lying on the floor. He is bleeding from a wound on the forehead, and his indwelling catheter is dislodged and hanging from the side of the bed. Where do you begin? Do you call for help? Do you return him to bed? Do you apply pressure to the cut? Do you reinsert the catheter? Do you call the doctor? What do you do *first*? This is why establishing priorities is so important.

Your nursing faculty recognized the importance of teaching you how to establish priorities. They required you to establish priorities both in clinical situations and when answering test questions. These are the type of questions that practical/vocational nursing students find most controversial.

Here is an example of a nursing school test question:

> Which of the following would most concern the LPN/LVN during a client's recovery from surgery?
>
> (1) Safety
> (2) Hemorrhage
> (3) Infection
> (4) Pain control

A conversation in class with your instructor may then go something like this:

Instructor: "The correct answer is (2)."

Student: "Why isn't infection the correct answer? It says right here *[pointing to textbook]* that infection is a major complication after surgery!"

Instructor: "Yes, infection is an important concern after surgery. But, if the client has a life-threatening hemorrhage, then the fact that the wound is infected is immaterial."

Student: "But it says here on page 106 that infection is a major complication after surgery. You can't count this answer wrong!"

In some situations, the faculty member will give you partial credit for your answer, or will "throw the question out" because there is more than one right answer. But you won't get the opportunity to argue about questions on the NCLEX-PN® exam. You either select the answer the test makers are looking for, or you get the question wrong. In the question above, all of the answers listed are important when caring for a postoperative client, but only one answer is the *best*.

The critical thinking required for priority questions is for you to recognize patterns in the answer choices. By recognizing these patterns, you will know which path you need to choose to correctly answer the question. This chapter will present several strategies to help you establish priorities on the NCLEX-PN® exam:

- Maslow strategy
- Nursing process strategy
- Safety strategy

We will outline each strategy, describe how and when it should be used, and show you how to apply these strategies to exam-style questions. By using these strategies, you will be able to eliminate the second-best answer and correctly identify the highest priority.

STRATEGY ONE: MASLOW

Maslow's hierarchy of needs (Figure 1) is crucial to establishing priorities on the NCLEX-PN® exam. Maslow identifies five levels of human needs: physiological, safety and security, love and belonging, self-esteem, and self-actualization.

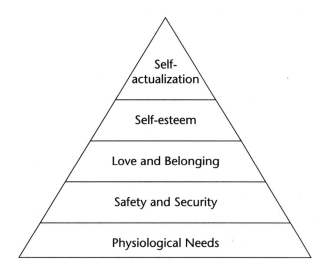

Figure 1: Maslow's Hierarchy of Needs

Because *physiological needs* are necessary for survival, they have the highest priority and must be met first. Physiological needs include oxygen, fluid, nutrition, temperature, elimination, shelter, rest, and sex. If you don't have oxygen to breathe or food to eat, you really don't care if you have stable psychosocial relationships!

Safety and security needs can be both physical and psychosocial. Physical safety includes decreasing what is threatening to the client. The threat may be an illness (myocardial infarction), accidents (a parent transporting a newborn in a car without using a car seat), or environmental threats (the client with COPD who insists on walking outside in 10° F [-12° C] temperatures).

To attain psychological safety, the client must have the knowledge and understanding about what to expect from others in his environment. For example, it is important to teach the client and his family what to expect after a "cerebrovascular accident (CVA)". It is also important that you allow a woman preparing for a mastectomy to verbalize her concerns about changes that might occur in her relationship with her partner.

To achieve *love and belonging,* the client needs to feel loved by family and accepted by others. When a client feels self-confident and useful, he will achieve the need of *self-esteem* as described by Maslow.

The highest level of Maslow's hierarchy of needs is *self-actualization.* To achieve this level the client must experience fulfillment and recognize his or her potential. In order for self-actualization to occur, all of the lower-level needs must be met. Because of the stresses of life, lower-level needs are not always met, and many people never achieve this high level of functioning.

The Maslow Four-Step Process

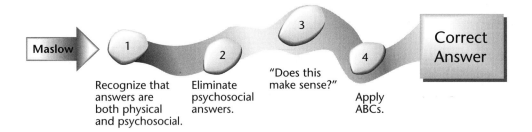

The first strategy to use in establishing priorities is a four-step process, beginning with Maslow's hierarchy. To use the Maslow strategy, you must first recognize the pattern in the answer choices.

Step 1. Look at your answer choices.

Determine if the answer choices are both physical and psychosocial. If they are, apply the Maslow strategy detailed in Step 2.

Step 2. Eliminate all psychosocial answer choices. If an answer choice is physiological, don't eliminate it yet. Remember, Maslow states that physiological needs must be met first. Although pain certainly has a physiological component, reactions to pain are considered "psychosocial" on this exam and will become a lower priority.

Step 3. Look at each of the answer choices that you have not yet eliminated and ask yourself if the answer choice makes sense with regard to the disease or situation described in the question. If it makes sense as an answer choice, keep it for consideration and go on to the next choice.

Step 4. Can you apply the ABCs?

Look at the remaining answer choices. Can you apply the ABCs? The ABCs stand for airway, breathing, and circulation. If there is an answer that involves maintaining a patent airway, it will be correct. If not, is there a choice that involves breathing problems? It will be correct. If not, go on with the ABCs. Is there an answer pertaining to the cardiovascular system? It will be correct. What if the ABCs don't apply? Compare the remaining answer choices and ask yourself, "What is the highest priority?" This is your answer.

Let's apply this technique to a few sample exam-style test questions.

> A woman is admitted to the hospital with a ruptured ectopic pregnancy. A laparotomy is scheduled. Preoperatively, which of the following goals is *MOST* important for the LPN/LVN to include on the client's plan of care?
>
> 1. Fluid replacement
> 2. Pain relief
> 3. Emotional support
> 4. Respiratory therapy

Look at the stem of the question. The words *most important* mean:

- This is a priority question.
- There probably will be more than one answer choice that is a correct nursing action, but it will not be the most important or highest priority action.

Step 1. Look at the answer choices.

You see that both physical and psychosocial interventions are included. Apply the Maslow strategy.

Step 2. Eliminate the answer choices that are psychosocial interventions.

Answer choice (2), which is pain relief, should be discarded. Remember, pain is considered a psychosocial problem on the NCLEX-PN® exam. Answer choice (3), emotional support, is also a psychosocial concern. Eliminate this answer. You have now eliminated two of the possible choices. You are halfway there!

Step 3. Now look at the remaining answer choices and ask yourself whether they make sense.

Answer choice (1), fluid replacement makes sense, because this client has a ruptured ectopic pregnancy. An ectopic pregnancy is implantation of the fertilized ovum in a site other than the endometrial lining, usually the fallopian tube. Initially, the pregnancy is normal, but as the embryo outgrows the fallopian tube, the tube ruptures, causing extensive bleeding into the abdominal cavity. Answer choice (4), respiratory therapy, does not make sense with a ruptured ectopic pregnancy. The obstetrical client is not likely to need respiratory care prior to surgery. Eliminate this answer choice.

You are left with the correct answer, (1). After reading this question, many students select answer choices (2) or (3) as the correct answer. They justify this by emphasizing the importance of managing this woman's pain, or addressing her grief about losing the pregnancy. Neither answer choice takes priority over the physiological demand of fluid replacement prior to surgery.

Ready for another question? Try this one.

The LPN/LVN implements care for a 14-year-old girl admitted with an eating disorder. On admission, the girl weighs 82 lbs. and is 5'4" tall. Lab tests indicate severe hypokalemia, anemia, and dehydration. The LPN/LVN should give which of the following nursing diagnoses the HIGHEST priority?

1. Body image disturbance related to weight loss
2. Self-esteem disturbance related to feelings of inadequacy
3. Altered nutrition: less than body requirements related to decreased intake
4. Decreased cardiac output related to the potential for dysrhythmias

---

The first thing you should notice in this question stem is the phrase *"highest priority"*. This alerts you that there may be more than one answer that could be considered correct.

Step 1. Look at the answer choices.

You will see that both physical and psychosocial interventions are included. Apply the Maslow strategy.

Step 2. Eliminate all answer choices that involve psychosocial concerns.

It is easy to see that body image disturbance is a psychosocial concern. The same is true of answer choice (2), self-esteem disturbance. Answer choices (3) and (4) are physiological. You have now eliminated all but two answer choices:

Step 3. Ask yourself whether the remaining answer choices make sense.

Answer choice (2) "Altered nutrition: less than body requirements related to decreased intake" does make sense. Remember, the client has anorexia and is 5'4" tall and weighs 82 lbs. Answer choice (4) "Decreased cardiac output related to the potential for dysrhythmias" also makes sense. Dysrhythmias are a concern for a client with severe hypokalemia, which often occurs with anorexia.

You still have work to do.

Step 4. Now use the ABCs to establish priorities.

Decreased cardiac output is a higher priority than altered nutrition. One answer choice remains: (4).

When you first read this question, you probably identified each of the answer choices as appropriate for a client with anorexia. Only one nursing diagnosis can be the highest priority. Using strategies involving Maslow and the ABCs will enable you to choose the correct answer on your NCLEX-PN® exam.

STRATEGY TWO: NURSING PROCESS (DATA COLLECTION VERSUS IMPLEMENTATION)

A second strategy that will assist you in establishing priorities involves the data collection and implementation steps of the nursing process. As a practical/vocational nursing student, you have been drilled so that you can recite the steps of the nursing process in your sleep—data collection, planning, implementation, and evaluation. In practical/vocational nursing school, you did have some test questions about the nursing process, but you probably did not use the nursing process to assist you in selecting a correct answer on an exam. On the NCLEX-PN® exam, you will be given a clinical situation and asked to establish priorities. The possible answer choices will include both the correct data collection action and implementation for this clinical situation. How do you choose the correct answer when both the correct mode of data collection and implementation are given? Think about these two steps of the nursing process.

Data collection is the process of establishing a data profile about the client and his or her health problems. The nurse obtains subjective and objective data in a number of ways: talking to clients, observing clients and/or significant others, taking a health history, evaluating lab results, and collaborating with other members of the healthcare team.

Once you collect the data you compare it to the client's baseline or normal values. On the NCLEX-PN® exam, the client's baseline may not be given, but as a practical/vocational nursing student you have acquired a body of knowledge. On this exam, you are expected to compare the client information you are given to the "normal" values learned from your nursing textbooks.

Data collection is the first step of the nursing process and takes priority over all other steps. It is essential that you complete the data collection phase of the nursing process before you implement nursing activities. This is a common mistake made by NCLEX-PN® exam takers: don't implement before you collect data. For example, when performing cardiopulmonary resuscitation (CPR), if you don't access the airway before performing mouth-to-mouth resuscitation, your actions may be harmful!

Implementation is the care you provide to your clients. Nursing interventions may be independent, dependent, and interdependent. Independent nursing interventions are generally *not* within the scope of the LPN/LVN's nursing practice. However, the LPN/LVN can follow established care plans, standards of care, and established protocols. For example, the LPN/LVN can instruct a client to turn, cough, and deep breathe after surgery. Dependent interventions are based on the written orders of a physician. On the NCLEX-PN® exam, you should assume that you have an order for all dependent interventions that are included in the answer choices.

This may be a different way of thinking from the way you were taught in practical/vocational nursing school. Many students select an answer on a nursing school test (that is later counted wrong) because the intervention requires a physician's order. Everyone walks away from the test review muttering "trick question." It is important for you to remember that there are no trick questions on the NCLEX-PN® exam. You should base your answer on an understanding that you have a physician's order for any nursing intervention described.

Interdependent interventions are shared with the RN and other members of the healthcare team. For instance, nutrition education would be directed and supervised by the RN and may be shared with the LPN/LVN and the dietician. Chest physiotherapy may be directed and supervised by the RN and shared with a respiratory therapist and an LPN/LVN.

The following strategy, utilizing the data collection and implementation phases of the nursing process, will assist you in selecting correct answers to questions that ask you to identify priorities.

Step 1. Read the answer choices to establish a pattern.

If the answer choices are a mix of data collection/validation and implementation, use the Nursing Process (Data Collection vs. Implementation) strategy.

Step 2. Refer to the question.

Determine whether you should be collecting data or implementing.

Step 3. Eliminate answer choices, and then choose the best answer.

If after Step 2 you find that, for example, it is a data collection question, eliminate any answers that clearly focus on implementation. Then choose the best data collection answer.

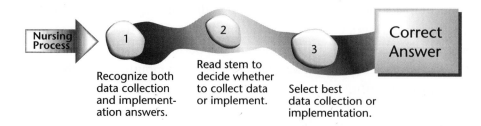

Data vs. implementation

Try this strategy on the following question.

> The LPN/LVN is caring for a client who underwent abdominal surgery 6 hours ago. Which of the following actions by the LPN/LVN is *MOST* important?
>
> 1. Have the client use a pillow to splint the incision.
> 2. Instruct the client how to safely get out of bed.
> 3. Reinforce the dry dressing to provide more padding.
> 4. Turn the client to check for bleeding underneath her.

} implementation

data collection

THE REWORDED QUESTION: What nursing priority should the LPN/LVN identify in this scenario? What are the risks for a client after abdominal surgery?

Step 1. Read the answer choices to establish a pattern.

There is one data collection answer, (4), and three implementation answers, (1), (2), and (3). You can use the Nursing Process (Data Collection vs. Implementation) strategy.

Step 2. Refer to the question to determine if you should be collecting data or implementing care.

You know that bleeding is a risk for all surgical abdominal wounds. According to the nursing process, you should collect data first.

Step 3. Eliminate answer choices, and then choose the best answer.

Eliminate answers (1), (2), and (3), which are implementation answers. You are left with only one answer choice, (4). Clients with abdominal surgical wounds often find their most comfortable position lying on their backs in bed. Fluid, namely blood, flows via gravity to dependent areas. A cursory look at the top of the dressing may reveal no drainage; however, when the client is rolled to her side, a pool of blood could be noted if the wound is hemorrhaging. Even if this had not occurred to you, you are still able to correctly answer this question using the data collection versus implementation strategy.

Let's look at another question.

> A boy was riding his bike to school when he hit the curb. He fell and hurt his leg. The LPN/LVN was called and found him alert and conscious but in severe pain with a possible fracture of the right femur. Which of the following is the *FIRST* action that the LPN/LVN should take?
>
> 1. Immobilize the affected limb with a splint and ask him not to move.
> 2. Make a thorough assessment of the circumstances surrounding the accident.
> 3. Put him in semi-Fowler's position for comfort.
> 4. Check the pedal pulse and blanching sign in both legs.

The words *"first action"* tell you that this is a "priority" question.

THE REWORDED QUESTION: What is the highest priority for a fractured femur?

Step 1. Read the answer choices to establish a pattern.

The answer choices are a mix of data collection and implementation, so use the Nursing Process (Data Collection vs. Implementation) strategy.

Step 2. Determine whether you should be collecting data or implementing.

According to the question, the LPN/LVN has determined that the boy has a possible fracture. This implies that the LPN/LVN has completed the data-collection step. It is now time to implement.

Step 3. Eliminate answer choices, and then choose the best answer.

Eliminate answers (2) and (4) because they involve data collection. This leaves you with choices (1) and (3). Which takes priority: immobilizing the affected limb, or placing the boy in a semi-Fowler's position to facilitate breathing? The question does not indicate the boy is experiencing any respiratory distress. The correct answer is (1), immobilize the affected limb.

Some students will choose an answer involving the ABCs without thinking it through. Students, beware. Use the ABCs to establish priorities, but make sure that the answer is appropriate to the situation. In this question, breathing was mentioned in one of the answer choices. If you thought of the ABCs immediately without looking at the context of the question, you would have answered this question incorrectly.

Look at this question in another form.

> A boy was riding his bike to school when he hit the curb. The boy tells the LPN/LVN, "I think my leg is broken." Which of the following is the *FIRST* action the LPN/LVN should take?
>
> 1. Immobilize the affected limb with a splint and ask the client not to move.
> 2. Ask the client to explain what happened.
> 3. Put the client in semi-Fowler's position to facilitate breathing.
> 4. Check the appearance of the client's leg.

Step 1. Determine whether you should be collecting data or implementing. In this question, the client has stated, "My leg is broken." This statement is not the LPN/LVN's assessment. This alerts the LPN/LVN that there is a problem, and the LPN/LVN should begin the steps of the nursing process. The first step is data collection.

Step 2. Eliminate answers (1) and (3). These are implementations.

Step 3. What takes priority? Examination of the leg takes priority over investigation into what happened to cause the accident. The correct answer is (4).

STRATEGY THREE: SAFETY

LPN/LVNs have the primary responsibility of ensuring the safety of clients. This includes clients in healthcare facilities, in the home, at work, and in the community. Safety includes: meeting basic needs (oxygen, food, fluids, etc.), reducing hazards that cause injury to clients (accidents, obstacles in the home), and decreasing the transmission of pathogens (immunizations, sanitation).

Remember that the NCLEX-PN® exam is a test of minimum competency to determine that you are able to practice safe and effective nursing care. Always think *safety* when selecting correct answers on the exam. When answering questions about procedures, this strategy will help you to establish priorities.

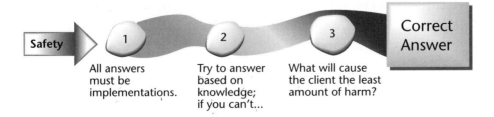

Safety

1. All answers must be implementations.
2. Try to answer based on knowledge; if you can't...
3. What will cause the client the least amount of harm?

Correct Answer

Step 1. Are all the answer choices implementations? If so, use the Safety strategy illustrated above.

Step 2. Can you answer the question based on your knowledge? If not, continue to Step 3.

Step 3. Ask yourself, "What will cause my client the least amount of harm?" and choose the best answer.

Apply this strategy to the following question.

A child undergoes a tonsillectomy for treatment of chronic tonsillitis unresponsive to antibiotic therapy. After surgery, the child is brought to the clinical unit. Which of the following actions should the LPN/LVN include in his plan of care?

1. Institute measures to minimize crying.
2. Perform postural drainage every 2 hours.
3. Cough and deep-breathe every hour.
4. Give ice cream as tolerated.

THE REWORDED QUESTION: What should you do after a tonsillectomy?

Step 1. Are all the answer choices implementations?

Yes.

Step 2. Can you answer the question based on your knowledge of a tonsillectomy?

If not, continue to Step 3.

Step 3. Ask yourself, "What will cause my client the least amount of harm?"

Answer choice (1), minimizing crying, will help prevent bleeding. Keep in consideration. Answer choice (2), postural drainage, may cause bleeding. Eliminate. Coughing and deep-breathing (3) may cause bleeding. Eliminate. Giving ice cream (4) may cause the child to clear his throat, causing bleeding. Eliminate. The correct answer is (1). The nurse must prevent postoperative hemorrhage, a complication seen after this type of surgery. Crying would irritate the child's throat and increase the chance of hemorrhage.

Let's try another question.

> The LPN/LVN doubts the accuracy of a drug order on the medication administration record. Which of the following actions should the LPN/LVN take *FIRST*?
>
> 1. Compare the drug order on the medication administration record with the physician's order sheet.
> 2. Contact the prescribing physician.
> 3. Consult with the pharmacist.
> 4. Look up the medication in a nursing drug book.

THE REWORDED QUESTION: What should you do if you think the Medication Administration Record (MAR) is incorrect?

Step 1. Are all the answers implementations?

Yes.

Step 2. Ask yourself the question, "What will protect my client the most?"

(1) Comparing the MAR with the original physician's order would certainly provide clarification regarding the questioned medication. Leave this choice for consideration.

(2) Calling the prescribing physician would certainly help clarify the order, but this should not be the first step. Eliminate.

(3) Consulting the pharmacist can shed light on a medication, but the LPN/LVN first needs to know what the original order said. Eliminate.

(4) Looking up the medication in a nursing drug book is a good idea, but will this step help the LPN/LVN if the original order was incorrectly written on the MAR? Eliminate.

Only choice (1) is left for consideration and is the correct answer. The NCLEX-PN® test makers want to know what decision you are going to make to protect your client, not what decision the physician will make.

Let's look at another question.

> A client is admitted with a diagnosis of dementia. He attempts several times to pull out his nasogastric tube. An order for cloth wrist restraints is received by the LPN/LVN. Which of the following actions by the LPN/LVN is *MOST* appropriate?
>
> 1. Attach the ties of the restraints to the bed frame.
> 2. Perform range of motion to the restrained extremities once a shift.
> 3. Remove the restraints when the client is up in a wheelchair.
> 4. Explain the need for restraints only to the family because the client is confused.

THE REWORDED QUESTION: "What is the safest way to apply restraints?"

Step 1. Are all answers implementations?

Yes.

Step 2. Can you answer this based on your knowledge?

If not, proceed to Step 3.

Step 3. Ask yourself, "What will cause the least amount of harm to the client?"

(1) Attaching the ties of the restraint to the bed frame will not harm the client. Retain this answer.

(2) Performing range of motion once a shift will not harm the client. However, it should be performed more frequently. Retain this answer.

(3) Removing the restraints when the client is up in a wheelchair will be harmful to the client. Restraints should not be removed when the client is unattended. Eliminate.

(4) Explaining the need for restraints only to the family can cause harm to the client. Restraints can increase the confusion or combativeness of the client. Even though the client is confused, he needs to receive an explanation. Eliminate.

You are now considering answer choices (1) and (2). What will cause the least amount of harm to the client—attaching the ties of the restraint to the bed frame or performing range of motion to the extremities once a shift? Range of motion should be performed every 2–4 hours to prevent loss of joint mobility. Eliminate (2). The correct answer is (1). Attaching the ties of the restraint to the bed frame will allow the nurse to raise and lower the side rail without injury to the client.

Priority questions are an important component of the NCLEX-PN® exam. To help you select correct answers, think:

- Maslow
- The Nursing Process
- Safety

Answer the following three questions using the appropriate priority strategy. The explanations follow the questions.

Question 1

The LPN/LVN cares for a client with a diagnosis of cerebrovascular accident (CVA). The LPN/LVN is feeding the client in a chair when he suddenly begins to choke. Which of the following actions should the LPN/LVN take *FIRST*?

1. Check for breathlessness by placing an ear over the client's mouth and observing the chest.
2. Leave the client in the chair and apply vigorous abdominal or chest thrusts from behind the client.
3. Ask the client, "Are you choking?"
4. Return the client to the bed and apply vigorous abdominal or chest thrusts while straddling the client's thighs.

Question 2

A client with a history of bipolar disorder is admitted to the psychiatric hospital. She was found by the police attempting to climb onto the wing of a plane at the airport. Her husband reports that she has not eaten or slept in 2 days, and he suspects she has stopped taking lithium. On admission, the LPN/LVN should place the HIGHEST priority on which of the following client care needs?

1. Teaching the client about the importance of taking lithium as prescribed
2. Providing the client with a safe environment with few distractions
3. Arranging for food and rest for the client
4. Setting limits on the client's behavior

Question 3

> The physician orders a nasogastric (NG) tube inserted and connected to low intermittent suction for a client with an intestinal obstruction. Two hours after the insertion of the NG tube, the client vomits 200 mL. While irrigating the NG tube, the LPN/LVN notes resistance. Which of the following actions should the LPN/LVN take FIRST?
>
> 1. Replace the NG tube with a larger one.
> 2. Turn the client on his left side.
> 3. Change the suction from intermittent to continuous.
> 4. Continue the irrigation.

Let's see if you were able to correctly determine which strategy you should use to determine priorities.

Question 1

Look at your answer choices to determine a pattern. Choices (1) and (3) involve data collection; (2) and (4) are implementations. Use the nursing process to select the correct answer.

Step 1. Determine whether you should be collecting data or implementing.

According to the situation, the client has begun to choke. This alerts the nurse that there is a problem. The first step of the nursing process is data collection.

Step 2. Eliminate (2) and (4) because they are implementations.

Step 3. What takes priority—assessing for breathlessness by placing an ear over the client's mouth or assessing the client by asking, "Are you choking?" Inability to speak or cough indicates the airway is obstructed. Breathlessness should be checked only in an unconscious client. The correct answer is (3).

Question 2

Look at the answer choices. They include both physiological and psychosocial interventions. Apply the Maslow strategy.

Step 1. Eliminate all answer choices that are psychosocial—(1) and (4).

Step 2. Look at the remaining answer choices and ask yourself if they make sense.

Choice (2), providing the client with a safe environment, does make sense. Retain this answer.

Choice (3), arranging for food and rest, also makes sense. Retain this answer.

Step 3. Answer the question, "What takes highest priority—providing for a safe environment or providing for food and rest?" According to Maslow, food and rest take highest priority. The correct answer is (3).

Question 3

This question is about a procedure. Read the answer choices to establish a pattern. All of the answers are interventions. If you are unsure about a procedure, think *safety*.

Step 1. What is the question? What should the LPN/LVN do when resistance is met while irrigating an NG tube? If you're not sure, think safety.

Step 2. Answer this question: "What will cause the client the least amount of harm?"

(1) Replacing the NG tube with a larger one could harm the client by damaging the mucosa. Eliminate.

(2) Turning the client to his left side would not hurt the client. Retain this answer.

(3) Changing the suction from intermittent to continuous is never done because it will erode the mucosa. Eliminate.

(4) Continuing the irrigation when there is resistance might be harmful. Never force an irrigation. Eliminate.

The correct answer is (2). The tip of the tube may be against the stomach wall. Repositioning the client might allow the tip to lie unobstructed in the stomach.

Using the critical thinking strategies outlined in this chapter will help you unlock the secrets of correctly answering priority questions.

CHAPTER 6

STRATEGIES FOR COORDINATION OF CARE QUESTIONS

The delivery of healthcare in the United States is an ever more integrated system, utilizing the skills of physicians; advanced practice nurses (e.g., nurse practitioners [NPs]); registered nurses (RNs); licensed practical nurses (LPNs), also called licensed vocational nurses (LVNs); certified nursing assistants (CNAs); and unlicensed assistive personnel (UAPs), such as nursing assistants and home health aides. Each position carries its own duties and responsibilities, but coordination of all the members of the healthcare team is essential for the delivery of optimal care to the client. This chapter discusses the coordination of care, especially as it pertains to LPN/LVNs.

Many healthcare settings, including hospitals, clinics, and physician and NP private practices, are staffed by RNs and LPN/LVNs, in addition to NPs, CNAs, and UAPs. In most situations, it is the responsibility of the RN to coordinate the care ordered by the physician and to assign specific duties to LPN/LVNs, CNAs, and UAPs, according to the level of knowledge and skills they possess and their legal scope of practice as set by state regulations. (In those situations in which NPs are present, the task of assigning duties to RNs and/or LPN/LVNs may fall to them.) The individual state boards of nursing set the standards that, for the most part, vary little and comply with the National Council of State Boards of Nursing (NCSBN).

In this chapter, we'll discuss the responsibilities and duties that the LPN/LVN is qualified to perform. We'll also review, in general, the scope of practice of LPN/LVNs and RNs, as well as the roles of NPs and UAPs. You'll see questions interspersed in the discussion to help make the general guidelines concrete in specific cases.

LICENSED PRACTICAL NURSE/LICENSED VOCATIONAL NURSE (LPN/LVN)

An LPN/LVN has specific education and skills and is licensed to work in a healthcare setting under the supervision of a physician, dentist, podiatrist, or, most commonly, an RN (or NP). The role of the LPN/LVN is defined by the theoretical and clinical content taught in practical/vocational nursing programs within each state and approved by the individual state board of nursing.

Scope of Practice/Role of the LPN/LVN

Each state has a specific scope of practice for LPN/LVNs under which they may practice. Under the supervision of an RN, licensed practical/vocational nurses provide care for which they are specifically trained. They care for stable clients and perform procedures with predictable outcomes.

The LPN/LVN is often the bedside nurse, providing care to stable clients. LPN/LVNs monitor vital signs; perform head-to-toe assessments; monitor intake and output; check blood sugars; apply dressings; insert and care for urinary catheters as well as nasogastric tubes; empty Jackson-Pratt (JP) drains; administer enemas; maintain oxygen protocols; and administer prescribed medications. Some states restrict the administration of IV medications and solutions by LPN/LVNs.

Many of the duties of an LPN/LVN involve data collection. The LPN/LVN is taught to distinguish normal from abnormal when observing clients (for example, normal versus abnormal heart sounds) and to recognize changes from previously recorded data (for example, a sudden drop in blood pressure). The data, especially abnormal findings and changes in clinical findings, are reported to an RN (or MD) to provide the necessary information for client care.

The LPN/LVN does not perform an initial client assessment: that is the responsibility of the supervising RN (or MD). However, after the initial assessment has been made and a plan of care initiated, the LPN/LVN may perform ongoing head-to-toe assessments, reporting the findings to the supervising RN. In general, the LPN/LVN carries out the plan of care developed by the RN.

LPN/LVNs may also be involved in client teaching, such as educating pregnant women about childbirth and the care of an infant. LPN/LVNs may also practice "telephone nursing," using protocols developed by a licensed practitioner (e.g., an MD or an NP). The protocols state what information to request of a caller, what to tell the caller, and how to direct the caller to proceed, depending on the condition for which she is calling.

In some states, LPN/LVNs, with additional education and certification, may have an expanded role in intravenous (IV) therapy and hemodialysis under the supervision of an on-site RN. The specific situations, medications, and procedures that the LPN/LVN may perform are strictly limited and outlined by state regulations. However, in most states, LPN/LVNs are responsible for assessing IV infusions and administration sites on their assigned clients, but they do not initiate, manage, or deliver IV therapy. LPN/LVNs also cannot pronounce a client dead in most states.

Also, in some states, LPN/LVNs assume the care of specific clients utilizing an overall plan of care developed by the RN. This situation most often arises in cases where rapid changes are not expected in the client's condition. The LPN/LVN may be assigned to monitor the client regularly while the RN is available for consultation and periodic monitoring. In long-term care facilities, the LPN/LVN may assume the "charge nurse" role with consultation of an in-house supervising RN.

Specifically, LPN/LVNs:

- Provide emotional and physical comfort for the client.
- Carry out the client plan of care initiated by the RN.
- Observe a client's signs and symptoms and report any changes to the supervising RN.
- Perform nursing procedures for which the LPN/LVN has the necessary skills and training, such as routine bedside care, head-to-toe assessments, dressing changes, urinary catheter insertion and care, respiratory care and suctioning, ostomy care, and non-IV medication administration.
- May help RNs in the care of seriously ill clients in intensive care units or in delivery rooms or neonatal units.
- Assist with the rehabilitation of clients according to the client's plan of care.

Let's look at a question that focuses on the scope of practice and roles of the LPN/LVN.

Which of the following client-care activities would it be appropriate for an LPN/LVN to perform?

1. Ask a client newly admitted with a suspected eating disorder for a detailed 24-hour diet recall.
2. Obtain a catheterized urine sample from a client with a low-grade fever and slight lower abdominal discomfort.
3. Assess a 12-year-old child experiencing an acute asthma attack.
4. Care for a 4-year-old child with laryngotracheal bronchitis with a new tracheostomy.

Strategy: Remember that LPN/LVNs perform activities concerning stable clients with predictable outcomes.

(1) A 24-hour diet history is an important part of the initial assessment of a client with suspected anorexia nervosa or other eating disorder and can guide the treatment plan. RNs, not LPN/LVNs, provide the initial clinical assessment. Eliminate this answer choice.

(2) LPN/LVNs routinely collect catheterized urine samples. It is an unchanging routine procedure that the LPN/LVN is qualified to perform. Keep this answer choice for consideration.

(3) A 12-year-old child with an acute asthma attack is not stable, especially because of the small airway of a child. The care of such an unstable client with an uncertain outcome would not normally be assigned to an LPN/LVN. Eliminate this answer choice.

(4) A 4-year-old child with a new tracheostomy for laryngotracheal bronchitis is not stable and therefore needs the assessment and care of an RN. Eliminate this answer choice.

The correct answer is (2).

REGISTERED NURSE (RN)

The RN is responsible for the quality of nursing care, including the assessment of nursing needs, the planning of nursing care and its implementation, the monitoring and evaluation of the plan, and the supervision of LPN/LVNs.

Scope of Practice/Roles of the RN

The RN is responsible and accountable for making decisions based on her knowledge, competency, experience, and use of nursing processes; compliance with state laws and regulations; practice within the scope of practice for RNs in her specific state and awareness of the scope of practice for LPN/LVNs. The decisions made must afford quality nursing care to clients and may include the assignment of specific duties to other qualified personnel (e.g., LPN/LVNs) and the appraisal of the care given by these assigned caregivers. Assignment of specific duties is essential if proper care is to be provided.

Specific responsibilities of the RN include:

- Assessing, evaluating, and making nursing judgments. These tasks cannot be delegated or assigned to LPN/LVNs or other members of the healthcare team.
- Assigning specific tasks to LPN/LVNs and other personnel for stable clients with predictable outcomes. If the client is unstable or the outcome of a specific procedure is unknown, the RN should personally monitor the client.
- Assigning standard activities involving unchanging procedures, such as feeding and bathing a stable client, to the appropriate member of the healthcare team. Feeding, bathing, and dressing a stable client are usually assigned to a UAP, while bedside monitoring following the client's individual plan of care is usually assigned to an LPN/LVN.

Coordination with LPN/LVNs

RNs and LPN/LVNs have a unique and delicate relationship within the healthcare setting. Although the RN assigns the LPN/LVN specific care or tasks for a specific client, the RN is ultimately responsible for the work of the LPN/LVN and how it affects the client. At the same time, the RN must recognize that LPN/LVNs are licensed by their state board of nursing and have completed a program of study that qualifies them to perform certain tasks and to have certain responsibilities. The LPN/LVN provides client care based on his or her own license.

The degree of supervision the RN exercises over the LPN/LVN is based on an evaluation of the condition of the client; of the education, skill, and training of the LPN/LVN; and of the nature of the tasks being assigned to the LPN/LVN. The supervision of the RN, physically present in the healthcare facility, may be a direct continuing presence or an intermittent observation and direction.

The next question may help you understand how this works in practice.

> **The LPN/LVN should question which of the following assignments?**
>
> 1. Obtain a stool sample for occult blood.
> 2. Provide information on nutrition to a new mother.
> 3. Adjust the position of a client who has received medication for pain relief.
> 4. Assess a client who has just returned to the room following abdominal surgery.

(1) Obtaining a stool sample is a routine procedure and thus can be performed by an LPN/LVN. Eliminate this answer choice.

(2) Providing information on nutrition to a new mother is within the scope of practice of an LPN/LVN. Eliminate this answer choice.

(3) Positioning a client is within the scope of practice of an LPN/LVN. Eliminate this answer choice.

(4) An LPN/LVN cannot perform the initial assessment of a client following surgery. This is outside the scope of practice of an LPN/LVN.

The correct answer is (4).

ROLES OF OTHER MEMBERS OF THE HEALTHCARE TEAM

Let's briefly mention the roles of other possible members of the healthcare team. As an LPN/LVN, you may find yourself working with any or all of the following professionals:

- **Nurse practitioners (NPs)** are RNs with advanced education and training; in most states, NPs can diagnose illnesses and prescribe medications. If present in the healthcare setting, the NP would supervise the RN and the LPN/LVN, or just the RN who, in turn, would assign duties to the LPN/LVN.
- **Certified nursing assistants (CNAs)** are regulated by the state boards of nursing.
- **Nursing assistants** are unlicensed assistive personnel, or UAPs. CNAs and UAPs aid RNs and LPN/LVNs by performing routine duties, such as feeding and bathing stable clients. Obtaining specific supplies requested by the LPN/LVN or RN for the care of a client would also be part of the duties of a nursing assistant.

Based on what you have learned about coordination of care and the duties of each member of the healthcare team, answer the next question.

> The nursing unit contains an RN, an LPN/LVN, and a nursing assistant. Which of the following client-care activities would be *MOST* appropriate for the LPN/LVN to perform?
>
> 1. Obtain vital signs for a 6-year-old child who was admitted with several fractures.
> 2. Monitor a 45-year-old woman, who had an ovarian tumor removed 2 days ago, for signs of infection.
> 3. Teach a client recently diagnosed with diabetes mellitus to perform an insulin injection.
> 4. Bathe a child who is recovering from an appendectomy and change his clothes.

(1) A child admitted with several fractures is not in a stable condition and needs assessment, part of which is obtaining vital signs. An RN needs to provide the initial assessment. Eliminate this answer choice.

(2) LPN/LVNs are trained to observe a client for changes in signs and symptoms, such as an increase in temperature or other signs of infection, and to report the changes to the supervising RN. Keep this answer choice for consideration.

(3) Teaching a client with newly diagnosed diabetes mellitus to perform injection techniques is not within the scope of practice of an LPN/LVN. An RN performs this type of teaching. Eliminate this answer choice.

(4) While an LPN/LVN could be asked to help in this situation, a nursing assistant is more likely to be asked to perform this duty. An LPN/LVN is licensed, with specific education and training, so her services could probably be better used in another way. Eliminate this answer choice.

The correct answer is (2). Although the LPN/LVN could be asked to perform the duties listed in answer choice (4), that assignment would not be the most appropriate.

The following is another question to help you understand coordination of care.

> Which of the following client-care assignments is *BEST* for an LPN/LVN?
>
> 1. Help a client who is recovering from surgery with bathing, linen change, and ambulation to the bathroom.
> 2. Perform a head-to-toe assessment, including breath sounds, for a client admitted yesterday with pneumonia.
> 3. Assess a newly admitted client with a high fever and productive cough.
> 4. Change the dressing for a stasis ulcer in a 65-year-old client with diabetes.

(1) A nursing assistant would normally be the person to help bathe and ambulate a client as well as change bed linen. Eliminate this answer choice.

(2) LPN/LVNs routinely perform head-to-toe assessments, including breath sounds, for stable clients. As this client is recently admitted, the RN should do the assessment. Eliminate this answer choice.

(3) RNs provide initial clinical assessment for newly admitted clients. Eliminate this answer choice.

(4) LPN/LVNs are qualified to change dressings in stable clients. This is the best client-care assignment.

The correct answer is (4).

COORDINATION OF CARE QUESTIONS

Here are a few more questions to test your understanding of coordination of care.

> **Which of the following client-care activities should be assigned to an LPN/LVN?**
>
> 1. Listening for breathing sounds and collecting a sputum sample from a man with a long history of respiratory problems
> 2. Immediate post-op assessment of a 9-year-old child who has undergone surgery to correct a spinal deformity
> 3. Emergency care to a 16-year-old football player who suffered cardiac arrhythmia during a football practice
> 4. Care of a 17-year-old stabbing victim who is unconscious and bleeding profusely

(1) A LPN/LVN can listen for breathing sounds, report the findings to the RN, and collect a sputum sample for analysis. Keep this answer choice for consideration.

(2) Immediate post-op assessment is the responsibility of the RN, especially in such a serious case as spinal surgery. The RN may subsequently ask the LPN/LVN to monitor the client, requesting that he be alert for specific signs/symptoms. Eliminate this answer choice.

(3) LPN/LVNs are not usually employed in emergency departments, but if they are, they help the RN (or MD), following specific instructions. Eliminate this answer choice.

(4) An unconscious 17-year-old stabbing victim with profuse bleeding is in unstable condition and has an unpredictable outcome. An LPN/LVN does not routinely provide care for such an unstable client. Eliminate this answer choice.

The correct answer is (1).

> **Which of the following client-care activities should be assigned to an LPN/LVN?**
>
> 1. Assess a new admission who is complaining of severe abdominal pain.
> 2. Review the education on birthing methods provided to a pregnant woman.
> 3. Provide bedside care for a 6-week-old with a fever and obvious discomfort.
> 4. Change the dressing of a woman who has undergone a partial mastectomy.

(1) Obtaining a complete assessment on a newly admitted client is the responsibility of an RN. Eliminate this answer choice.

(2) While an LPN/LVN may provide education to a pregnant woman on birthing methods, only an RN can evaluate the effectiveness of the teaching. Eliminate this answer choice.

(3) Fever in a newborn is always a serious concern. It requires careful assessment and frequent monitoring, tasks that should be performed by an RN. Eliminate this answer choice.

(4) LPN/LVNs are qualified to look for changes in the appearance of a wound and to change dressings as part of their overall monitoring of a stable client recovering from surgery. Keep this answer choice for consideration.

The correct answer is (4).

As stated earlier, healthcare in the United States, with its ever more sophisticated tests, techniques, and treatments, in combination with budget constraints and frequent understaffing, requires the coordination of care among licensed and unlicensed members of the healthcare team. Each member of the team must be called upon to contribute specific knowledge and skills so that an integrated personalized plan of care for each client is implemented. It is very important to utilize the specific education, training, and skills of an LPN/LVN, who provides bedside care for stable clients under the supervision of an RN. Doing so frees the RN to perform assessment, nursing diagnosis, development and implementation of a plan of care, and evaluation. At the same time, the assignment of time-consuming routine tasks, such as bathing and feeding stable clients, to a nursing assistant or other UAP allows the licensed members of the team to maximize the use of their skills.

An understanding of the coordination of care is essential for an LPN/LVN and for other members of the healthcare team. The efficient use of each member's specific knowledge and skills allows the pursuit of a common goal—the best care possible for the client.

CHAPTER 7

STRATEGIES FOR POSITIONING QUESTIONS

Because many illnesses affect body alignment and mobility, you must be able to safely care for these clients in order to be an effective LPN/LVN. These topics are also important on the NCLEX-PN® exam. The successful test taker must correctly answer questions about impaired mobility and positioning.

Immobility occurs when a client is unable to move about freely and independently. To answer questions on positioning, you need to know the hazards of immobility, normal anatomy and physiology, and the terminology for positioning.

Many graduate LPN/LVNs are not comfortable answering these questions because:

- They don't understand the "whys" of positioning.
- They don't know the terminology.
- They have difficulty imaging the various positions.

If you have difficulty answering positioning questions, the following strategy will assist you in selecting the correct answer.

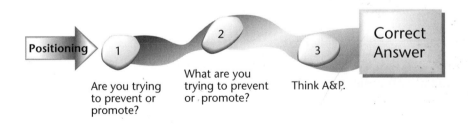

Step 1. Decide if the position for the client is designed to prevent something or promote something.

Step 2. Identify what it is you are trying to prevent or promote.

Step 3. Think about anatomy, physiology, and pathophysiology ("A & P").

Step 4. Which position best accomplishes what you are trying to prevent or promote?

Does this sound a little confusing? Hang in there. Let's walk through a question using this strategy.

> Immediately after a percutaneous liver biopsy, the LPN/LVN should place the client in which of the following positions?
>
> 1. Supine
> 2. Right side-lying
> 3. Left side-lying
> 4. Semi-Fowler's

Before you read the answers, let's go through the four steps outlined above.

Step 1. By positioning the client after a liver biopsy, are you trying to prevent something or promote something? Think about what you know about a liver biopsy. You position a client after this procedure to prevent something.

Step 2. What are you trying to prevent? The most serious and important complication after a percutaneous liver biopsy is hemorrhage.

Step 3. Think about the principles of anatomy, physiology, and pathophysiology. What do you do to prevent hemorrhage? You apply pressure. Where would you apply pressure? On the liver. Where is the liver? On the right side of the abdomen under the ribs.

Step 4. How should the client be positioned to prevent hemorrhage from the liver, which is on the right side of the body? Look at your answer choices.

(1) Supine. If you lay the client flat on his back, no pressure will be applied to the right side. Eliminate.

(2) Right side-lying. If you lay the client in a right side-lying position, will pressure be applied to the right side? Yes. Keep it in for consideration.

(3) Left side-lying. No pressure is applied to the right side. Eliminate.

(4) Semi-Fowler's. If you lay the client on his back with head partially elevated, no pressure is applied to the right side. Eliminate.

The correct answer is (2). Some students select (3) because they don't know normal anatomy and physiology. Some students select (4) because semi-Fowler's position is used for a lot of reasons.

THINGS TO REMEMBER

- Even if you didn't memorize what position to use before, during, and after a procedure, think about the question for a moment. You can figure out what position is needed.

- You cannot figure out the correct position if you do not know what the terms (such as *supine* or *Fowler's*) mean.

- You cannot figure out a correct position if you do not know anatomy and physiology. If you think the liver is on the left side of the body, you are in trouble!

- You cannot figure out a correct position if you do not know what you are trying to accomplish. If you couldn't remember that a complication after a liver biopsy is hemorrhage, you will simply be taking a random guess at the correct answer.

- If you think in images, you should form a mental image of each position. Picture yourself placing the client in each position, and then see if the position makes sense.

Let's try another question using the strategies for positioning.

> An angiogram is scheduled for a client with decreased circulation in her right leg. After the angiogram, the LPN/LVN should place the client in which of the following positions?
>
> 1. Semi-Fowler's with right leg bent at the knee
> 2. Side-lying with a pillow between her knees
> 3. Supine with her right leg extended
> 4. High Fowler's with her right leg elevated

Let's go through the steps.

Step 1. By positioning the client after an angiogram, are you trying to prevent something or promote something? You are trying to promote something.

Step 2. What are you trying to promote? Adequate circulation of the right leg.

Step 3. Think about the principles of anatomy, physiology, and pathophysiology. What promotes adequate circulation in the right leg? Keeping the leg at or below the level of the heart so blood flow is not constricted.

Step 4. How will the client be positioned after an angiography to prevent constriction of vessels and keep the right leg at or below the level of the heart? Look at the answer choices.

(1) Semi-Fowler's with the right leg bent at the knee. The head of the bed is elevated 30 to 45 degrees in this position. The leg is lower than the heart. If the right leg is bent at the knee, this could constrict arterial blood flow. Eliminate.

(2) Side-lying with a pillow between her knees. Use of a pillow in this position could create pressure points in the right leg. You don't want the knees bent. Eliminate.

(3) Supine with leg extended. In this position, the leg is at the level of the heart. Circulation will not be constricted because the leg is straight. Keep this answer in for consideration.

(4) High Fowler's with her right leg elevated. The head of the bed is elevated 60 to 90 degrees in this position. Elevating the leg promotes venous return. Eliminate.

The correct answer is (3). The client is on bed rest for 8 to 12 hours in a supine position after an angiogram.

If you didn't know the specific positioning needed after an angiogram, you could apply your knowledge to select the correct answer by just thinking about it.

Let's look at another question.

> The LPN/LVN cares for a client after a lumbar laminectomy. Which of the following statements *BEST* describes the method of turning a client following a lumbar laminectomy?
>
> 1. The head of the bed is elevated 30 degrees; the client locks her knees when turning.
> 2. A pillow is placed between the client's legs; her body is turned as a unit.
> 3. The client straightens her back and grasps the side rail on the opposite side of the bed.
> 4. The head of the bed is flat; the client bends her knees and rolls to the side.

This question isn't about positioning after a procedure. It asks how to turn the client after surgery.

Step 1. When turning the client after a laminectomy, are you trying to prevent or promote something? Promote.

Step 2. What are you trying to promote? A straight back. The client can't bend or twist the torso.

Step 3. Think about the principles of anatomy, physiology, and pathophysiology. A laminectomy is removal of one or more vertebral laminae. After a laminectomy, the back should be kept straight.

Step 4. How should the client be turned in order to keep the back straight?

(1) If the head of the bed is elevated 30 degrees, the back will not be straight. Eliminate.

(2) If a pillow is placed between the legs and the body is rolled as a unit, the client's back will be kept straight. Keep in for consideration.

(3) If the client grabs the opposite side rail, the client's torso will twist. The back will not be straight even though the client straightened her back before turning and twisting. Eliminate.

(4) If the head of the bed is flat, the client's back will be straight. If the client bends her knees and rolls to her side, her back will not be kept straight. Eliminate.

The correct answer is (2). That is a textbook description of log-rolling. But if you didn't recall log-rolling, you were able to select the correct answer by thoughtfully considering each answer choice.

Sometimes a positioning question will be difficult to identify, such as in the following example.

> The LPN/LVN cares for a client after an appendectomy. The client continues to complain of discomfort to the nurse shortly after receiving an analgesic. Which of the following measures by the LPN/LVN would be *MOST* appropriate?
>
> 1. Notify the physician.
> 2. Place the client in Fowler's position.
> 3. Massage his abdomen.
> 4. Provide him with reading material.

As you can see, not all of the answer choices involve positioning. How should you approach this question?

First, reword the question so that you know what to focus on in the answer choices. The question really being asked is, "What should the LPN/LVN do to help this client with pain relief?" Let's look at the answer choices.

(1) Calling the doctor, as you know, is almost never the right answer. See if another answer choice is more appropriate.

(2) Fowler's position. Why change this client's position? To promote pain relief. Will Fowler's position decrease the client's pain? Yes, by relieving pressure on the client's abdomen. This answer is a possibility.

(3) Massaging his abdomen will increase the client's pain. Eliminate.

(4) Providing him with reading materials might distract him from his discomfort, but this is not an appropriate intervention for a client in pain. Eliminate.

The correct answer is (2).

Positioning is an important part of the NCLEX-PN® exam. You must be able to answer these questions correctly in order to prove your competence. If you use the strategies just discussed, you will be thinking about nursing principles and you will select correct answers!

ESSENTIAL POSITIONS TO KNOW FOR THE NCLEX-PN® EXAM

POSITION	THERAPEUTIC FUNCTION
Flat (supine)	Avoids hip flexion, which can compress arterial flow
Dorsal recumbent	Supine with knees flexed; more comfortable
Side lateral	Allows drainage of oral secretions
Side with leg bent (Sims')	Allows drainage of oral secretions; decreases abdominal tension
Head elevated (Fowler's)	Increases venous return; allows maximal lung expansion • High Fowler's: 60 to 90 degrees • Fowler's: 45 to 60 degrees • Semi-Fowler's: 30 to 45 degrees • Low Fowler's: 15 to 30 degrees
Feet and legs elevated	Increases blood return to heart; relieves pressure on lumbosacral area
Feet elevated and head lowered (Trendelenburg)	Used to insert central venous pressure (CVP) line, or for treatment of umbilical cord compression
Feet elevated 20 degrees, knees straight, trunk flat, and head slightly elevated (modified Trendelenburg)	Increases venous return; used for shock
Elevation of extremity	Increases venous return; increases blood volume to extremity
Flat on back, thighs flexed, legs abducted (lithotomy)	Increases vaginal opening for examination
Prone	Promotes extension of hip joint; not well tolerated by persons with respiratory or cardiovascular difficulties
Knee-chest	Provides maximal visualization of rectal area

CHAPTER 8

STRATEGIES FOR COMMUNICATION QUESTIONS

Communication is emphasized on the NCLEX-PN® exam because it is critical to your success as a beginning practitioner. Therapeutic communication means listening to and understanding the client while promoting clarification and insight. It enables the practical/vocational nurse to form a working relationship with both the client and the healthcare team, using both verbal and nonverbal communication. Remember that nonverbal communication is the most accurate reflection of attitude.

Therapeutic responses include the following.

Response	Goal/Purpose
Using silence	Allows the client time to think and reflect; conveys acceptance. Allows the client to take the lead in conversation.
Using general leads or broad opening	Encourages the client to talk. Indicates your interest in the client. Allows the client to choose the subject.
Clarification	Encourages recall and details of a particular experience. Encourages description of feelings. Seeks explanation; pinpoints specifics.
Reflecting	Paraphrases what client says. Reflects on what client says, especially the feelings conveyed.

ELIMINATING ANSWER CHOICES

There are many questions on the NCLEX-PN® exam that require you to select the correct therapeutic communication response. As with other NCLEX-PN® exam questions, one of the biggest errors that students commit when trying to answer this type of question is to look for the correct answer. Remember, you are selecting the *best* answer from the four possible answers that you are given. To select the best answer, you must eliminate answer choices. Let's look at some of the different answer choices you can eliminate:

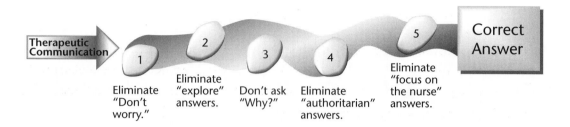

Therapeutic Communication

1 — Eliminate "Don't worry."

2 — Eliminate "explore" answers.

3 — Don't ask "Why?"

4 — Eliminate "authoritarian" answers.

5 — Eliminate "focus on the nurse" answers.

Correct Answer

- **"Don't Worry" Answers:** Eliminate answer choices that offer false reassurance. These type of responses discourage communication between the LPN/LVN and the client by not allowing the client to explore his or her own ideas and feelings. False reassurance also discounts what the client is feeling. Examples include:
  - "It is going to be OK."
  - "Don't worry. Your doctors will do everything necessary for your care."

- **"Let's Explore" Answers:** Another incorrect answer choice that many graduate practical/vocational nurses select is the choice that includes the word "explore." On the NCLEX-PN® exam, avoid being a junior psychiatrist. It isn't the practical/vocational nurse's role to delve into the reasons why the client is feeling a particular way. The client must be allowed to verbalize the fact that he or she is sad, angry, fearful, or overwhelmed. Examples include:
  - "Let's talk about why you didn't take your medication."
  - "Tell me why you really injured yourself."

- **"Why" Questions:** Eliminate answer choices that include "why" questions: ones that seek reasons or justification. "Why" questions imply disapproval of the client, who may become defensive. A "why" question can come in many forms and need not always begin with "why." Any response that puts the client on the defensive is nontherapeutic and therefore incorrect. Examples include:
  - "What makes you think that?"
  - "Why do you feel this way?"

- *Authoritarian Answers:* Eliminate answer choices in which the LPN/LVN is telling the client what to do without regard to the client's desires or feelings. Examples include:
  - Insisting that the client follow unit rules
  - Insisting that the client do what you command, immediately

- *Nurse-Focused Answers:* Eliminate answer choices in which the focus of the comment is on the LPN/LVN. Be careful, because these answer choices may sound very empathetic. The focus of your communication should always be on the client. Examples include:
  - "That happened to me once."
  - "I know from experience this is hard for you."

- *Close-Ended Questions:* Eliminate answer choices that include close-ended questions that can be answered with yes, no, or another monosyllabic response. Close-ended questions discourage the client from sharing thoughts and feelings. Examples include:
  - "Are you feeling guilty about what happened?"
  - "How many children do you have?"

Eliminating these types of nontherapeutic responses that appear as answer choices is a very effective strategy when answering therapeutic communication questions. Don't simply look for the specific words that you see here; you may need to "translate" the answer choices into the above errors of therapeutic communication.

SELECTING THE CORRECT RESPONSE

So, how do you select the correct response? By choosing from the answer choices that are left! The correct response will usually contain one or both of the following elements:

- *Gives correct information.* Offering information encourages further communication from the client. Examples of giving correct information include:
  - "You are experiencing acute alcohol withdrawal; you may see and feel things that aren't real."
  - "There are many reasons for memory loss; tell me more about what you have noticed."

- *Is empathetic and reflects the client's feelings.* *Empathy* is the ability to perceive what another person experiences using that person's frame of reference. *Reflection* communicates to the client that the LPN/LVN has heard and understands what the client is trying to communicate. When reflecting feelings, the LPN/LVN focuses on the feelings and not the content of what is said. Examples of empathetic, reflective statements include:
  - "I can see that you are frightened about being here."
  - "You seem very upset. Tell me how you're feeling."

Let's practice with a few exam-style test questions.

> A client is admitted to the telemetry unit with a diagnosis of acute myocardial infarction. The client tells the LPN/LVN, "I'm scared, I think I'm going to die." Which of the following responses by the LPN/LVN would be *MOST* appropriate?
>
> 1. "Everything is going to be fine. We'll take good care of you."
> 2. "I know what you mean. I thought I was having a heart attack once."
> 3. "I'll call your doctor so you can discuss it with him."
> 4. "It's normal to feel frightened. We're doing everything we can for you."

Step 1. Eliminate incorrect answer choices.

(1) This is a "don't worry" response. There is no acknowledgment of the client's fears. Eliminate it.

(2) The focus of this response is on the LPN/LVN, not the client. Eliminate it.

(3) It is within the scope of nursing practice for the LPN/LVN to respond to the client's feelings. Don't pass the responsibility to the physician. Eliminate it.

(4) This answer choice responds to feelings and provides information.

Step 2. Select an answer from the remaining choices.

One answer was not eliminated: (4). This is the correct answer. The LPN/LVN both acknowledges that the client feels frightened and provides information.

Let's try another question.

> A mother is to undergo a breast biopsy. She tells the LPN/LVN, "If I lose my breast, I know my husband will no longer find me attractive." Which of the following responses by the LPN/LVN would be *MOST* appropriate?
>
> 1. "You don't know if you are going to lose your breast. They are just doing the biopsy now."
> 2. "You should focus on your children. They are young and they need you."
> 3. "You seem to be concerned that your relationship with your husband might change."
> 4. "Why don't you wait and see what your husband's reaction is before you get upset."

Step 1. Eliminate answer choices.

(1) This response gives false reassurance and discounts the client's feelings. Eliminate it.

(2) This response is authoritarian: the LPN/LVN tells the client what to do. Eliminate it.

(3) This response reflects the fears of the client. The response is open-ended and allows the client to express what she is feeling. Keep it in for consideration.

(4) This response dismisses the feelings that the client is experiencing and gives advice. Eliminate it.

Step 2. Select an answer from the remaining choices.

You have eliminated three of the four answer choices. The correct answer is the only answer choice remaining, (3).

Let's look at one more question.

> A client in the psychiatric unit asks the LPN/LVN, "Am I in a special radioactive shelter? When was it last checked for radioactivity?" Which of the following responses by the LPN/LVN would be *MOST* appropriate?
>
> 1. "This is a hospital, and we do not have a nuclear medicine department here."
> 2. "Don't worry, you're safe. There's no radioactivity here."
> 3. "I'm sure your safety is of concern to you, but this is a hospital."
> 4. "Please share with me what makes you think there is radioactivity here."

Step 1. Eliminate answer choices.

(1) This response provides information. Leave it in for consideration.

(2) This response offers false reassurances. Eliminate it.

(3) This response reflects the client's concern about safety and provides information. Keep it in for consideration.

(4) This response allows the client to verbalize, but you don't want to encourage a client with psychological problems to talk about hallucinations or delusions. Rather, you want your discussion to focus on the feelings that accompany them. Eliminate this choice.

Step 2. Select an answer from the remaining choices.

You have more than one possible answer choice: (1) and (3). Look for the answer choice that reflects feelings and gives information. The correct answer is (3).

Some things to remember about selecting correct answers to therapeutic communication questions are:

- No matter how confident you are about an answer choice, read all of the choices before selecting an answer.
- Even if you would never say any of the responses given in the answer choices, choose the "textbook" answer.

- When you first read the answer choices, don't look for the correct answer. Always eliminate answer choices first.

If you follow the Kaplan strategies for therapeutic communication, you will be able to select the correct answers to this question type on the NCLEX-PN® exam.

CHAPTER 9

HOW TO STUDY FOR THE NCLEX-PN® EXAM

Now that you've read about the various Kaplan test-taking strategies, you are probably thinking, "Wow! This is great!" Most of you have started identifying why you are having difficulty answering application/analysis-level test questions. Some of you have already formulated a plan to master your NCLEX-PN® exam questions using the strategies outlined in this book, and are confident that you will pass the exam. Others are thinking, "This sounds great, but can I really answer questions using these strategies?"

The authors of this book work for Kaplan, the oldest test prep company in the nation. We have been preparing graduate nurses and international nurses for licensure exams for more than 25 years. We know what works to prepare for the exam and what doesn't work.

INEFFECTIVE WAYS TO PREPARE

Here are a few of the biggest mistakes some NCLEX-PN® exam test takers make before Test Day.

Relying on False Hopes

Some students use what is knows as the "hope" method of study. "I hope that I don't have questions about chest tubes on the test." "I hope that I don't have questions about medication on my test." "I hope that I have questions about electrolytes because I did great on that test in school." The "hope" method usually doesn't work very well. The test pool contains thousands of questions. How many topics do you "hope" won't be on your test?

Lacking Respect for the Exam

Many candidates for the NCLEX-PN® exam are good students in school. Because of their school success, they expect to pass the exam with minimal preparation. After all, it's just a test of minimum competency. These students do some studying, but they really believe there is no chance they might fail this exam. You might think that you can't possibly fail, but if you do not respect this exam and prepare for it correctly, you run the risk of failure!

All students know why they take the NCLEX-PN® exam. However, after interviewing hundreds of students, we have discovered that many have no idea what the exam content is. How can you effectively study for a test if you don't know what content the exam tests? Learn what is on the NCLEX-PN® exam and then you will realize that preparation with a planned method of study is essential.

Cramming

Some students completed nursing school with a minimal understanding of nursing content. These students studied long and hard on the night before a nursing school test, cramming as many facts into their heads as they could remember. Because the test questions primarily involved recognition and recall, cramming worked for tests in nursing school. But as we said earlier, the NCLEX-PN® exam is not an exam about facts. It tests your ability to apply the knowledge that you have learned and to think critically. Recognition and recall will not work!

Poor Planning

As with all standardized exams, you must work on your areas of weakness. This is hard to do because there's usually a reason you're weak in an area. Some graduate practical/vocational nurses, for example, profess a weakness in or dislike for obstetrical nursing. Some students didn't understand the theory, while other students had a poor clinical experience or didn't get to see many deliveries; still other students simply didn't like this rotation. Whatever the reason, it causes you to have a weakness in a particular area. In order to pass a standardized test, you must work on your areas of weakness.

Some students don't establish a plan of study. Other students establish a plan of study but don't follow it. You can buy review books, but if you don't apply yourself, they will do you no good.

EFFECTIVE METHODS OF PREPARATION

To pass the NCLEX-PN® exam, you not only need to know nursing content, you also need to be able to apply the critical thinking skills we've just reviewed. Next, you need to be an expert on the content of the exam. What topics are usually included on the NCLEX-PN® exam? How is the content organized? And finally, you need to create a study plan, and make sure that you are able to cope with the testing experience.

So let's start by talking about some of the issues that you may be asking yourself.

Question: "I'm terrible at standardized tests. Is this really going to help me?"

Answer: Yes, these strategies will help you choose more correct responses when you take the NCLEX-PN® exam. Read this book—more than once if necessary—to learn the strategies. Then practice, practice, practice. Use the strategies to answer many, many test questions, and you will find yourself answering more and more questions correctly. Tear out the Chart of Critical Thinking Paths in Appendix A and consult it while you are answering practice test questions. This will help you become more comfortable with putting the strategies into practice. As you answer more and more questions, put the diagram aside and rely on your memory to identify and implement a critical thinking strategy.

Question: "Am I going to have enough time when I take the NCLEX-PN® exam to figure out which strategy to use?"

Answer: Timing is a concern on the NCLEX-PN® exam. You need to maximize your efforts on each test question. Practice answering test questions using the various strategies we've outlined. As you get more proficient, you will discover that it takes you less time to identify the strategy or path that will lead you to the correct answer.

Question: "I don't have to use these strategies on every question, do I? I think I'll use them only when I can't figure out the correct answer on my own."

Answer: Wrong! You should use critical thinking to answer every question on the NCLEX-PN® exam to make sure that you pass. Follow the steps that we have outlined for every practice question that you answer as you prepare for the exam. If you practice these steps, you will not need to randomly guess the correct answer on the NCLEX-PN® exam.

Question: "So all I have to do is memorize the strategies, right?"

Answer: Just memorizing the various strategies will not ensure your success on the NCLEX-PN® exam. Remember, the exam does not test your ability to memorize either critical thinking strategies or the nursing content. The NCLEX-PN® exam tests your ability to think critically and use the nursing knowledge that you have. It's relatively easy to just memorize nursing content. The hard part is to figure out how to use this knowledge to make nursing decisions. It's relatively easy to memorize the critical thinking strategies. The hard part is to figure out which strategy to use on each and every question. That takes practice.

Question: "What if I use the strategies but still can't figure out the correct answer?"

Answer: It's not unusual that students will read a question, read the answers, and think "Huh? Something is missing." If you feel like something is missing, reread the question to determine if you have correctly identified what the question is asking. If you have identified the question correctly, then read the answer choices to make sure that you haven't missed the nursing concept contained in the answer choices.

Question: "Will these strategies work on every practice question that I answer?"

Answer: The critical thinking strategies discussed in this book will enable you to answer all kinds of multiple-choice test questions. The critical thinking strategies apply to test questions written at the application/analysis level and do not work with knowledge-based test questions. If you feel that the strategies don't work with the practice questions you are answering, determine the level of difficulty of the questions you are working with. Are the practice questions knowledge-based, or are they at the application/analysis level of difficulty? Remember, the majority of questions that are of a passing level of difficulty on the NCLEX-PN® exam are at the application/analysis level of difficulty.

It's time for you to start your successful preparation for the NCLEX-PN® exam. Begin by identifying your strengths and weaknesses, as follows:

- Take as many diagnostic exams as you can.
- Identify your weaknesses in nursing content.
- Identify your weaknesses in test-taking skills.

Next, decide if you need to take a review course. If you decide that this is the best way for you to prepare, ask yourself these questions:

- Is the course mainly a review of nursing content or memory techniques? This type of review won't help you put it all together on Test Day. You can know everything about heart failure, but if you don't know how to use this information to answer a question about heart failure correctly on the NCLEX-PN® exam, you will have difficulty on the exam. Are the strategies specific for the NCLEX-PN® exam?
- Are there plenty of opportunities for practice testing? You need to prove your competence by answering NCLEX-PN® exam-style test questions, so you should practice answering these questions. If the exam were about opening a sterile pack, what would you spend your time doing to prepare for the exam? Reading about opening a sterile pack or practicing opening a sterile pack? Are there exam-style questions included in the course? Do the questions require recall and recognition of facts or application of nursing care principles? Remember, your NCLEX-PN® exam will consist mainly of analysis/application-level questions.
- What do students who have taken the course have to say about how it helped them prepare for the exam? If a review course boasts of a particularly high pass rate, ask to see their statistics. Be an informed consumer.
- Is there a guarantee? There are guarantees and there are empty promises. Make sure the course you are considering puts the guarantee in writing. Study the small print. Is your total tuition refunded? Do you have to fail the exam more than once?
- How much does it cost? This sounds easy, but "extras" can add up. Are there additional charges for books? Software? Registration fees?
- Is this course right for me?

And finally, create a realistic study schedule that works for you. Then make a vow to stick to that plan and reward yourself when you do. Spend at least 3 weeks before your exam date preparing. Don't cram! Your content focus should be in understanding the principles of nursing care, not memorizing facts.

Stay away from people who are "prophets of doom." You know the type. With the proper preparation you can and will pass the NCLEX-PN® exam. Keep a positive attitude.

You may need to consider some techniques for battling stress and managing the Test Day experience. Do any of these statements apply to you?

> *"I always freeze up on tests."*
> *"I need to pass to get my new job/promotion/commission."*
> *"My best friend/girlfriend/sister/brother did really well, but I won't."*
> *"My hospital/family/parents won't like it if I fail."*
> *"I'm afraid of losing concentration."*
> *"I'm afraid I'm not spending enough time preparing."*

If these sound familiar, you may want to mentally prepare yourself by understanding ways to manage test stress. Forcing yourself to identify and face fears may make you edgy at first but will significantly alleviate test stress in the long run by adding another dimension to your preparation.

MENTAL PREPARATION*

1. Visualize

You have probably learned how to do this with clients; now it's your turn. Sit back and let your shoulders and arms relax. Close your eyes and imagine yourself in a relaxing situation—it can be fictional, but a real-life memory is best. Make it as detailed as possible. Think about the sights, the sounds, the smells, even the tastes that you associate with the relaxing situation. Keep your eyes shut; keep sinking back into your chair. Now that you're in that situation, start bringing your test in—think about the experience of taking the test while *in* that relaxing situation. Imagine how much easier it would be if you could take your test in that situation. Notice how much easier your test seems in that situation.

Here's another variation. Close your eyes and think about a situation in which you did well on a test. If you can't come up with one, pick a situation in which you did some good academic work that you were really proud of, or some other kind of genuine accomplishment. Not a fiction, mind you: it has to be from real life. Make it as detailed as possible. Think about the

---

* Some of these methods were originally conceptualized by Dr. Emile Coué, who in the 1920s told everyone that the key to a happy life was to constantly repeat the phrase, "Every day in every way I am getting better and better." As advice to test takers, that isn't bad at all!

sights, the sounds, the smells, even the tastes, that you associate with this experience of academic success. Now think about your test in line with that experience. Don't make comparisons between them. Just imagine taking your test with that same feeling of relaxed control.

2. Exercise

Whether it be jogging, walking, yoga, push-ups, or a pickup basketball game, physical exercise is a great way to stimulate the mind and body and improve one's ability to think and concentrate. A surprising number of those who prepare for standardized tests don't exercise regularly because they spend so much time preparing. Sedentary people—this is a medical fact—get less oxygen in the blood, and therefore to the brain, than active people.

3. Do the Following on Exam Day:

- *Keep moving forward.* By Test Day, do enough preparation with practice questions that it becomes an instinct to keep moving forward instead of getting bogged down in a difficult question. You don't need to get everything right to pass, so don't linger on a question that is going nowhere. The best test takers don't get bothered by difficult questions because they accept that everyone encounters them on the NCLEX-PN® exam.

- *Don't listen to negative words or behavior.* Don't be distracted by the ignorant babble or the behavior of other, less-prepared, less-skilled candidates around you. Negative thoughts lead to negative feelings and may interfere with performing your best on Test Day.

- *Don't be anxious if other test takers seem to be working harder or answering questions more quickly.* Continue to spend your time patiently but doggedly thinking through your answers; it's going to lead to higher-quality test taking and better results. Set your own pace and stick to it.

- *Keep breathing!* Weak standardized test takers tend to share one major trait: forgetting to breathe steadily as the test proceeds. They do not know the value of proper breathing. They start holding their breath without realizing it, or begin breathing erratically or arrhythmically. This can hurt confidence and accuracy. Do what you can to instill an awareness of proper breathing before and during each study or testing section.

- *Do some quick isometrics during the test.* This is helpful especially if your concentration is wandering or energy is waning. For example, put your palms together and press intensely for a few seconds.

To effectively prepare for the NCLEX-PN® exam, first identify your strengths and weaknesses, and then choose an effective method of study that works for you. Then use mental preparation techniques to alleviate stress and manage your Test Day experience.

CHAPTER 10

THE LICENSURE PROCESS

The process of obtaining an American nursing license requires a definite sequence of actions by the candidate. Because this may be your first experience with the LPN/LVN licensure process, and because there are no established test dates, you may have difficulty knowing exactly how to complete the paperwork and go through the process. This chapter will give you a checklist to follow when planning to take the NCLEX-PN® exam. This is a general list, so you must individualize it according to the requirements for the state in which you wish to become licensed; see Appendix D, State Licensing Requirements, for information on individual state requirements. We will outline the questions that you need to ask, and the steps you need to take to complete the licensure process.

HOW TO APPLY FOR THE NCLEX-PN® EXAM

During your last semester of nursing school, you will be given the following applications:

(1) Application for licensure that goes to your state board of nursing.

(2) Application for the NCLEX-PN® exam that goes to Pearson VUE.

On a predetermined date, you will submit the completed forms and the required licensure fees to your nursing school.

Application Fees

- The NCLEX-PN® examination fee is $200. Additional licensure fees are determined by each state nursing board; see Appendix D, State Licensing Requirements, to determine your state's fee.
- You are responsible for mailing the completed test application and the $200 fee to Pearson VUE.

The Registration Process

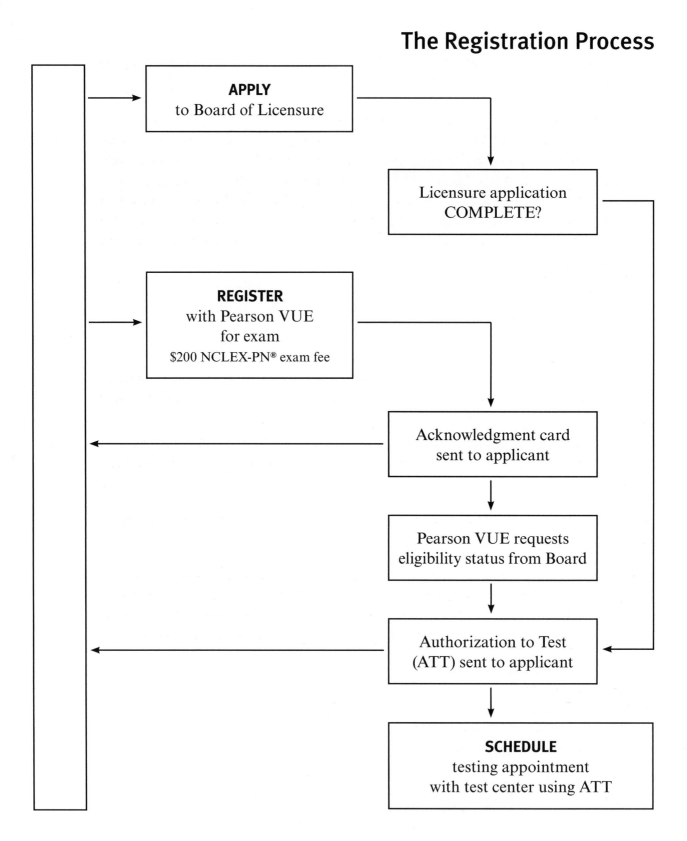

APPLY
to Board of Licensure

Licensure application
COMPLETE?

REGISTER
with Pearson VUE
for exam
$200 NCLEX-PN® exam fee

Acknowledgment card
sent to applicant

Pearson VUE requests
eligibility status from Board

Authorization to Test
(ATT) sent to applicant

SCHEDULE
testing appointment
with test center using ATT

Applicant must APPLY, REGISTER, and SCHEDULE

Registration

You can register for the NCLEX-PN® with Pearson VUE using any one of the following three methods:

(1) *Internet Registration:* To register online, go to *vue.com/nclex* or *pearsonvue.com/nclex* (the "NCLEX Candidate Website"). There are two general payment options: credit or debit card (using VISA, MasterCard or American Express), or money order, cashier's check, or certified check. If you choose the latter, upon completion of the registration information, you will be provided with directions to print a confirmation document that should be mailed with a certified check, cashier's check, or money order (made payable to the National Council of State Boards of Nursing) in U.S. currency drawn on a bank in the United States to:

> NCLEX Operations
> P.O. Box 64950
> St. Paul, MN 55164-0950

(2) *Mail-in Registration:* Obtain a registration scan form by contacting your state board of nursing and mail a certified check, cashier's check, or money order to the address noted above.

(3) *Telephone Registration:* Call NCLEX Candidate Services at 1-866-496-2539 (1-866-49-NCLEX). To register by phone, you must pay using a VISA, MasterCard, or American Express credit or debit card.

Some states require that the testing application form and fee be sent along with the licensure application and fee.

For more information, visit *ncsbn.org* and download the *2010 NCLEX Candidate Bulletin*. For questions regarding registering to take the NCLEX -PN® exam, your Authorization to Test (ATT), a lost ATT, acceptable forms of identification, or comments about the test center, visit the NCLEX Candidate Website (*pearsonvue.com/nclex* or *vue.com/nclex*) or contact:

> NCLEX Candidate Services
> 1-866-49-NCLEX
>
> NCLEX-PN® Examination Program
> Pearson Professional Testing
> 5601 Green Valley Drive
> Bloomington, MN 55437
> pvamericascustomerservice@pearson.com

How Do You Know Your Application Has Been Received?

You will receive a card from your state board confirming that all of your information has been received.

Potential Problems with Licensure Application

Some states require that your permanent transcript be mailed with your application.

Here is a checklist to follow to avoid problems with your application:

- Have you met all requirements for graduation? Do you have any electives still outstanding?
- Has your nursing school received a permanent transcript for any credits that you transferred from another institution?
- Do you owe any fines or have any unpaid parking tickets? (This can delay the release of your permanent transcript. Check at your nursing school office, just to be sure.)
- Some states require that a statement be sent from your nursing school stating that you have met all requirements for graduation.
- Did you change your mind about the state to which you want to apply for licensure? If so, you must apply to the new state—and forfeit the original application fee.

What If You Want to Apply for Licensure in a Different State?

If you plan to apply for licensure in a different state from the one in which you are attending practical/vocational nursing school, contact the state board of nursing in the state in which you wish to become licensed (refer to Appendix D, State Licensing Requirements).

Here's a checklist for obtaining a license in another state:

- Call or write the state board of nursing of that state and find out what their requirements are for licensure.
- Find out what their fees are.
- Request a new candidate application for licensure.

After you pass the NCLEX-PN® exam, you will receive your nursing license from the state in which you applied for licensure regardless of where you took your exam. For example, if you applied for licensure in Michigan, you can take the test in Florida if you wish. You would then receive a license to practice as an LPN in Michigan because that is where you applied for licensure.

When Can You Schedule Your NCLEX-PN® Exam?

Pearson VUE will send you a document entitled "Authorization to Test" (ATT). The ATT will be sent to you by mail, and via email if you listed an email address on your registration. You will be unable to schedule your test date until you receive this form.

On the ATT is your assigned candidate number; you will need to refer to this when scheduling your exam. Your ATT is valid for a time determined by the individual state board of nursing, and you must test before your ATT expires. If you don't, you will need to reapply to take the exam and pay the testing fees again. With your ATT, you will receive a list of test centers (see Appendix E for a current listing). You can schedule your NCLEX-PN® exam using the following procedures:

- Log on to the NCLEX Candidate Website at *pearsonvue.com/nclex* or *vue.com/nclex*
- Call NCLEX Candidate Services

    United States: 1-866-496-2539 (1-866-49-NCLEX) (toll-free)

    Asia Pacific Region: +603-8314-9605 (pay number)

    India: 91-120-439-7837 (pay number)

    Europe, Middle East, Africa (EMEA): +44-161-855-7445 (pay number)

    All other countries not listed above: 1-952-681-3815 (pay number)

Candidates with hearing impairments who use a Telecommunications Device for the Deaf (TDD) can call the U.S.A. Relay Service at 1-800-627-3529 (toll-free) or the Canada & International Inbound relay service at 1-605-627-3527 (pay)

Those with special testing requests, such as persons with disabilities, must call the NCLEX-PN® Program Coordinator at NCLEX Candidate Services at one of the numbers listed above. If you require special accommodations, you cannot schedule your exam through the NCLEX Candidate Website.

There is a space on the ATT for you to record the date and time of your scheduled exam. You will also receive confirmation of your scheduled date and time.

Potential Rescheduling Problems

- You must test prior to the expiration date of your ATT. If you miss your appointment, you forfeit your testing fees and must reapply to both the state board of nursing and Pearson VUE.
- If you wish to change your appointment, you must notify Pearson VUE 24 hours prior to your scheduled appointment. Call one of the numbers listed above or go the NCLEX Candidate Website (*vue.com/nclex* or *pearsonvue.com/nclex*). If your test date is on a Saturday, Sunday, or Monday, make sure to call on or before Friday.

Do not call the test site directly or leave a message on an answering machine if you are unable to take your test on the scheduled date. You must follow the procedure listed above.

When Will You Take the Exam?

The earliest date on which you can take the NCLEX-PN® exam varies depending on your state, but the majority of students test approximately 45 days after the date of their graduation. Variables include: when you submit the applications and fees, the length of time the ATT is valid, personal factors (weddings, births, vacations), and job requirements. Each state determines the requirements for graduate practical/vocational nurses, licensure pending. If you are working as a graduate practical/vocational nurse, you must be knowledgeable about the rules in your state.

TAKING THE EXAM

What Happens on the Day of My NCLEX-PN® Exam?

Arrive at the test center at least 30 minutes before your scheduled test time. Wear layered clothing—the rooms may be cool in the morning but can warm up as the day progresses.

Here's a checklist of things to bring on the day of the exam:

- Your Authorization to Test (ATT).
- One form of signed identification that includes a picture. If you have changed your hair color, lost weight, or grown a beard, have a new picture ID made before Test Day. The name on your ID must match exactly the name on your ATT. Acceptable forms of identification include driver's license, state/province identity card, passport, and U.S. military ID.
- A snack and something to drink.
- *Do not* bring any study materials to the test center.

Check-in procedure:

- Present your ATT.
- Present your picture ID.
- Sign in.
- A computer picture will be taken of you.
- You will be fingerprinted and may have your palm vein pattern scanned.
- All of your belongings will be placed in a locker outside the testing room.
- Earplugs are available on request. Request them, in case you find yourself distracted by background noise.

Where Will I Take My Test?

You will be in a room separate from the rest of the test center. Many testing sites consist of a room with 10 to 15 computers placed around the outside walls. Each computer sits on a full-size desk, with an adjustable chair for you to sit on. There are dividers between desks, but you will be able to see the person sitting next to you. There is a picture window from which the proctor will observe each person testing. There are also video cameras and sound sensors mounted on the walls to monitor each candidate.

What Will the Computer Screen Look Like?

The number of the question you are answering is located in the lower-right side of your computer screen. In the upper-right corner is a digital clock that counts down from 5:00—representing the five hours you have to complete the short tutorial that begins the exam, the exam itself, and all breaks.

If the question is a traditional four-option, text-based, multiple-choice question, the question stem is located in the top half of the screen and the four answer choices are located in the lower half of the screen (Figure 1). Radio buttons are in front of each answer choice.

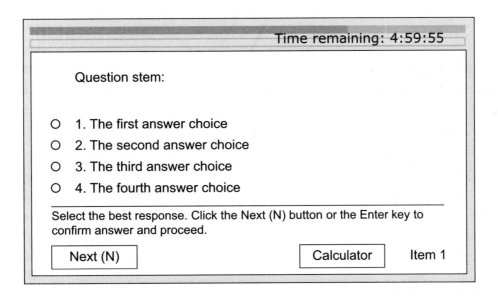

Figure 1

You will notice that there are two buttons at the bottom of the computer screen. You use the Next (N) button to confirm your answer selection and move to the next question. Click the Calculator button to display a drop-down calculator that can be used to perform computations.

If the question is an alternate question that may have more than one correct answer, you will see the phrase, "Select all that apply" between the stem of the question and five or six answer choices. A small box is in front of each answer choice. The Next (N) button and Calculator button are at the bottom of the computer screen.

If the question is a hot spot alternate question, the screen will contain a graphic or a picture. The Next (N) button and Calculator button are at the bottom of the computer screen.

If the question is a fill-in-the-blank alternate question, a text box will be under the question. The Next (N) button and Calculator button are at the bottom of the computer screen.

If the question is a drag-and-drop/ordered response alternate question, the unordered options will be under the question and to the left. The space for the ordered response will be to the right of the unordered options. The Next (N) button and Calculator button are at the bottom of the computer screen.

If the question is a chart/exhibit alternate question, it will include the following prompt after the question stem: "Click on the exhibit button below for additional client information." The Exhibit button is located at the bottom of the computer screen between the Next (N) button and the Calculator button. Click on the Exhibit button to display a pop-up box containing 3 tabs. Click on each of the tabs to display information needed to answer the question.

If the question is an audio alternate question, the question will contain an audio clip that you must listen to in order to answer the question. Click on the Play button (a right-pointing arrow) to listen to the clip. A slider bar allows you to adjust the volume at which you hear the clip. If you want to listen to the audio clip more than once, you can click on the Play button again.

If the question is a graphics alternate question, each of the four answer choices will be a graphic instead of text.

How Do I Use the Calculator?

Using the mouse, click on the Calculator button, and a drop-down calculator will appear on the computer screen. Use the mouse to click on the calculator keys. Remember, the diagonal or slash (/) key is used for division. When you are through with your calculations, click on the Calculator button again, and the calculator will disappear.

How Do I Select an Answer Choice for Traditional Four-Option, Multiple-Choice Questions?

You will use a two-step process to answer each question. Read the question and select an answer by using the mouse to click on the radio button preceding your answer choice. Your answer is now highlighted. When you are certain of your answer, click on the Next (N) button or press the Enter key to confirm your answer. Your answer is now locked in and a new question will appear on the screen. *You are not able to change your answer after clicking on the Next (N) button or pressing the Enter key, so be certain of your answer before you do so.*

After your answer is entered into the computer, the computer selects a new question for you based on the accuracy of your previous answer and the components of the NCLEX-PN® exam test plan. If you answer a question correctly, the next question selected by the computer is more difficult. If you answer a question incorrectly, the next question selected by the computer is easier.

What If I Want to Change the Answer That I Have Highlighted?

If you want to change the highlighted answer, click on a different answer choice. Your answer is not locked in until you click on the Next (N) button or press the Enter key.

Even if you've never used a computer before, don't panic. You will be given instructions at the beginning of the test, and you will have to answer three tutorial questions before your test begins. These questions allow you to practice using the mouse to select an answer.

How Do I Select an Answer Choice for Select All That Apply Questions?

Read the question and click on the small box in front of the answer choice you want. A small check will appear in the box. Click on each answer choice that answers the question.

What If I Want to Change an Answer That I Have Checked?

If you change your mind and don't want an answer choice that you have selected, just click again on the small box in front of that answer choice and the check will disappear. When you are certain of your answer, click on the Next (N) button or press the Enter key to confirm your answer. Your answer is now locked in and a new question appears on the screen.

How Do I Select an Answer Choice for Hot Spot Questions?

To answer a hot spot alternate question, just click on the area of the graphic or picture that answers the question.

What If I Want to Change the Area That I Have Selected?

If you change your mind and want to select another area of the graphic or picture, just use your mouse to click on the area that you want and the original selection disappears. When you are certain of your answer, click on the Next (N) button or press the Enter key to confirm your answer. Your answer is now locked in and a new question appears on the screen.

How Do I Enter an Answer Choice for Fill-in-the-Blank Questions?

To enter an answer for a fill-in-the-blank question, just use the keyboard to select the numbers or letters you want. If a unit of measurement already appears next to the answer box on the screen, be sure you enter *numbers* only into the answer box; adding a unit of measurement may cause your answer to be wrong.

What If I Want to Change What I Have Entered in the Text Box?

If you change your mind and want to enter another answer in the text box, just backspace over the answer you entered and then use the keyboard to enter another answer. When you are certain of your answer, click on the Next (N) button or press the Enter key to confirm your answer. Your answer is now locked in and a new question appears on the screen.

How Do I Select Options for Drag-and-Drop/Ordered Response Questions

To put the responses in the correct order, click on the option you think should come first, hold down the button on the mouse, and drag the option over to the box on the right side of the screen. You may also highlight the option in the box on the left side and then click the arrow key that points to the box on the right side to move the option. Do the same with each response in the proper order.

What If I Want to Change the Order of My Responses?

If you change your mind about the order of a response, click on it with the mouse and drag it back to the left side of the screen or use the arrow key as described above. To complete the question, you must move all options from the box on the left side of the screen to the box on the right side. When you are certain of your answer, click on the Next (N) button or press the Enter key to confirm your answer. Your answer is now locked in and a new question appears on the screen.

How Do I Enter or Change an Answer Choice for Chart/Exhibit, Audio, and Graphics Alternate Questions?

Chart/exhibit, audio, and graphics alternate questions all use a four-option, multiple-choice format, so you can enter or change your answer choices just as you would for a traditional text-based, four-option, multiple-choice question.

Do I Get Any Breaks?

You will receive an optional break at the end of two hours of testing. There will be a pre-programmed prompt offering you a break. Leave the testing room, stretch your legs, and eat your snack. Take some deep, cleansing breaths and get yourself ready to go back into the testing room. The computer will offer you another optional break after 3½ hours of testing. We recommend that you take it unless you feel you're on a roll.

You may take a break at any time during your test, but the time that you spend away from your computer is counted as a part of your five hours of total testing time. Kaplan recommends that you take a short (2–5 minute) break if you are having trouble concentrating. Take time to go to the restroom, eat your snack, or get a drink. This will enable you to maintain or regain your concentration for the test. Remember, every question counts! If you need to take a break, raise your hand to notify the test administrator. You must leave the testing room, and you will be re-fingerprinted before you are allowed to resume your test.

How Will I Know When My Test Ends?

A screen will appear on your computer that states, "Your test is concluded." You will then be required to answer several exit questions. These are a few multiple-choice questions about your response to the examination experience. They do not count toward your results.

How Long Will It Take to Receive My Results?

Your results are sent to you by your state board of nursing. Each state board determines when the NCLEX-PN® exam results are released. In the following jurisdictions, you may access your "unofficial" results two business days after taking your examination via the NCLEX® Candidate Website (for a $7.95 fee) or through the NCLEX® Quick Results Line (1-900-776-2539 (1-900-77-NCLEX) (for a $9.95 fee):

Arizona, Colorado, Connecticut, District of Columbia, Florida, Georgia, Illinois, Idaho, Indiana, Iowa, Kansas, Kentucky, Louisiana, Maine, Maryland, Massachusetts, Michigan, Minnesota, Missouri, Montana, Nebraska, Nevada, New Jersey, New Mexico, New York, North Carolina, North Dakota, Ohio, Oklahoma, Oregon, Pennsylvania, South Carolina, South Dakota, Tennessee, Texas, Utah, Vermont, Washington, Wisconsin, Wyoming

For most states, you will receive your official results approximately 2–6 weeks after your test date.

CHAPTER 11

TAKING THE TEST MORE THAN ONCE

Some people may never have to read this chapter, but it's a certainty that others will. The most important advice we can give to repeat test takers is: Don't despair. There is hope. We can get you through the NCLEX-PN® exam.

You Are Not Alone

Think about that awful day when the big brown envelope arrived. You just couldn't believe it. You had to tell family, friends, your supervisor, and coworkers that you didn't pass the NCLEX-PN® exam. When this happens, each unsuccessful candidate feels like he or she is the only person who has failed the exam.

How to Interpret Unsuccessful Test Results

Most unsuccessful candidates on the NCLEX-PN® exam will usually say, "I almost passed." Some of you *did* almost pass, and some of you weren't very close. If you fail the exam, you will receive a diagnostic profile from the NCSBN. In this profile, you will be told how many questions you answered on the exam. The more questions you answered, the closer you came to passing. The only way you will continue to get questions after you answer the first 85 is if you are answering questions close to the level of difficulty needed to pass the exam. If you are answering questions far above the level needed to pass or far below the level needed to pass, your exam will end at 85 questions.

Figure 1 on the next page shows a representation of what happens when a candidate fails in 85 questions. This student does not come close to passing. In 85 questions, this student demonstrates an inability to consistently answer questions correctly at or above the level of difficulty needed to pass the exam. This usually indicates a lack of nursing knowledge, considerable difficulties with taking a standardized test, or a deficiency in critical thinking skills.

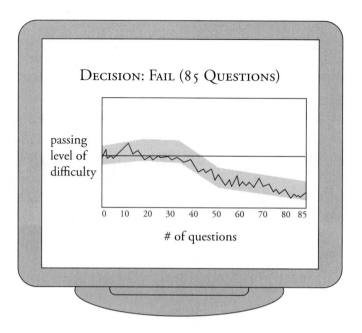

Figure 1

Figure 2 shows what happens when a candidate takes all 205 questions and fails. This candidate "almost passed." The candidate answers question 204 and the computer does not make a determination when it selects the last question. If the last question is below the level of difficulty needed to pass, the candidate fails.

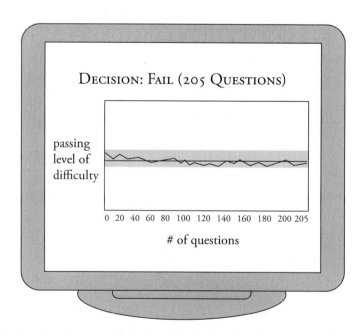

Figure 2

If the last question is above the level of difficulty needed to pass, the candidate passes. If you took a test longer than 85 questions and failed, you were probably familiar with most of the content you saw on the exam but you may have difficulty using critical thinking skills or taking standardized tests.

The information contained on the diagnostic profile helps you identify your strengths and weaknesses on this particular NCLEX-PN® exam. This knowledge will help you identify where to concentrate your study when you prepare to retake the NCLEX-PN® exam.

SHOULD YOU TEST AGAIN?

Absolutely! You completed your nursing education to become an LPN/LVN. The initial response of many unsuccessful candidates is to declare, "I'm never going back! That was the worst experience of my life! What do I do now?"

When you first received your results, you went through a period of grieving— the same stages that you learned about in nursing school. Three to four weeks later, you find that you want to begin preparing to retake the NCLEX-PN® exam.

HOW SHOULD YOU BEGIN?

You should prepare in a different way this time. Whatever you did to prepare last time didn't work well enough. The most common mistake made by candidates who failed is to assume that they did not study hard enough or learn enough content. For some of you, that's true. But for the majority of you, memorizing more content does not mean more right answers. It could simply mean more frustration for you.

The first step in preparing for your next exam is to make a commitment that you will test again. Decide when you want to schedule your test and allow yourself enough time to prepare. Mark this test date on your calendar. You can do all of this before you send in your fees and receive your authorization to test. Remember, you cannot retake the NCLEX-PN® exam for 45 to 90 days, depending on your state board of nursing, so you may as well use this time wisely.

The next step is to figure out why you failed the NCLEX-PN® exam. Check off any reasons that pertain to you:

- ☐ I didn't know the nursing content.
- ☐ I memorized facts without understanding the principles of client care.
- ☐ I had unrealistic expectations about the NCLEX-PN® exam test questions.
- ☐ I had difficulty correctly identifying THE REWORDED QUESTION.
- ☐ I had difficulty staying focused on THE REWORDED QUESTION.

- ☐ I found myself predicting answer choices.
- ☐ I did not carefully consider each answer choice.
- ☐ I am not good at choosing answers that require me to establish priorities of care.
- ☐ I answered questions based on my real-world experiences.
- ☐ I did not cope well with the computer-adaptive experience.
- ☐ I thought I would complete the exam in 85 questions.
- ☐ When I got to question 180 I totally lost my concentration, and just answered questions to get through the rest of the exam.

After determining why you failed, the next step is to establish a plan of action for your next test. Remember, you should prepare differently this time. Consider the following when setting up your new plan of study:

You've seen the test.

You may wish that you didn't have to walk back into the testing center again, but if you want to be a licensed practical/vocational nurse, you must go back. This time you will have an advantage over the first-time test taker: you've seen the test! You know exactly what you are preparing for, and there are no unknowns. The computer will remember what questions you took before, and you will not be given any of the same questions. However, the content of the questions, the style of the questions, and the kinds of answer choices will not change. You will not be surprised this time!

Study both content and test questions.

By the time you retest, you will be out of nursing school for 6 months or longer. Remember that old saying, "What you are not learning, you are forgetting." Because this is a content-based test about safe and effective nursing care, you must remember all you can about nursing theory in order to select correct answers. You must study content that is integrated and organized like the NCLEX-PN® exam.

You must also master exam-style test questions. It is essential that you be able to correctly identify what each question is asking. You will *not* predict answers. You will *think* about each and every answer choice to decide if it answers the reworded question. In order to master test questions, you must practice answering them. We recommend that you answer hundreds of exam-style test questions, especially at the application level of difficulty.

Know all of the words and their meanings.

Some students who have to learn a great deal of material in a short period of time have trouble learning the extensive vocabulary of the discipline. For example, difficulty with terminology is a problem for many good students who study history. They enjoy the concepts but find it hard to memorize all of the names and dates that allow them to do well on history tests. If you are one of those students who have trouble memorizing terms, you may find it useful to review a list of the terminology that you must know to pass the NCLEX-PN® exam. There is a list of those words at the end of this book.

Practice test-taking strategies.

There is no substitute for mastering the nursing content. This knowledge, combined with test-taking strategies, will help you to select a greater number of correct answers. For many students, the strategies mean the difference between a passing test and a failing test. Using strategies effectively can also determine whether you take a short test (85 questions) or a longer test (up to 205 questions).

Evaluate your testing experience.

Some students attribute their failure to the testing experience. Comments we have heard include:

"I didn't like answering questions on the computer."

"I found the background noise distracting. I should have taken the earplugs!"

"I looked up every time the door opened."

"I should have taken a snack. I got so hungry!"

"After 2½ hours I didn't care what I answered. I just wanted the computer to shut off!"

"I didn't expect to be there for four hours!"

"I should have rescheduled my test, but I just wanted to get it over with!"

"I wish I had taken aspirin with me. I had such a headache before it was over!"

Do any of these comments sound familiar? It is important for you to take charge of your testing experience. Here's how:

- Choose a familiar testing site.
- Select the time of day that you test your best. (Are you a morning person or an afternoon person?)
- Accept the earplugs when offered.
- Take a snack and a drink for your break.
- Take a break if you become distracted or fatigued during the test.
- Contact the proctors at the test site if something bothers you during the test.
- Plan on testing for five hours. Then, if you get out early, it's a pleasant surprise.
- Say to yourself every day, "I will pass the NCLEX-PN® exam."

CHAPTER 12

ESSENTIALS FOR INTERNATIONAL NURSES

Many of you have years of nursing experience in your home country. Now you are preparing for the NCLEX-PN® exam so you can be licensed to practice your profession in the United States. Because of Kaplan's extensive experience preparing nurses who were educated in other countries, we are very aware of the special issues that you face when trying to pass the NCLEX-PN® exam. Your special concerns will be discussed in this chapter.

Many nurses educated outside of the United States have not had the experience of taking an objective multiple-choice test as well as answering newer alternate questions, including those that require you to select more than one response, fill-in-the-blank questions, and pictures and graphs that require you to identify a "hot spot" or specific area on an image. Your testing experience may have been limited to oral exams or writing answers to essay and short answer questions. Multiple-choice tests are used in the United States because they measure knowledge more objectively and are easier to administer to large groups of people. In order to pass the NCLEX-PN® exam, you must demonstrate that you are a safe and effective nurse by correctly answering a predominantly multiple-choice test as well as the newer innovative question types, including fill-in-the-blank and hot spot questions.

NCLEX-PN® EXAM ADMINISTRATION ABROAD

NCSBN administers the NCLEX-PN® exam in selected international locations including Australia, Canada, the United Kingdom, Germany, Hong Kong, India, Japan, Mexico, the Philippines, and Taiwan. Please see *ncsbn.org* for details and the NCLEX Candidate Website (*vue.com/nclex* or *pearsonvue.com/nclex*) to locate a test center near you.

International sites provide greater convenience for international nurses to take the NCLEX-PN® exam. The international administration does not circumvent any regulations posed by the state boards of nursing, and the test sites are subject to the same security and procedures followed in U.S. test sites. If you choose to take the test at one of these sites, you must pay an additional $150 scheduling fee plus a Value Added Tax (VAT) where applicable.

THE CGFNS® CERTIFICATE

In order to apply for licensure as an LPN/LVN in the United States, many U.S. state boards of nursing require internationally educated LPN/LVNs to obtain a certificate from the Commission on Graduates of Foreign Nursing Schools (CGFNS®). The process of obtaining a CGFNS® certificate includes (1) a review of your nursing education credentials and original nursing program, (2) passing the CGFNS® exam that tests nursing knowledge, and (3) obtaining a minimum score on a designated English language proficiency exam.

The CGFNS® exam is a two-part test of nursing knowledge. Nurses who pass this exam have been shown to be more likely to pass the NCLEX-PN® exam on the first try than nurses who have not passed the CGFNS®. This exam can be taken overseas at a number of international testing sites run by CGFNS® or at selected sites in the United States.

Applications for the CGFNS® exam are free and can be obtained by calling CGFNS® at 1-215-349-8767, or you may apply online at *cgfns.org*. On the CGFNS® website, you will also find application deadlines and test dates. With an online application, you can submit your educational and professional documentation, choose a location and date for your exam, and pay fees by credit card.

To find out about a particular state's requirements for international nurses, call that state's board of nursing and request an application packet for initial licensure as an internationally educated LPN/LVN. You can also visit your chosen state's website using the key words "Board of Nursing" and the state name. The phone numbers and addresses for each of the state boards of nursing in the United States are listed in Appendix D.

Regarding the CGFNS® English proficiency requirements, the following information will help you register for the appropriate exams. Remember that these exam results are usually only valid for two years, so plan accordingly to avoid retakes. For more information about preparing for these exams, see the Kaplan English Programs section at the end of this chapter.

TOEFL®, TWE®, and TSE®
Educational Testing Service
P.O. Box 6151
Princeton, NJ 08541-6151
1-877-863-3546 (United States, U.S. Territories, Canada)
1-609-771-7100 (all other locations)
Fax: 1-610-290-8972
Email: *toefl@ets.org*

TOEIC® Testing Program
Educational Testing Service
Rosedale Road
Princeton, NJ 08540
Phone: 1-609-771-7170
Fax: 1-609-771-7111
Email: *toeic@ets.org*

IELTS® International
825 Colorado Boulevard, Suite 112
Los Angeles, CA 90041
Phone 1-323-255-2771
Fax 1-323-255-1261
Email: *ielts@ieltsintl.org*

WORK VISAS

For the most current information on visa requirements, contact the nearest U.S. embassy or consulate in your home country or the nearest regional office of the Immigration and Naturalization Service if you already live in the United States. You can also contact CGFNS® by telephone at 1-215-349-6735, or by mail at 3600 Market Street, Suite 400, Philadelphia, PA 19104-2651.

NURSING PRACTICE IN THE UNITED STATES

Some international LPN/LVNs find nursing in the United States similar to nursing as they learned it in their country. For others, nursing in the United States is very different from what they learned or experienced in their home country. The NCLEX-PN® exam may ask you questions about procedures that are unfamiliar to you. You may be asked questions about diets and foods that are new to you. In order to be successful on the NCLEX-PN® exam, you must be able to correctly answer questions about nursing as it is practiced in the United States.

Here is an overview of services and skills that LPN/LVNs are expected to perform:

- LPN/LVNs are involved with prevention, early detection, and treatment of illness for people of all ages.
- LPN/LVNs care for the whole person, not just an illness. Their focus is on client needs; that is, how a client will respond to an illness.

- LPN/LVNs are professionals who are responsible for their actions.
- LPN/LVNs must communicate with clients and all the members of the healthcare team: RNs, unlicensed assistive personnel, physicians, dietitians, and social workers.
- LPN/LVNs serve as clients' advocates; that is, they counsel clients and make sure their rights are protected.
- LPN/LVNs help clients understand the healthcare system, and assist them to make decisions about their healthcare.
- LPN/LVNs are assertive and ask questions of other healthcare professionals when necessary, including physicians. Their style of communication is polite but very direct.
- LPN/LVNs are responsible for meeting the needs of clients whose care involves high-tech equipment.
- LPN/LVNs are responsible for basing their actions on knowledge and acceptable nursing practice.
- LPN/LVNs, not families, are responsible for all the hands-on nursing care for clients in the hospital setting.
- LPN/LVNs are responsible for teaching clients and their families how to manage their healthcare needs.

U.S.-STYLE NURSING COMMUNICATION

An issue of special concern for international nurses is therapeutic communication. Correctly answering the questions about communication can be difficult for some nurses educated in the United States. These questions become a special challenge to test takers for whom English is a second language, or for test takers who do not yet fully understand American-style communication.

Key features of U.S.-style communication in nursing:

- *Validate the client's experience and feelings by responding to the client verbally.* Ask questions that relate directly to what the client says.
- *Direct the client's behavior to promote comfort and well-being.* Do not patronize or reject the client by imposing a value judgment.
- *Maintain eye contact with the client, especially during conversation.* Lean forward to face the client. Nod, smile, or frown to demonstrate agreement or disagreement while listening.

Responses used in U.S. nursing are based on an assessment of the client's needs and are designed to foster growth and establish mutually formulated goals.

NCLEX-PN® exam questions concerning communication are best answered by:

- Conveying *respect* and *warmth*, making the client feel accepted and respected as an individual regardless of his or her words, actions, or behavior. This means that the LPN/LVN:
    - Assumes that all client behavior is purposeful and has meaning even though it may not make sense to others
    - Defines the social, physical, and emotional boundaries of the nurse-client relationship
    - Develops a contract with the client
    - Structures time to develop a nurse-client relationship
    - Creates a safe and secure environment
    - Accepts the dependency needs of the client while encouraging, assisting, and supporting movement toward health and independence
    - Intervenes when a client behaves inappropriately to directly reject the behavior but not the client
    - Intervenes directly to respond to the client, not to reinforce an inappropriate behavior

- Demonstrating *active listening* and *genuineness*. This means that the LPN/LVN:
    - Asks questions that relate directly to what the client says
    - Maintains good eye contact
    - Leans forward in the chair to face the client
    - Nods, smiles, or frowns to show agreement or disagreement
    - Understands that the personal feelings and past experiences of the nurse can negatively or positively affect relationships with clients

- Communicating *interest* and *empathy* by allowing the client to comfortably communicate concerns and behave in new ways. This means that the LPN/LVN:
    - Focuses conversation on the client's feelings
    - Understands that clients respond to the behavioral expectations of the nursing staff
    - Validates the client's feelings
    - Analyzes both verbal and nonverbal behavioral clues
    - Anticipates that there might be some difficulty as the client learns new behaviors

LPN/LVNs create barriers in the communication process when they demonstrate a poor understanding of the basics in therapeutic communication. They must convey respect, warmth, and genuineness through active listening and communicating interest and empathy about the concerns of clients, families, or staff.

Examples of barriers to communication:

- Minimizing concerns
- Giving false reassurance
- Giving approval
- Rejecting the person, not the behavior
- Choosing sides with the client, family member, or staff member in a conflict
- Blaming the external environment for the situation
- Disagreeing or arguing with the client or family member
- Offering advice about a situation
- Pressuring the client or family member for an explanation
- Defending one's own actions or behavior
- Belittling concerns of the client, family member, or staff
- Giving one-word responses to questions
- Using denial
- Interpreting or analyzing both verbal and nonverbal behavioral clues to the client in the situation
- Shifting the focus of the conversation away from the concerns of the client, family member, or staff
- Using jargon or medical terminology without explanation in conversation with the client and/or family
- Invalidating the client's, family member's, or staff's feelings
- Offering unrealistic hope for the future
- Ignoring client clues to help the client set appropriate limits on his or her behavior

The following are some questions that will allow you to practice the right approach.

SAMPLE QUESTIONS

Directions: Carefully read the question and all answer choices. Examine each answer choice and determine whether it is an appropriate response. Indicate your decision in the column labeled Correct/Incorrect and give the reason for your choice.

QUESTION	CORRECT/ INCORRECT	REASON
1. A client has been hospitalized for 2 days for treatment of hepatitis A. When the LPN/LVN enters the client's room, the client asks the LPN/LVN to leave him alone and stop bothering him. Which of the following responses by the LPN/LVN would be *MOST* appropriate? (1) "I understand and will leave you alone for now." (2) "Why are you angry with me?" (3) "Are you upset because you do not feel better?" (4) "You seem upset this morning."		
2. A client states she is afraid to have her cast removed from her fractured arm. Which of the following is the *MOST* appropriate response by the LPN/LVN? (1) "I know it is unpleasant. Try not to be afraid. I will help you." (2) "You seem very anxious. I will stay with you while the cast is removed." (3) "I don't blame you. I'd be afraid also." (4) "My aunt just had a cast removed and she's just fine."		

	QUESTION	CORRECT/ INCORRECT	REASON

3. A client comes to the clinic because she thinks she is pregnant. She tells the LPN/LVN that she wants the pregnancy terminated because she and her husband do not want to have children, and then begins to cry. Which of the following statements by the LPN/LVN is the *MOST* appropriate?

   (1) "Are you upset because you forgot to use birth control?"

   (2) "Why are you so upset? You're married. There's no reason not to have the baby."

   (3) "If you're so upset, why don't you have the baby and put it up for adoption?"

   (4) "You seem upset. Let's talk about how you're feeling."

4. A client is in the terminal stages of carcinoma of the lung. A family member asks the LPN/LVN, "How much longer will it be?" Which of the following responses by the LPN/LVN would be *MOST* appropriate?

   (1) "I cannot say exactly. What are your concerns at this time?"

   (2) "I don't know. I'll call the doctor."

   (3) "This must be a terrible situation for you."

   (4) "Don't worry, it will be very soon."

QUESTION	CORRECT/ INCORRECT	REASON

5. A client is admitted to the hospital with a diagnosis of manic-depressive disorder. The man approaches the nurse and says, "Hi, baby," and opens his robe, under which he is naked. Which of the following comments by the LPN/LVN would be *MOST* appropriate?

   (1) "This is inappropriate behavior. Please close your robe and return to your room."

   (2) "Please dress in your clothes and then join us for lunch in the dining room."

   (3) "I am offended by your behavior and will have to report you."

   (4) "Do you need some assistance dressing today?"

6. A client is placed in Buck's traction. The LPN/LVN assigned to her prepares to assist her with a bath. The woman says, "You're too young to know how to do this. Get me somebody who knows what they're doing." Which of the following responses by the LPN/LVN would be *MOST* appropriate?

   (1) "I am young, but I graduated from nursing school."

   (2) "If I don't bathe you now, you'll have to wait until I'm finished with my other clients."

   (3) "Can you be more specific about your concerns?"

   (4) "Your concerns are unnecessary. I know what I'm doing."

	QUESTION	CORRECT/ INCORRECT	REASON

7. A client is admitted to the hospital with an abdominal mass and is scheduled for an exploratory laparotomy. She asks the LPN/LVN admitting her, "Do you think I have cancer?" Which of the following responses by the LPN/LVN would be *MOST* appropriate?

   (1) "Would you like me to call your doctor so that you can discuss your specific concerns?"

   (2) "Your tests show a mass. It must be hard not knowing what is wrong."

   (3) "It sounds like you are afraid that you are going to die from cancer."

   (4) "Don't worry about it now; I'm sure you have many healthy years ahead of you."

8. A client is admitted to the postpartum unit following a miscarriage. The next day the LPN/LVN finds the woman crying while looking at the babies in the newborn nursery. Which of the following approaches by the LPN/LVN would be *MOST* appropriate?

   (1) Assure the woman that the loss was "for the best."

   (2) Explain to her that she is young enough to have more children.

   (3) Ask her why she is looking at the babies.

   (4) Acknowledge the loss and be supportive.

	QUESTION	CORRECT/ INCORRECT	REASON
9.	An elderly client is hospitalized with Alzheimer's disease. His daughter tells the LPN/LVN that caring for him is too hard, but that she feels guilty placing him in a nursing home. Which of the following statements by the LPN/LVN is *MOST* appropriate?		
	(1) "It is hard to be caught between taking care of your needs and your father's needs."		
	(2) "Would you like me to help you find a nursing home?"		
	(3) "Don't feel guilty. The only solution is to place your father in a nursing home."		
	(4) "I think I would feel guilty too if I had to place my father in a nursing home."		

Read the explanations to these questions and make sure that the American approach to these communications questions is understandable to you. It will help you to choose the right answer on the NCLEX-PN® exam.

ANSWERS TO SAMPLE QUESTIONS

1. (4) **"You seem upset this morning,"** is the correct answer choice because the LPN/LVN seeks to verbally validate the client's behavior rather than simply respond to the behavior. This response promotes the nurse-client relationship by encouraging the client to share his feelings with the LPN/LVN.

   (1) *"I understand and will leave you alone for now,"* is not the best approach because it does not promote further communication between the LPN/LVN and the client about how the client is feeling. In order to interpret this client's behavior, the LPN/LVN must first validate it with the client.

   (2) *"Why are you angry with me?"* is incorrect. The LPN/LVN is drawing a conclusion about the client's behavior. This type of action is too confrontational. "Why" questions are considered nontherapeutic.

   (3) *"Are you upset because you do not feel better?"* is not the best choice. The LPN/LVN is drawing a conclusion about the client's behavior without validating it first. This type of response may also belittle the client's actual concerns.

2. (2) **"You seem very anxious. I will stay with you while the cast is removed,"** is the best response because the LPN/LVN responds to the client's feelings of fear. This is consistent with therapeutic communication used in American nursing. This response also provides an additional opportunity for the LPN/LVN to remain with the client in a supportive capacity enhancing the nurse-client relationship.

   (1) *"I know it is unpleasant. Try not to be afraid. I will help you,"* is not the best response. It is not clear what concerns the client has about this procedure. The LPN/LVN should establish this before responding. The LPN/LVN falsely reassures the client by saying, "I will help you." Because you do not know the nature of the client's concerns, you cannot honestly offer help.

   (3) *"I don't blame you. I'd be afraid also,"* is not the correct response because the LPN/LVN shifts the focus of the conversation from the client to the LPN/LVN. This sets up a barrier to further communication. The LPN/LVN concedes the issue too quickly, leaving the source of the client's fear unknown.

   (4) *"My aunt just had a cast removed and she's just fine,"* is not the best choice. The focus of the conversation is shifted from the client to the LPN/LVN's aunt, who is of no concern to the client. This response fails to explore the source of the client's anxiety and sets up a block to further communication.

3. (4) **"You seem upset. Let's talk about how you're feeling,"** is the best answer to this question. This promotes the nurse-client relationship and illustrates therapeutic communication used in American nursing. The LPN/LVN responds to the client's feelings in a nonjudgmental, empathetic way.

   (1) *"Are you upset because you forgot to use birth control?"* is inappropriate because it places blame on the client. The LPN/LVN should not assume that the client "forgot" to do something. This response also fails to respond to the client's feelings and does not encourage the client to discuss her concerns.

   (2) *"Why are you so upset? You're married. There's no reason not to have the baby,"* is inappropriate in terms of American therapeutic communication. This response is harsh and presumptive, and assumes that the purpose of every marriage is to have children. This is not always the case in American culture. With this response the LPN/LVN does not attempt to verify the reason for the client's tears, thereby discouraging further conversation about what the client is actually experiencing.

   (3) *"If you're so upset, why don't you have the baby and put it up for adoption?"* is also inappropriate. This is a value-laden assumption placing positive value on adoption. Again, the LPN/LVN fails to explore with the client the reason for the client's tears, thereby discouraging further communication. The LPN/LVN is also offering advice.

4. (1) **"I cannot say exactly. What are your concerns at this time?"** is the most appropriate response because it is unclear why the family member has approached the LPN/LVN at this point. Perhaps the client is in pain and the family member wants to discuss it with the LPN/LVN. This response allows for that possibility. This response is also direct and factually correct.

   (2) *"I don't know. I'll call the doctor,"* is not the most appropriate response. It shifts the focus of responsibility from the LPN/LVN to the physician, which prevents a nurse–family member relationship from developing.

   (3) *"This must be a terrible situation for you,"* is not the most appropriate response. It is a value-laden statement that fails to explore the family member's reason for approaching the LPN/LVN.

   (4) *"Don't worry, it will be very soon,"* is inappropriate because the LPN/LVN offers the family member false reassurance. It also offers advice by telling the family member not to worry. This statement is demeaning and may sound as if the nurse is too busy to discuss the family member's concerns.

5. (1) **"This is inappropriate behavior. Please close your robe and return to your room,"** is the correct answer choice. This statement by the LPN/LVN responds to the client's behavior, sets limits on the behavior, and directs the client towards more appropriate social behavior in the milieu. This statement rejects the client's behavior, not the client as a person.

(2) *"Please dress in your clothes and then join us for lunch in the dining room,"* is incorrect. It ignores the behavior of the client exposing himself. Instead it directs the client to dress and report to the dining room for lunch as though nothing has happened. This is inappropriate and nontherapeutic.

(3) *"I am offended by your behavior and will have to report you,"* is incorrect. It shifts the focus from the client to the LPN/LVN and the LPN/LVN's feelings. The LPN/LVN's personal feelings are irrelevant. Also, the LPN/LVN goes on to threaten the client with reporting him. This is nontherapeutic.

(4) *"Do you need some assistance dressing today?"* is incorrect. This question fails to respond to the client's behavior. It is also a yes/no question, which is nontherapeutic.

6. (3) **"Can you be more specific about your concerns?"** is the correct answer. This is the best answer choice because it seeks to validate the client's message. It is direct, is not defensive, and allows the client to express her point of view.

(1) *"I am young, but I graduated from nursing school,"* is incorrect. It responds to only part of the message that the client sent to the LPN/LVN. It assumes that the LPN/LVN knows what the client's concerns are and agrees that there is some problem associated with being too young. Further clarification is necessary in this situation.

(2) *"If I don't bathe you now, you'll have to wait until I'm finished with my other clients,"* is a nontherapeutic response. It fails to explore the client's concerns about the LPN/LVN. It is an uncaring and punitive statement by the LPN/LVN that is inappropriate in a nurse-client relationship.

(4) *"Your concerns are unnecessary. I know what I'm doing,"* is incorrect. The LPN/LVN dismisses the client's concerns by telling her that she shouldn't be concerned. The LPN/LVN should not tell a client how he or she should be feeling. It may sound as if the LPN/LVN is trying to reassure the client by telling her that the LPN/LVN knows what he or she is doing; however, the LPN/LVN has yet to validate the concerns that underlie the client's statement.

7. (2) **"Your tests show a mass. It must be hard not knowing what is wrong,"** is the correct answer choice. This is the best answer choice because it responds to the client's feelings. It allows the client to continue to identify and express her concerns regarding surgery, hospitalization, and the possibility of having a potentially life-threatening illness. The LPN/LVN validates that the client has appropriate concerns and invites her to elaborate on them.

(1) *"Would you like me to call your doctor so that you can discuss your specific concerns?"* This response is incorrect because it shifts the focus of responsibility from the LPN/LVN to the doctor, thereby reducing the possibility of developing an ongoing nurse-client relationship.

(3) *"It sounds like you are afraid that you are going to die from cancer,"* is inappropriate. It fails to validate with the client that "dying from cancer" is in fact the issue. The

LPN/LVN inappropriately concludes this on the basis of a brief statement made by the client without giving the client a chance to elaborate.

(4) *"Don't worry about it now; I'm sure that you have many healthy years ahead of you,"* is inappropriate. The LPN/LVN is telling the client how she should feel and then goes on to offer false reassurance. This response fails to address or explore the actual concerns of the client.

8. (4) **"Acknowledge the loss and be supportive,"** is the best answer choice. It promotes the nurse-client relationship and allows for the identification of feelings and the expression of sadness. The client is in an acute stage of grief. This type of response addresses this issue.

(1) *"Assure the woman that the loss was "for the best,"* is incorrect. This statement is insensitive to the client, offers false reassurance, and belittles the client's most immediate concerns.

(2) *"Explain to her that she is young enough to have more children,"* is inappropriate because it is insensitive to the grief that the client is experiencing. The LPN/LVN offers false reassurance by telling the woman that she can have other children.

(3) *"Ask her why she is looking at the babies,"* is also incorrect. This is inappropriate because it is a "why" question and because the woman may become defensive when answering such a question. This response also fails to respond to the client's immediate grief.

9. (1) **"It is hard to be caught between taking care of your needs and your father's needs,"** is the correct response. This is the most therapeutic response as it allows for continued development of a relationship with the family member of the client. This response allows the LPN/LVN to explore and validate the daughter's feelings about the nursing home placement.

(2) *"Would you like me to help you find a nursing home?"* is not the best answer choice. It is a yes/no question and doesn't encourage discussion of the daughter's feelings.

(3) *"Don't feel guilty. The only solution is to place your father in a nursing home,"* is not the best therapeutic response. The daughter's concerns are minimized when the LPN/LVN tells the daughter not to worry. While it may be true that the daughter has done all that she can, this response cuts off an opportunity for further conversation with the LPN/LVN.

(4) *"I think I would feel guilty too if I had to place my father in a nursing home,"* is also incorrect. This statement is value-laden and judgmental, and could block further communication between the LPN/LVN and the client's daughter. It is not important what the LPN/LVN thinks about the daughter's decision, nor is it the LPN/LVN's role to make the daughter feel more guilty about her decision.

LANGUAGE

English is the predominant language spoken and written in the United States, and the NCLEX-PN® exam is administered only in English. With the exception of the medical terminology, the reading level of the NCLEX-PN® exam is that of a sophomore in an American high school. In order to be successful on the NCLEX-PN® exam, you must understand English—and the terminology—as it is used in the United States.

Vocabulary

Vocabulary can be a challenge for international nurses on the NCLEX-PN ® exam. Not only must you know what each word means, but sometimes a word may have more than one meaning. You need to be able to correctly identify words as they are used in context. Refer to the NCLEX-PN® Exam Resources section in the back of this book for some of the commonly found words on the NCLEX-PN® exam. Some other ways to increase your vocabulary and learn how the words are used in everyday English include:

- Talking with Americans
- Watching American movies and television
- Reading American newspapers and magazines

Abbreviations

Many of you are unfamiliar with the abbreviations used in the United States. When studying, always look up unknown words in a medical dictionary. Consult Appendix C for a list of abbreviations used by nurses in American healthcare settings.

As an internationally educated nurse, you face special challenges in preparing for the NCLEX-PN® exam. Following the tips and guidelines outlined in this book will increase your chances of passing the NCLEX-PN® exam and will allow you to reach your career goals.

KAPLAN PROGRAMS FOR INTERNATIONAL NURSES

Knowing something about U.S. culture and how U.S. nurses fit into the overall healthcare industry is important for nurses trained outside the United States. If you are not from the United States but are interested in learning more about U.S. nursing, wish to practice in the United States, or are exploring the possibilities of attending a U.S. nursing school for graduate study, Kaplan is able to help you.

CGFNS® (Commission on Graduates of Foreign Nursing Schools) Preparation for International Nurses

Many U.S. state boards of nursing require internationally educated nurses to obtain a CGFNS® certificate before applying for initial licensure as an LPN/LVN. The certification process requires that a candidate pass a two-part test of nursing knowledge and demonstrate English language proficiency on the TOEFL® exam. Kaplan offers a comprehensive course of study to help you pass this exam. To obtain information, please call 1-800-533-8850. Outside the United States, please call 1-213-452-5700 or log on to the website at *kaplannursing.com*.

Preparation for the NCLEX-PN® (National Council Licensure Examination) Examination for International Nurses

An internationally educated nurse must pass the NCLEX-PN® exam in order to obtain a license to practice as an LPN/LVN in the United States. Kaplan has a comprehensive course and review products to help international nurses pass this exam. To obtain information, please call 1-800-533-8850. Outside the United States, please call 1-213-452-5700 or log on to the website at *kaplannursing.com*.

Kaplan English Programs

In addition to Kaplan Nursing programs, Kaplan also offers English programs to help you improve your English skills and score on the TOEFL® exam. Kaplan's English programs are designed to help students and professionals from outside the United States meet their educational and career goals. At locations throughout the United States, international students take advantage of Kaplan's programs to help them improve their academic and conversational English skills, raise their scores on the TOEFL® and other standardized exams, and gain admission to the schools of their choice. Our staff and instructors give international students the individualized instruction they need to succeed. The following sections provide brief descriptions of some of Kaplan's programs for non-native English speakers.

English Language Programs

Kaplan offers a wide range of English language programs to help you improve your English quickly and effectively, regardless of your current level. Each of our programs has a special focus, allowing you to direct your study in a way that suits your particular language needs. All of the essential language skills are covered, and your fluency and confidence will increase rapidly thanks to Kaplan's communicative teaching method.

TOEFL® and Academic English

Kaplan has updated its world-famous TOEFL® course to prepare students for the TOEFL® iBT. Designed for high-intermediate to advanced-level English speakers, our course focuses on the academic English skills you will need to succeed on the test. The course includes

TOEFL®-focused reading, writing, listening, and speaking instruction and hundreds of practice items similar to those on the exam. Kaplan's expert instructors help you prepare for the four sections of the TOEFL® iBT, including the Speaking section. Our simulated online TOEFL® tests help you monitor your progress and provide you with feedback on areas where you require improvement. We will teach you how to get a higher score!

Other Kaplan Programs

Since 1938, more than 3 million students have come to Kaplan to advance their studies, prepare for entry to American universities, and further their careers. In addition to the above programs, Kaplan offers courses to prepare for the SAT®, ACT®, GMAT®, GRE®, LSAT®, MCAT®, DAT®, USMLE®, and other standardized exams at locations throughout the United States.

Applying to Kaplan English Programs*

To get more information, or to apply for admission to any of Kaplan's programs for non-native English speakers, contact us at:

Kaplan English Programs
700 South Flower Street, Suite 2900
Los Angeles, CA 90017 USA
Phone: 1-213-452-5800
Fax: 1-213-892-1360
Website: *kaplaninternational.com*
Email: *northamerica@kaplaninternational.com*

*Kaplan is authorized under federal law to enroll nonimmigrant alien students.
Test names are registered trademarks of their respective owners.

FREE Services for International Students

Kaplan now offers international students many services online—free of charge! Students may assess their TOEFL® skills and gain valuable feedback on their English language proficiency in just a few hours with Kaplan's TOEFL® Skills Assessment. Log on to *kaplaninternational.com* today.

PART 2

THE PRACTICE TEST

PRACTICE TEST

> **Directions:** Each question or incomplete statement below is followed by four suggested answers or completions. In each case, select the statement that best answers the question or completes the statement.

1. The LPN/LVN is gathering data from a client who is being treated for obsessive-compulsive disorder. Which of the following is the *MOST* important question the LPN/LVN should ask this client?

   1. "Do you find yourself forgetting simple things?"
   2. "Do you find it hard to stay on a task?"
   3. "Do you have trouble controlling upsetting thoughts?"
   4. "Do you experience feelings of panic in a closed area?"

2. The LPN/LVN is caring for a client who states, "I just want to die." The LPN/LVN should examine the client's medical record for which of the following documents?

   1. Advance directives
   2. Power of attorney
   3. "Do not resuscitate" order
   4. Living will

3. A newly admitted client with a history of convulsions suddenly says to the LPN/LVN, "I hear drums." Which of the following should the LPN/LVN do *FIRST*?

   1. Tell the client to ignore the drums.

2. Place the client in a darkened room away from the nurses' station.
3. Continue to question the client.
4. Insert an oral airway in the client.

4. A client diagnosed with multiple myeloma is admitted to the unit after developing pneumonia. When the LPN/LVN enters the client's room wearing a mask, the client says, in an irritated tone of voice, "Why are you wearing that mask?" Which of the following responses by the LPN/LVN is *BEST*?

   1. "The chest X-ray taken this morning indicates you have pneumonia."
   2. "What have you been told about the X-rays that were taken this morning?"
   3. "You have been placed on contact precautions due to your infection."
   4. "I am trying to protect you from the germs in the hospital."

5. A nursing team consists of an RN, an LPN/LVN, and a nursing assistant. The LPN/LVN should be assigned to which of the following clients?

   1. A 72-year-old client with diabetes who requires a dressing change for a stasis ulcer

2. A 42-year-old client who has cancer of the bone and is complaining of pain

3. A 55-year-old client with terminal cancer who is being transferred to hospice home care

4. A 23-year-old client who has a fracture of the right leg and asks to use the urinal

6. To determine the structural relationship of one hospital department with another, the LPN/LVN should consult which of the following?

1. Organizational chart
2. Job descriptions
3. Personnel policies
4. Policies and Procedures Manual

7. A client complains of pain in his right lower extremity. The physician orders codeine 60 mg and aspirin grains X PO every 4 hours, as needed for pain. Each codeine tablet contains 15 mg of codeine. Each aspirin tablet contains 325 mg of aspirin. Which of the following should the LPN/LVN administer?

1. 2 codeine tablets and 4 aspirin tablets
2. 4 codeine tablets and 3 aspirin tablets
3. 4 codeine tablets and 2 aspirin tablets
4. 3 codeine tablets and 3 aspirin tablets

8. The LPN/LVN cares for a client receiving paroxetine (Paxil). It is *MOST* important for the LPN/LVN to report which of the following to the physician?

1. The client states there is no change in her appetite.
2. The client states she has started taking digoxin (Lanoxin).
3. The client states she applies sunscreen before going outside.
4. The client states she drives her car to work.

9. A client with a DNR (do not resuscitate) physician's order experiences a cardiac arrest. Which of the following is the *FIRST* action the LPN/LVN should take?

1. Administer lifesaving medications.
2. Assess the client for signs of death.
3. Open the airway and give 2 breaths.
4. Summon the emergency code team.

10. An LPN/LVN is working in the newborn nursery. Which of the following client-care assignments should the LPN/LVN question?

1. A 2-day-old infant lying quietly alert with a heart rate of 185
2. A 1-day-old infant crying with the anterior fontanel bulging
3. A 12-hour-old infant being held; respirations 45 breaths per minute and irregular
4. A 5-hour-old infant sleeping with hands and feet blue bilaterally

11. While inserting a nasogastric tube, the LPN/LVN should use which of the following protective measures?

1. Gloves, gown, goggles, and surgical cap
2. Sterile gloves, mask, plastic bags, and gown
3. Gloves, gown, mask, and goggles
4. Double gloves, goggles, mask, and surgical cap

12. The LPN/LVN is caring for clients in the outpatient clinic. Which of the following clients should the LPN/LVN see *FIRST*?

1. A client with hepatitis A who states, "My arms and legs are itching."
2. A client with a cast on the right leg who states, "I have a funny feeling in my right leg."

3. A client with osteomyelitis of the spine who states, "I am so nauseous that I can't eat."

4. A client with rheumatoid arthritis who states, "I am having trouble sleeping."

13. Which of the following client assignments should an LPN/LVN question?

    1. A client with a chest tube who is ambulating in the hall

    2. A client with a colostomy who requires assistance with a colostomy irrigation

    3. A client with a right-sided cerebrovascular accident (CVA) who requires assistance with bathing

    4. A client who is refusing medication to treat cancer of the colon

14. The LPN/LVN is caring for a client with hepatitis B. The client is to be discharged the next day. The LPN/LVN would be *MOST* concerned if the client made which of the following statements?

    1. "I must not share eating utensils with my family."

    2. "I must use my own bath towel."

    3. "I'm glad that my husband and I can continue to have intimate relations."

    4. "I must eat small, frequent feedings."

15. The LPN/LVN carries out the plan for care of a client with anemia who is complaining of weakness. Which of the following tasks could be assigned to the nursing assistant?

    1. Listen to the client's breath sounds.

    2. Set up the client's lunch tray.

    3. Obtain a diet history.

    4. Instruct the client on how to balance rest and activity.

16. The LPN/LVN is caring for clients on the surgical floor and has just received report from the RN. Which of the following clients should the LPN/LVN see *FIRST*?

    1. A 35-year-old admitted 3 days ago with a gunshot wound; 1.5-cm area of dark drainage noted on the dressing

    2. A 43-year-old who had a mastectomy 2 days ago; 23 mL of serosanguinous fluid noted in the Jackson-Pratt drain

    3. A 59-year-old with a collapsed lung due to an accident; no drainage noted in the previous 8 hours

    4. A 62-year-old who had an abdominal-perineal resection 3 days ago; client complains of chills

17. A client scheduled for a cardiac catheterization says to the LPN/LVN, "I know you were in here when the doctor had me sign the consent form for the test. I thought I understood everything, but now I'm not so sure." Which of the following responses by the LPN/LVN is *BEST*?

    1. "Why didn't you listen more closely?"

    2. "You sound as if you would like to ask more questions."

    3. "I'll get you a pamphlet about cardiac catheterization."

    4. "That often happens when this procedure is explained to clients."

18. A 1-day-old newborn diagnosed with intrauterine growth retardation is observed by the LPN/LVN to be restless, irritable, and fist-sucking, and has a high-pitched, shrill cry. Based on this data, which of the following actions should the LPN/LVN take *FIRST*?

    1. Massage the infant's back.

    2. Tightly swaddle the infant in a flexed position.

    3. Schedule feeding times every 3–4 hours.

4. Encourage eye contact with the infant during feedings.

19. The LPN/LVN visits a neighbor who is at 20 weeks' gestation. The neighbor complains of nausea, headache, and blurred vision. The LPN/LVN notes that the neighbor appears nervous, is diaphoretic, and is experiencing tremors. It would be *MOST* important for the LPN/LVN to ask which of the following questions?

   1. "Are you having menstrual-like cramps?"
   2. "When did you last eat or drink?"
   3. "Have you been diagnosed with diabetes?"
   4. "Have you been lying on the couch?"

20. The LPN/LVN notes that a child newly admitted to the pediatric unit is scratching her head almost constantly. It would be *MOST* important for the LPN/LVN to take which of the following actions?

   1. Discuss basic hygiene with the parents.
   2. Instruct the child not to sleep with her dog.
   3. Inform the parents that they must contact an exterminator.
   4. Observe the scalp for small white specks.

21. A suicidal client who was admitted to the psychiatric unit for treatment and observation a week ago suddenly appears cheerful and motivated. The LPN/LVN should be aware of which of the following?

   1. The client is probably sleeping well because of the medication.
   2. The client has made new friends and has a support group.
   3. The client may have finalized a suicide plan.
   4. The client is responding to treatment and is no longer depressed.

22. The LPN/LVN is caring for clients in the GYN clinic. A client complains of an off-white vaginal discharge with a curdlike appearance and vulvar itching. It would be *MOST* important for the LPN/LVN to ask which of the following questions?

   1. "Do you douche?"
   2. "Are you sexually active?"
   3. "What kind of birth control do you use?"
   4. "Have you taken any cough medicine?"

23. The physician orders an Ace bandage wrap for a client's left leg from toes to mid-thigh. The LPN/LVN should do which of the following?

   1. Increase friction between the skin and bandage surfaces.
   2. Leave a small distal part of the extremity exposed.
   3. Use multiple pins to secure the bandage.
   4. Position the left leg in abduction.

24. A client recovering from a laparoscopic laser cholecystectomy says to the LPN/LVN, "I hate the thought of eating a low-fat diet for the rest of my life." Which of the following responses by the LPN/LVN is *MOST* appropriate?

   1. "I will ask the dietician to come talk to you."
   2. "What do you think is so bad about following a low-fat diet?"
   3. "It may not be necessary for you to follow a low-fat diet for that long."
   4. "At least you will be alive and not suffering that pain."

25. The LPN/LVN is caring for clients in a pediatric clinic. The mother of a 14-year-old male privately tells the LPN/LVN that she is worried about her son because she unexpectedly walked into his room and discovered him masturbating. Which of the following responses by the LPN/LVN is *MOST* appropriate?

    1. "Tell your son he could go blind doing that."
    2. "Masturbation is a normal part of sexual development."
    3. "He's really too young to be masturbating."
    4. "Why don't you give him more privacy?"

26. A client begins to breathe very rapidly. Which of the following actions by the LPN/LVN would be the *MOST* appropriate?

    1. Assess the apical pulse.
    2. Measure blood pressure and pulse.
    3. Notify the physician.
    4. Obtain an oxygen saturation.

27. The LPN/LVN plans morning care for a client hospitalized after a cerebrovascular accident (CVA) resulting in left-sided paralysis and homonymous hemianopia. During morning care, the LPN/LVN should do which of the following?

    1. Provide care from the client's right side.
    2. Speak loudly and distinctly when talking with the client.
    3. Reduce the level of lighting in the client's room to prevent glare.
    4. Provide all of the client's care to reduce his energy expenditure.

28. A primigravid woman comes to the clinic for her initial prenatal visit. She is at 32 weeks' gestation and says that she has just moved from out of state. The client says that she has had periodic headaches during her pregnancy, and that she is continually bumping into things. The LPN/LVN notes numerous bruises in various stages of healing around the client's breasts and abdomen. Vital signs are: BP 120/80, pulse 72, resp 18, and FHT 142. Which of the following responses by the LPN/LVN is *BEST*?

    1. "Are you battered by your partner?"
    2. "How do you feel about being pregnant?"
    3. "Tell me about your headaches."
    4. "You may be more clumsy due to your size."

29. The LPN/LVN is providing care for a client with chronic lung disease who is receiving oxygen through a nasal cannula. The LPN/LVN should expect which of the following to occur?

    1. Arterial blood gases will be drawn q 2 hours.
    2. The client's oral intake will be restricted.
    3. The client will be on strict bed rest.
    4. The oxygen flow rate will be set at 3 L/min or less.

30. The LPN/LVN cares for a child who is in a leg cast for treatment of a fractured right ankle. It is *MOST* important for the LPN/LVN to reinforce which of the following activities after discharge?

    1. The child performs isometric exercises of the right leg.
    2. The mother gently massages the child's right foot with emollient cream.
    3. The mother cleans the leg cast with mild soap and water.

4. The mother elevates the right leg on several pillows.

31. The LPN/LVN is caring for a client who had a thyroidectomy 12 hours ago for treatment of Graves' disease. The LPN/LVN would be *MOST* concerned if which of the following were observed?

   1. The client's blood pressure is 138/82, pulse 84, respirations 16, oral temp 99° F (37.2° C).
   2. The client supports his head and neck when turning his head to the right.
   3. The client spontaneously flexes his wrist when the blood pressure is obtained.
   4. The client is drowsy and complains of a sore throat.

32. A client is admitted with complaints of severe pain in the right lower quadrant of the abdomen. To assist with pain relief, the LPN/LVN should take which of the following actions?

   1. Encourage the client to change positions frequently in bed.
   2. Massage the right lower quadrant of the abdomen.
   3. Apply warmth to the abdomen with a heating pad.
   4. Use comfort measures and pillows to position the client.

33. Which of the following actions by the LPN/LVN would be considered negligence?

   1. Administering subQ (subcutaneous) heparin into a client's abdomen without first aspirating for blood.
   2. Crushing furosemide (Lasix) and adding to a teaspoon of applesauce for an elderly client.

   3. Lowering the bed side rails after administering meperidine (Demerol) and hydroxyzine (Vistaril) to a client preoperatively.
   4. Placing a used syringe and needle in a sharps container in a client's room.

34. The LPN/LVN teaches an elderly client with right-sided weakness how to use a cane. Which of the following behaviors by the client indicates that the teaching was effective?

   1. The man holds the cane with his right hand, moves the cane forward followed by the right leg, and then moves the left leg.
   2. The man holds the cane with his right hand, moves the cane forward followed by his left leg, and then moves the right leg.
   3. The man holds the cane with his left hand, moves the cane forward followed by the right leg, and then moves the left leg.
   4. The man holds the cane with his left hand, moves the cane forward followed by his left leg, and then moves the right leg.

35. The LPN/LVN has been caring for a 72-year-old client for the past 2 days. The client's vital signs have been within normal limits. This morning her vital signs are: tympanic temperature 103.6° F (39.77° C), pulse 82 regular and strong, respirations 14 shallow and unlabored, BP 134/88. What should the LPN/LVN's next action be?

   1. Call the physician immediately to report the vital signs.
   2. Proceed with the client's care.
   3. Record the vital signs on the graphic record in the chart.

4. Retake the temperature with a different thermometer.

36. A 46-year-old man is admitted to the hospital with a fractured right femur. He is placed in balanced suspension traction with a Thomas splint and Pearson attachment. During the first 48 hours, the LPN/LVN should gather data related to which of the following complications?

    1. Pulmonary embolism
    2. Fat embolism
    3. Avascular necrosis
    4. Malunion

37. The LPN/LVN is helping a nursing assistant provide a bed bath to a comatose client who is incontinent. The LPN/LVN should intervene if which of the following actions is noted?

    1. The nursing assistant answers the phone while wearing gloves.
    2. The nursing assistant log-rolls the client to provide back care.
    3. The nursing assistant places an incontinence diaper under the client.
    4. The nursing assistant positions the client on the left side, head elevated.

38. A 70-year-old woman is transferred to the orthopedic unit from the emergency room for treatment after being found on the floor by her daughter. X-rays reveal a displaced subcapital fracture of the left hip and osteoarthritis. When comparing the legs, the LPN/LVN would most likely make which of the following observations?

    1. The client's left leg is longer than the right leg and externally rotated.
    2. The client's left leg is shorter than the right leg and internally rotated.
    3. The client's left leg is shorter than the right leg and adducted.
    4. The client's left leg is longer than the right leg and is abducted.

39. The LPN/LVN is caring for a client with a cast on the left leg. The LPN/LVN would be *MOST* concerned if which of the following is observed?

    1. Capillary refill time is less than 3 seconds.
    2. Client complains of discomfort and itching.
    3. Client complains of tightness and pain.
    4. Client's foot is elevated on a pillow.

40. The LPN/LVN is assisting with discharging a client from an inpatient alcohol treatment unit. Which of the following statements by the client's wife indicates that the family is coping adaptively?

    1. "My husband will do well as long as I keep him engaged in activities that he likes."
    2. "My focus is learning how to live my life."
    3. "I am so glad that our problems are behind us."
    4. "I'll make sure that the children don't give my husband any problems."

41. An LPN/LVN is caring for clients in the mental health clinic. A woman comes to the clinic complaining of insomnia and anorexia. The client tearfully tells the LPN/LVN that she was laid off from a job that she had held for 15 years. Which of the following responses by the LPN/LVN is *MOST* appropriate?

    1. "Did your company give you a severance package?"
    2. "Focus on the fact that you have a healthy, happy family."
    3. "Tell me what happened."
    4. "Losing a job is common nowadays."

42. A client with a history of alcoholism is transferred to the unit in an agitated state. He is vomiting and diaphoretic. He says he had his last drink 5 hours ago. The LPN/LVN would expect to administer which of the following medications?

    1. Chlordiazepoxide hydrochloride (Librium)
    2. Disulfiram (Antabuse)
    3. Methadone hydrochloride (Dolophine)
    4. Naloxone hydrochloride (Narcan)

43. An elderly client is admitted to a long-term care setting. The client is occasionally confused and her gait is often unsteady. Which of the following actions by the LPN/LVN is *MOST* appropriate?

    1. Ask the client's family to provide personal items such as photos or mementos.
    2. Select a room with a bed by the door so the client can look down the hall.
    3. Suggest the client eat her meals in the room with her roommate.
    4. Encourage the client to ambulate in the halls twice a day.

44. The LPN/LVN reinforces how to use a standard aluminum walker with an elderly client. Which of the following behaviors by the client indicates that the teaching was effective?

    1. The client slowly pushes the walker forward 12 inches, then takes small steps forward while leaning on the walker.
    2. The client lifts the walker, moves it forward 10 inches, and then takes several small steps forward.
    3. The client supports his weight on the walker while advancing it forward, then takes small steps while balancing on the walker.
    4. The client slides the walker 18 inches forward, then takes small steps while holding onto the walker for balance.

45. An LPN/LVN is providing care for a group of elderly clients in a residential home setting. The LPN/LVN knows that the elderly are at greater risk of developing sensory deprivation for which of the following reasons?

    1. Increased sensitivity to the side effects of medications
    2. Decreased visual, auditory, and gustatory abilities
    3. Isolation from their families and familiar surroundings
    4. Decreased musculoskeletal function and mobility

46. The LPN/LVN would expect which of the following clients to be able to sign a consent form for nonemergent medical treatment?

    1. A 10-year-old with a right tibia and fibula fracture
    2. A 21-year-old requiring surgery for acute appendicitis
    3. A 35-year-old who is confused after an automobile accident
    4. A 73-year-old who has been legally declared incompetent

47. An LPN/LVN is assisting with the discharge of a client with a diagnosis of hepatitis of unknown etiology. The LPN/LVN knows that teaching has been successful if the client makes which of the following statements?

    1. "I am so sad that I am not able to hold my baby."
    2. "I will eat after my family eats."
    3. "I will make sure that my children don't eat or drink from my dishware."

4. "I'm glad that I don't have to get help taking care of my children."

48. The LPN/LVN checks the IV flow rate for a postoperative client. The client is to receive 3,000 mL of Ringer's lactate solution IV to run over 24 hours. The IV infusion set has a drop factor of 10 drops per milliliter. The LPN/LVN would expect the client's IV to be running at how many drops per minute?

    1. 18
    2. 21
    3. 35
    4. 40

49. A client with emphysema becomes restless and confused. Which of the following actions should the LPN/LVN take next?

    1. Encourage the client to perform pursed-lip breathing.
    2. Check the client's temperature.
    3. Assess the client's potassium level.
    4. Increase the client's oxygen flow rate to 5 L/min.

50. The LPN/LVN cares for a client following surgery for removal of a cataract in the right eye. The client complains of severe eye pain in her right eye. Which of the following activities should the LPN/LVN do *FIRST*?

    1. Administer an analgesic to the client.
    2. Recheck the client in 30 minutes.
    3. Document the finding in the client's chart.
    4. Report the finding to the RN.

51. The LPN/LVN is caring for a client 4 hours after intracranial surgery. Which of the following actions should the LPN/LVN take immediately?

    1. Turn, cough, and deep-breathe the client.

2. Place the client with the neck flexed and head turned to the side.
3. Perform passive range-of-motion exercises.
4. Move client to the head of the bed using a turning sheet.

52. A 6-year-old child with a congenital heart disorder is admitted with congestive heart failure. Digoxin (Lanoxin) 0.12 mg is ordered for the child. The bottle of Lanoxin contains 0.05 mg of Lanoxin in 1 mL of solution. Which of the following amounts should the LPN/LVN administer to the child after validating the dose with the RN?

    1. 1.2 mL
    2. 2.4 mL
    3. 3.5 mL
    4. 4.2 mL

53. The LPN/LVN is caring for a client diagnosed with chronic lymphocytic leukemia, hospitalized for treatment of hemolytic anemia. The LPN/LVN should expect to implement which of the following actions?

    1. Encourage activities with other clients in the day room.
    2. Isolate the client from visitors.
    3. Provide a diet high in vitamin C.
    4. Maintain a quiet environment.

54. The LPN/LVN is caring for a client with cervical cancer. The LPN/LVN notes that the radium implant has become dislodged. Which of the following actions should the LPN/LVN take *FIRST*?

    1. Stay with the client and contact radiology.
    2. Wrap the implant in a blanket and place it behind a lead shield.

3. Pick up the implant with long-handled forceps and place it in a lead container.

4. Obtain a dosimeter reading on the client and report it to the physician.

55. The LPN/LVN comes to the home of a client with cellulitis of the left leg to perform a daily dressing change. The client tells the LPN/LVN that the nursing assistant changed the dressing earlier that morning. Which of the following actions by the LPN/LVN is *BEST*?

1. Tell the client that the nursing assistant did a good job with the dressing change.

2. Notify the RN supervisor of the situation.

3. Ask the client to describe the dressing change.

4. Report the nursing assistant to the home care agency.

56. The LPN/LVN is caring for a client with pernicious anemia. The LPN/LVN reinforces teaching about the plan of care. The LPN/LVN should report which of the following statements to the RN?

1. "In order to get better, I will need to take iron pills."

2. "I am going to attend smoking cessation classes."

3. "I will learn how to perform IM injections."

4. "I need to eat a balanced diet."

57. The LPN/LVN is caring for clients on a general medical/surgical unit of an acute care facility. Four clients have been admitted in the last 20 minutes. Which of the admissions should the LPN/LVN see *FIRST*?

1. A client complaining of vomiting and diarrhea

2. A client with third-degree burns to the face

3. A client with a fractured left hip

4. A client complaining of epigastric pain

58. The LPN/LVN is caring for a client with a diagnosis of COPD, bronchitis-type, in the long-term care facility. The client is wheezing, and his oxygen saturation is 85 percent. Four hours ago, the oxygen saturation was 88 percent. It is *MOST* important for the LPN/LVN to take which of the following actions?

1. Administer beclomethasone (Vanceril), 2 puffs per metered-dose inhaler.

2. Listen to breath sounds.

3. Increase oxygen to 4 L per mask.

4. Administer albuterol (Proventil), 2 puffs per metered-dose inhaler.

59. The LPN/LVN is caring for a client hospitalized for observation following a fall. The client states, "My friend fell last year, and no one thought anything was wrong. She died 2 days later!" Which of the following responses by the LPN/LVN is *BEST*?

1. "This happens to quite a few people."

2. "We are monitoring you, so you'll be okay."

3. "Don't you think I'm taking good care of you?"

4. "You're concerned that it might happen to you?"

60. The LPN/LVN is caring for clients on the pediatric unit. An 8-year-old client with second- and third-degree burns on the right thigh is being admitted. The LPN/LVN should expect the new client to be placed with which one of the following roommates?

1. A 2-year-old with chickenpox

2. A 4-year-old with asthma

3. A 9-year-old with acute diarrhea

4. A 10-year-old with methicillin-resistant *Staphylococcus aureus* (MRSA)

61. In order to evaluate the effectiveness of a client's heparin therapy, the LPN/LVN should monitor which of the following laboratory values?

1. Platelet count

2. Partial thromboplastin time

3. Bleeding time

4. Prothrombin time

62. The LPN/LVN is reinforcing teaching with a client who is scheduled for a paracentesis. Which of the following statements by the client indicates that teaching has been successful?

1. "I will be in surgery for less than 1 hour."

2. "I must not void prior to the procedure."

3. "The physician will remove 2–3 liters of fluid."

4. "I will lie on my back and breathe slowly."

63. The LPN/LVN is performing chest physiotherapy on an elderly client in long-term care with chronic airflow limitations (CAL). Which of the following actions should the nurse take *FIRST?*

1. Perform chest physiotherapy prior to meals.

2. Auscultate the chest prior to beginning the procedure.

3. Administer bronchodilators after the procedure.

4. Percuss each lobe prior to asking the client to cough.

64. In which of the following situations would it be *MOST* appropriate for the LPN/LVN to wear a protective gown and clean gloves?

1. Administering oral medications to a client with AIDS

2. Assisting in the care of a car-accident victim who is bleeding

3. Bathing a client with an abdominal wound infection

4. Changing the linen of a client with sickle-cell anemia

65. A client is receiving 1,000 mL of 5% dextrose in 0.45 NaCl intravenous solution in an 8-hour period. The intravenous set delivers 15 drops per milliliter. The LPN/LVN should expect the flow rate to be how many drops per minute?

1. 15

2. 31

3. 45

4. 60

66. A client is admitted to the hospital with complaints of seizures and a high fever. A brain scan is ordered. Before the scan, the client asks the LPN/LVN what position he will be in while the procedure is being done. Which of the following statements by the LPN/LVN is *MOST* accurate?

1. "You will be in a side-lying position, with the foot of the bed elevated."

2. "You will be in a semi-upright sitting position, with your knees flexed."

3. "You will be lying on your back with a small pillow under your head."

4. "You will be flat on your back, with your feet higher than your head."

67. A client with a diagnosis of delirium is admitted to the hospital. To evaluate the cause of the client's delirium, blood is sent to the laboratory for analysis. The results are as follows: Na^+ 156, Cl^- 100, K^+ 4.0, HCO_3 21, BUN 86, glucose 100. Based on these laboratory results, the LPN/LVN would expect to see which of the following nursing diagnoses on the client's care plan?

1. Alteration in patterns of urinary elimination
2. Fluid volume deficit
3. Nutritional deficit: less than body requirements
4. Self-care deficit: feeding

68. A client is to receive 3,000 mL of 0.9% NaCl IV in 24 hours. The intravenous set delivers 15 drops per milliliter. The LPN/LVN would expect the flow rate to be how many drops of fluid per minute?

1. 21
2. 28
3. 31
4. 42

69. The LPN/LVN cares for a client diagnosed with asthma. The physician orders neostigmine (Prostigmin) IM. Which of the following actions by the LPN/LVN is *MOST* appropriate?

1. Administer the medication.
2. Check the blood pressure and pulse.
3. Ask the pharmacy if the medication can be given orally.
4. Notify the physician.

70. The LPN/LVN cares for a client with a history of Addison's disease who has received steroid therapy for several years. The LPN/LVN would expect the client to exhibit which of the following changes in appearance?

1. Buffalo hump, girdle-obesity, gaunt facial appearance
2. Tanning of the skin, discoloration of the mucous membranes, alopecia, weight loss
3. Emaciation, nervousness, breast engorgement, hirsutism
4. Truncal obesity, purple striations on the skin, moon face

71. The LPN/LVN is caring for a client who is jaundiced due to pancreatic cancer. The LPN/LVN should give the *HIGHEST* priority to which of the following needs?

1. Nutrition
2. Self-image
3. Skin integrity
4. Urinary elimination

72. An 8-year-old boy is seen in a clinic for treatment of attention deficit hyperactivity disorder (ADHD). Medication has been prescribed for the child along with family counseling. The LPN/LVN reinforces the teaching plan about the medication and discusses parenting strategies with the parents. Which of the following statements by the parents indicates that further teaching is necessary?

1. "We will give the medication at night so it doesn't decrease his appetite."
2. "We will provide a regular routine for sleeping, eating, working, and playing."
3. "We will establish firm but reasonable limits on his behavior."
4. "We will reduce distractions and external stimuli to help him concentrate."

73. A teenage client is admitted to the hospital with anorexia nervosa. Which of the following statements by the client requires immediate follow-up by the LPN/LVN?

1. "My gums were bleeding this morning."

2. "I'm getting fatter every day."

3. "Nobody likes me because I'm so ugly."

4. "I'm feeling dizzy and weak today."

74. A client is admitted to the hospital for treatment of *Pneumocystis carinii* pneumonia and Kaposi sarcoma. The client tells the LPN/LVN that he has been considering organ donation when he dies. Which of the following responses by the LPN/LVN is *BEST*?

    1. "What does your family think about your decision?"

    2. "You will help many people by donating your organs."

    3. "Would you like to speak to the Organ Donor Representative?"

    4. "That is not possible based on your illness."

75. The LPN/LVN is caring for a client 2 days after a pancreatectomy for cancer of the pancreas. The LPN/LVN notes that there is minimal drainage from the nasogastric (NG) tube. It is *MOST* important for the LPN/LVN to take which of the following actions?

    1. Notify the physician.

    2. Monitor vital signs q 15 minutes.

    3. Check the tubing for kinks.

    4. Replace the NG tube.

76. The LPN/LVN plans to administer furosemide (Lasix) 20 mg PO to a client diagnosed with renal failure. The client asks the LPN/LVN why he is receiving this medication. Which of the following responses by the LPN/LVN is *BEST*?

    1. "To increase the blood flow to your kidney."

    2. "To decrease your circulating blood volume."

    3. "To increase excretion of sodium and water."

    4. "To decrease the workload on your heart."

77. The LPN/LVN is reinforcing discharge teaching for a client with Parkinson's disease. To maintain safety, the LPN/LVN should make which of the following suggestions to the family?

    1. Install a raised toilet seat.

    2. Obtain a hospital bed.

    3. Instruct the client to hold his arms in a dependent position when ambulating.

    4. Perform an exercise program during the late afternoon.

78. The LPN/LVN is reinforcing discharge teaching for a client with chronic pancreatitis. Which of the following statements by the client indicates that further teaching is necessary?

    1. "I do not have to restrict my physical activity."

    2. "I should take pancrelipase (Viokase) before meals."

    3. "I will eat 3 meals per day."

    4. "I am not allowed to drink any alcoholic beverages."

79. Following a laparoscopic cholecystectomy, the client complains of abdominal pain and bloating. Which of the following responses by the LPN/LVN is *BEST*?

    1. "Increase your intake of fresh fruits and vegetables."

    2. "I'll give you the prescribed pain medication."

    3. "Why don't you take a walk in the hallway?"

    4. "You may need an indwelling catheter."

80. The nursing team consists of an RN, a nursing assistant, and an LPN/LVN. The LPN/LVN would expect to be assigned to which of the following clients?

 1. A client scheduled for an MRI
 2. An unconscious client who requires a bed bath
 3. A client with a fracture who is in balanced suspension traction
 4. A client with diabetes who needs help bathing

81. The physician orders 1 liter of D5 1/2 NS to run over 8 hours. The drip factor stated on the IV tubing is 15 gtt/mL. How many milliliters should the LPN/LVN expect to be infused every hour?

 _____ 31.25 _____ mL

82. A client has a vagotomy with antrectomy to treat a duodenal ulcer. Postoperatively, the client develops dumping syndrome. Which of the following statements by the client indicates to the LPN/LVN that further dietary teaching is necessary?

 1. "I should eat bread with each meal."
 2. "I should eat smaller meals more frequently."
 3. "I should lie down after eating."
 4. "I should avoid drinking fluids with my meals."

83. The LPN/LVN reinforces discharge teaching with a client with emphysema. Which of the following statements by the client indicates that teaching was successful?

 1. "Cold weather will help my breathing problems."
 2. "I should eat 3 balanced meals but limit my fluid intake."

 3. "My outside activity should be limited when pollution levels are high."
 4. "An intensive exercise program is important in regaining my strength."

84. A client has been taking aluminum hydroxide (Amphojel) daily for 3 weeks. The LPN/LVN should be alert for which of the following side effects?

 1. Nausea
 2. Hypercalcemia
 3. Constipation
 4. Anorexia

85. The LPN/LVN hears a client calling for help. The LPN/LVN enters the room and finds an elderly client in bilateral wrist restraints with a cool, pale right hand with no palpable radial pulse. Which of the following would be the most appropriate action for the LPN/LVN to take *FIRST*?

 1. Leave to find the client's nurse.
 2. Massage the client's wrist and hand.
 3. Remove the right wrist restraint.
 4. Reposition the client to reduce pressure.

86. The LPN/LVN is reinforcing discharge teaching for a client with a new colostomy. The LPN/LVN knows teaching was successful when the client chooses which of the following menu options?

 1. Sausage, sauerkraut, baked potato, and fresh fruit
 2. Cheese omelet with bran muffin and fresh pineapple
 3. Pork chop, mashed potatoes, turnips, and salad
 4. Baked chicken, boiled potato, cooked carrots, and yogurt

87. A client is admitted to the unit to rule out acute renal failure. The LPN/LVN would be *MOST* concerned if the client made which of the following statements?

    1. "My urine is often pink-tinged."
    2. "It is hard for me to start the flow of urine."
    3. "It is quite painful for me to urinate."
    4. "I urinate in the morning and again before dinner."

88. The LPN/LVN is implementing the protocol for teaching a new mother how to breastfeed her newborn. The LPN/LVN knows that teaching has been successful if the client makes which of the following statements?

    1. "My baby's weight should equal her birthweight in 5–7 days."
    2. "My baby should have at least 6–8 wet diapers per day."
    3. "My baby will sleep at least 6 hours between feedings."
    4. "My baby will feed for about 10 minutes per feeding."

89. A client is admitted to the telemetry unit for evaluation of complaints of chest pain. Eight hours after admission, the client goes into ventricular fibrillation. The physician defibrillates the client. The LPN/LVN understands that the purpose of defibrillation is to do which of the following?

    1. Increase cardiac contractility and cardiac output.
    2. Cause asystole so the normal pacemaker can recapture.
    3. Reduce cardiac ischemia and acidosis.
    4. Provide energy for depleted myocardial cells.

90. The LPN/LVN is caring for a client who suddenly complains of chest pain. The LPN/LVN knows that which of the following symptoms would be *MOST* characteristic of an acute myocardial infarction?

    1. Colic-like epigastric pain
    2. Sharp, well-localized, unilateral chest pain
    3. Severe substernal pain radiating down the left arm
    4. Sharp, burning chest pain moving from place to place

91. The physician orders packing for a nonhealing open surgical wound. Which of the following is the *FIRST* action by the LPN/LVN?

    1. Identify wound size, shape, and depth.
    2. Observe for wound drainage or discharge.
    3. Plan to set up for clean technique.
    4. Select the proper dressing material.

92. A client returns to the clinic 2 weeks after discharge from the hospital. He is taking wafarin sodium (Coumadin) 2 mg PO daily. Which of the following statements by the client to the LPN/LVN indicates that further teaching is necessary?

    1. "I have been taking an antihistamine before bed."
    2. "I take aspirin when I have a headache."
    3. "I use sunscreen when I go outside."
    4. "I take Mylanta if my stomach gets upset."

93. To enhance the percutaneous absorption of nitroglycerine ointment, it would be *MOST* important for the LPN/LVN to select a site that is which of the following?

1. Muscular
2. Near the heart
3. Non-hairy
4. Over a bony prominence

94. When assisting the RN in planning care for a postoperative client, which of the following should be the *FIRST* choice of the LPN/LVN to reduce the client's risk for pooled airway secretions and decreased chest wall expansion?

    1. Chest percussion
    2. Incentive spirometry
    3. Position changes
    4. Postural drainage

95. Which of the following actions by the LPN/LVN would be *MOST* helpful in preventing injury to elderly clients in a healthcare facility?

    1. Closely monitor the temperature of hot oral fluids.
    2. Keep unnecessary furniture out of the way.
    3. Maintain the safe function of all electrical equipment.
    4. Use safety protection caps on all medications.

96. Which of the following statements by a client during a group therapy session requires immediate follow-up by the LPN/LVN?

    1. "I know I'm a chronically compulsive liar, but I can't help it."
    2. "I don't ever want to go home; I feel safer here."
    3. "I don't really care if I ever see my girlfriend again."
    4. "I'll make sure that doctor is sorry for what he said."

97. A client newly diagnosed with Alzheimer's disease is admitted to the unit. Which of the following actions by the LPN/LVN is *BEST?*

    1. Place the client in a private room away from the nurses' station.
    2. Ask the family to wait in the waiting room while the nurse admits the client.
    3. Assign a different nurse daily to care for the client.
    4. Ask the client to state today's date.

98. A female client visits the clinic with complaints of right calf tenderness and pain. It would be *MOST* important for the LPN/LVN to ask which of the following questions?

    1. "Do you exercise excessively?"
    2. "Have you had any fractures in the last year?"
    3. "What type of birth control do you use?"
    4. "Are you under a lot of stress?"

99. Which of the following should be the LPN/LVN's *FIRST* priority in providing care for a client who has terminal ovarian cancer and has been weakened by chemotherapy?

    1. Assess if the client is experiencing pain.
    2. Determine if the client is hungry or thirsty.
    3. Explore the client's feelings about dying.
    4. Observe the client's self-care abilities.

100. The LPN/LVN in the postpartum unit cares for a client who delivered her first child the previous day. The LPN/LVN notes multiple varicosities on the client's lower extremities. Which of the following actions should the LPN/LVN perform?

1. Teach the client to rest in bed when the baby sleeps.

2. Encourage early and frequent ambulation.

3. Apply warm soaks for 20 minutes every 4 hours.

4. Perform passive range-of-motion exercises 3 times daily.

101. The LPN/LVN cares for a client with a fracture of the left femur. A cast is applied. The nurse knows that which of the following exercises would be *MOST* beneficial for this client?

    1. Passive exercise of the affected limb

    2. Quadriceps setting of the affected limb

    3. Active range-of-motion exercises of the unaffected limb

    4. Passive exercise of the upper extremities

102. In preparation for a dressing change, the LPN/LVN puts on sterile gloves. Where should the LPN/LVN initially grip the first sterile glove?

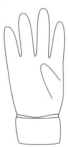

103. A client is being discharged from the hospital following a right total hip arthroplasty. The LPN/LVN reinforces discharge teaching. Which of the following statements by the client indicates that teaching was successful?

    1. "I can bend over to pick up something on the floor."

    2. "I should not cross my ankles when sitting in a chair."

3. "I need to lie on my stomach when sleeping in bed."

4. "I should spread my knees apart to put on my shoes."

104. The LPN/LVN cares for a client with continuous bladder irrigation. At 7 A.M., the LPN/LVN notes 4,200 mL of normal saline left in the irrigation bags. During the next shift (7 A.M. to 3 P.M.), the LPN/LVN hangs another 3,000 mL and empties a total of 5,625 mL from the urine drainage bag. At 3 P.M., there are 2,300 mL of irrigant left hanging. What is the actual urine output for the client from 7 A.M. to 3 P.M.?

    _____ mL

105. The LPN/LVN observes activities on a medical/surgical unit. The LPN/LVN should intervene if which of the following is observed?

    1. A client's wife disposes of her husband's used tissue in the bedside container before opening the roommate's milk carton.

    2. A nursing assistant removes her gloves and washes her hands for 15 seconds after emptying an indwelling urinary catheter.

    3. An LPN/LVN puts on a gown, gloves, mask, and goggles prior to inserting a nasogastric tube.

    4. A visitor talks with a client diagnosed with methicillin-resistant *Staphylococcus aureus* (MRSA) wound infection while he eats his lunch.

106. A client is admitted to the unit with complaints of nausea, vomiting, and abdominal pain. He is a type 1 diabetic (IDDM). Four days earlier, he reduced his insulin dose when flu symptoms prevented

him from eating. The LPN/LVN observes the client and finds poor skin turgor, dry mucous membranes, and fruity breath odor. The LPN/LVN should be alert for which of the following problems?

1. Hypoglycemia
2. Viral illness
3. Ketoacidosis
4. Hyperglycemic hyperosmolar nonketotic coma

107. The LPN/LVN knows that it is *MOST* important for which of the following clients to receive his scheduled medication on time?

1. A client diagnosed with myasthenia gravis receiving pyridostigmine bromide (Mestinon)
2. A client diagnosed with bipolar disorder receiving lithium carbonate (Lithobid)
3. A client diagnosed with tuberculosis receiving isonicotinic acid hydrazide (INH)
4. A client diagnosed with Parkinson's disease receiving levodopa (L-dopa)

108. An 11-year-old boy is admitted to the hospital for evaluation for a kidney transplant. The LPN/LVN learns that the client received hemodialysis for 3 years due to renal failure. The LPN/LVN knows that his illness can interfere with this client's achievement of which of the following?

1. Intimacy
2. Trust
3. Industry
4. Identity

109. The LPN/LVN notes that a 67-year-old client has an unsteady gait. The LPN/LVN should do which of the following? **Select all that apply.**

1. Apply a chest or vest restraint at night.
2. Help the client put on nonskid shoes for walking.
3. Keep the call light within the client's reach.
4. Lower the bed and raise all 4 side rails.
5. Provide adequate lighting.
6. Remove obstacles and room clutter.

110. Haloperidol (Haldol) 5 mg tid is ordered for a client with schizophrenia. Two days later, the client complains of "tight jaws and a stiff neck." The LPN/LVN should recognize that these complaints are which of the following?

1. Common side effects of antipsychotic medications that will diminish over time
2. Early symptoms of extrapyramidal reactions to the medication
3. Psychosomatic complaints resulting from a delusional system
4. Permanent side effects of Haldol

111. A client is receiving a continuous gastric tube feeding at 100 mL per hour. The LPN/LVN checks for feeding residual and finds 90 mL in the client's stomach. Which of the following actions should the LPN/LVN take?

1. Discard the residual and continue the tube feeding.
2. Discard the residual and stop the tube feeding.
3. Return the residual to the stomach and continue the tube feeding.
4. Return the residual to the stomach and stop the tube feeding.

112. The LPN/LVN opens several sterile 4 × 4s on the client's over-bed table. The LPN/LVN knows that the sterile dressings will be contaminated if she does which of the following?

    1. Does not allow the dressings prolonged exposure to the air.
    2. Keeps sterile 4 × 4s inside the border of the sterile packaging.
    3. Positions the top of the table at or above waist level.
    4. Pours sterile saline onto the opened sterile 4 × 4s on the table.

113. A client has adamantly refused all hygiene measures over the last 3 days. The LPN/LVN and the client are finally able to collaborate to achieve the hygiene goal of "self-administration of a complete bath once a day while in the hospital." To evaluate if this goal is met, the LPN/LVN should do which of the following?

    1. Ask the client if he has performed his daily bath.
    2. Bathe the client to be sure the hygiene goal is met.
    3. Observe the client performing portions of his daily bath.
    4. Remind the client to take his bath, providing the needed supplies.

114. The LPN/LVN is caring for a client in labor. The MD palpates a firm, round form in the uterine fundus, small parts on the woman's right side, and a long, smooth, curved section on the left side. Based on these findings, where should the LPN/LVN anticipate auscultating the fetal heart?

1. A
2. B
3. C
4. D

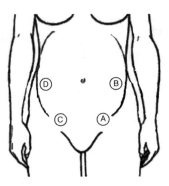

115. When completing data collection of an immobilized client, the LPN/LVN knows that he is most likely to observe edema in which of the following?

    1. Abdomen
    2. Feet and ankles
    3. Fingers and wrists
    4. Sacrum

116. A client is preparing to take her 1-day-old infant home from the hospital. The LPN/LVN discusses the test for phenylketonuria (PKU) with the mother. The LPN/LVN's teaching should be based on an understanding that the test is *MOST* reliable in which of the following circumstances?

    1. After a source of protein has been ingested
    2. After the meconium has been excreted
    3. After the danger of hyperbilirubinemia has passed
    4. After the effects of delivery have subsided

117. The LPN/LVN is caring for an Rh-negative mother who has delivered an Rh-positive child. The mother states, "The doctor told me about RhoGAM, but I'm still a little confused." Which of the following responses by the LPN/LVN is *MOST* appropriate?

1. "RhoGAM is given to your child to prevent the development of antibodies."

2. "RhoGAM is given to your child to supply the necessary antibodies."

3. "RhoGAM is given to you to prevent the formation of antibodies."

4. "RhoGAM is given to you to encourage the production of antibodies."

118. A woman is hospitalized with a diagnosis of bipolar disorder. While she is in the client activities room on the psychiatric unit, she flirts with male clients and disrupts unit activities. Which of the following approaches would be *MOST* appropriate for the LPN/LVN to take at this time?

1. Set limits on the client's behavior and remind her of the rules.

2. Distract the client and escort her back to her room.

3. Instruct the other clients to ignore this client's behavior.

4. Tell the client that she is behaving inappropriately and send her to her room.

119. A client is brought to the emergency room bleeding profusely from a stab wound in the left chest area. The client's vital signs are blood pressure 80/50, pulse 110, and respirations 28. The LPN/LVN should expect which of the following potential problems?

1. Hypovolemic shock

2. Cardiogenic shock

3. Neurogenic shock

4. Septic shock

120. A client is admitted to the hospital for surgical repair of a detached retina in the right eye. In implementing the plan of care for this client postoperatively, the LPN/LVN should encourage the client to do which of the following?

1. Perform self-care activities.

2. Maintain patches over both eyes.

3. Limit movement of both eyes.

4. Refrain from excessive talking.

121. The LPN/LVN cares for a client receiving a balanced complete food by tube feeding. The LPN/LVN knows that the *MOST* common complication of a tube feeding is which of the following?

1. Edema

2. Diarrhea

3. Hypokalemia

4. Vomiting

122. A 6-week-old infant is brought to the hospital for treatment of pyloric stenosis. The following nursing diagnosis is on the infant's care plan: "fluid volume deficit related to vomiting." The LPN/LVN would expect to see which of the following findings to support this diagnosis?

1. The infant eagerly accepts feedings.

2. The infant vomited once since admission.

3. The infant's skin is warm and moist.

4. The infant's anterior fontanel is depressed.

123. The LPN/LVN cares for a 4-year-old diagnosed with a fractured pelvis due to an auto accident. The LPN/LVN prepares the child for the application of a hip spica cast. It is *MOST* important for the LPN/LVN to take which of the following actions?

1. Obtain a doll with a hip spica cast in place.

2. Tell the child that the cast will feel cold when it is put on her skin.

3. Reassure the child that the cast application is painless.

4. Introduce the child to another child who has a hip spica cast.

124. A woman comes to the clinic because she thinks she is pregnant. Tests are performed and the pregnancy is confirmed. The client's last menstrual period began on September 8 and lasted for 6 days. The LPN/LVN calculates that her expected date of confinement (EDC) is which of the following?

1. May 15

2. June 15

3. June 21

4. July 8

125. A 2-month-old infant is brought to the pediatrician's office for a well-baby visit. During the examination, congenital subluxation of the left hip is suspected. The LPN/LVN would expect to see which of the following symptoms?

1. Lengthening of the limb on the affected side

2. Deformities of the foot and ankle

3. Asymmetry of the gluteal and thigh folds

4. Plantar flexion of the foot

126. After completing data collection, the LPN/LVN observes that a client is exhibiting early symptoms of a dystonic reaction related to the use of an antipsychotic medication. Which of the following actions by the LPN/LVN would be *MOST* appropriate?

1. Reality test with the client and assure her that her physical symptoms are not real.

2. Teach the client about common side effects of antipsychotic medications.

3. Explain to the client that there is no treatment that will relieve these symptoms.

4. Notify the physician and obtain an order for IM Benadryl.

127. The LPN/LVN is preparing to perform mouth care for an unconscious client. Which of the following actions should the LPN/LVN take *FIRST*?

1. Assess for the presence of a gag reflex.

2. Place the client into Sims' position.

3. Separate the teeth with a padded tongue blade.

4. Suction secretions from the oral cavity.

128. As a client nears death, the client's husband says, "I wish I could do something for her." Which of the following responses by the LPN/LVN is *MOST* appropriate?

1. "It may be comforting to your wife if you talk to her calmly and clearly."

2. "Your wife does not know that you are here, but you can sit here with her."

3. "Unfortunately, there is little that you can do at this point."

4. "Why don't you take a break? It is just a matter of time now."

129. The LPN/LVN provides care to clients in a long-term care facility. Four meal choices are available to the clients. The LPN/LVN should ensure that a client on a low-cholesterol diet receives which of the following meals?

1. Egg custard and boiled liver

2. Fried chicken and potatoes

3. Hamburger and french fries

4. Grilled flounder and green beans

130. The LPN/LVN removes a client's breakfast tray and notes that the client consumed 4 oz. of pudding, 4 oz. of gelatin, 6 1/2 oz. of tea, and 5 oz. of apple juice. How many milliliters should the LPN/LVN record for the client's breakfast intake?

_____ mL

131. The LPN/LVN cares for a client diagnosed with cholecystitis. The client says to the LPN/LVN, "I don't understand why my right shoulder hurts when the gallbladder is not by my shoulder!" Which of the following responses by the LPN/LVN is *BEST*?

1. "Sometimes small pieces of the gallstones break off and travel to other parts of the body."

2. "There is an invisible connection between the gallbladder and the right shoulder."

3. "The gallbladder is on the right side of the body and so is that shoulder."

4. "Your shoulder became tense because you were guarding against the gallbladder pain."

132. A woman comes to the clinic at 32 weeks' gestation. A diagnosis of pregnancy-induced hypertension (PIH) is made. The LPN/LVN reinforces teaching performed by the RN. Which of the following statements by the client indicates that further teaching is required?

1. "Lying in bed on my left side is likely to increase my urinary output."

2. "If the bed rest works, I may lose a pound or two in the next few days."

3. "I should be sure to maintain a diet that has a good amount of protein."

4. "I will have to keep my room darkened and not watch much television."

133. The LPN/LVN collects data about a client's fluid balance. Which of the following findings *MOST* accurately indicates to the LPN/LVN that the client has retained fluid during the previous 24 hours?

1. Edema is found in both ankles.

2. Fluid intake is equal to fluid output.

3. Intake of fluid exceeds output by 200 mL.

4. Weight gain of 4 pounds is noted.

134. The LPN/LVN cares for a group of residents in a dependent-living facility. The LPN/LVN determines which of the following clients is *MOST* at risk to develop pneumonia?

1. A 72-year-old female with left-sided hemiparesis after a cerebrovascular accident.

2. A 76-year-old male with a history of hypertension and type 2 diabetes.

3. An 80-year-old female who walks 1 mile every day and has a history of depression.

4. An 87-year-old male who smokes and has a history of lung cancer.

135. The LPN/LVN is caring for a client diagnosed with bipolar disorder. Which of the following behaviors by the client indicates that a manic episode is subsiding?

1. The client tells several jokes at a group meeting.

2. The client sits and talks with other clients at mealtimes.

3. The client begins to write a book about his life.

4. The client initiates an effort to start a radio station on the unit.

136. A mother brings her 4-year-old daughter to the pediatrician for treatment of chronic otitis media. The mother asks the LPN/LVN how she can prevent her child from getting ear infections so often. The LPN/LVN's response should be based on an understanding that the recurrence of otitis media can be decreased by which of the following?

1. Cover the child's ears while bathing.

2. Treat upper respiratory infections quickly.

3. Administer nose drops at bedtime.

4. Isolate her child from other children.

137. A man calls the Suicide Prevention Hotline and states that he is going to kill himself. Which of the following questions should the LPN/LVN ask FIRST?

1. "What happened to cause you to want to end your life?"

2. "How do you plan to kill yourself?"

3. "When did you start to feel as though you wanted to die?"

4. "Do you want me to prevent you from killing yourself?"

138. Prior to the client undergoing a scheduled intravenous pyelogram (IVP), it would be MOST important for the LPN/LVN to ask which of the following questions?

1. "Do you have difficulty voiding?"

2. "Do you have any allergies to shellfish or iodine?"

3. "Do you have a history of constipation?"

4. "Do you have frequent headaches?"

139. The LPN/LVN is assigned to a newly admitted elderly client in the hospital setting who states that she has no living relatives and only friends of her own age. One of the LPN/LVN's most immediate considerations for this client will be to help the RN implement which of the following?

1. A concept map

2. A critical pathway

3. A discharge plan

4. A utilization group

140. A woman delivers a 6 lb., 10 oz. baby girl. The mother observes the LPN/LVN in the delivery room place drops in her daughter's eyes. The mother asks the LPN/LVN why this was done. Which of the following responses by the LPN/LVN is BEST?

1. "The drops constrict your baby's pupils to prevent injury."

2. "The drops will remove mucus from your baby's eyes."

3. "The drops will prevent infections that might cause blindness."

4. "The drops will prevent neonatal conjunctivitis."

141. The LPN/LVN cares for a client admitted for a possible herniated intervertebral disk. Ibuprofen (Motrin), propoxyphene hydrochloride (Darvon), and cyclobenzaprine hydrochloride (Flexeril) are ordered PRN. Several hours after admission, the client complains of pain. Which of the following actions should the LPN/LVN take FIRST?

1. Administer Motrin.

2. Call the physician to determine which medication should be given.

3. Gather more information from the client about the complaint.

4. Allow the client some time to rest to see if the pain subsides.

142. The LPN/LVN is completing a client's preoperative checklist prior to an early morning surgery. The LPN/LVN obtains the client's vital signs: temperature 97.4° F (36° C), radial pulse 84 strong and regular, respirations 16 and unlabored, and blood pressure 132/74. Which of the following actions should the LPN/LVN take *FIRST*?

   1. Notify the physician of the client's vital signs.
   2. Obtain orthostatic blood pressures lying and standing.
   3. Lower the side rails and place the bed in its lowest position.
   4. Record the data on the client's preoperative checklist.

143. The LPN/LVN expects to see which of the following physiological changes in a client experiencing an episode of acute pain?

   1. Decreased blood pressure
   2. Decreased heart rate
   3. Decreased skin temperature
   4. Decreased respirations

144. A client is transferred to an extended-care facility following a cerebrovascular accident (CVA). The client has right-sided paralysis and has been experiencing dysphagia. The LPN/LVN observes an aide preparing the client to eat lunch. Which of the following situations would require an intervention by the LPN/LVN?

1. The client is in bed in high Fowler's position.
2. The client's head and neck are positioned slightly forward.
3. The aide puts the food in the back of the client's mouth on the unaffected side.
4. The aide waters down the pudding to help the client swallow.

145. During the LPN/LVN's morning data collection, a client's blood pressure is 146/92 with labored respirations of 24. There is red drainage on the client's IV dressing, and the client complains of pain in the left hip, depression, and hunger. The LPN/LVN identifies which of the following as subjective data? **Select all that apply.**

   1. Blood pressure
   2. Depression
   3. Hip pain
   4. Hunger
   5. IV drainage
   6. Respirations

YOUR PRACTICE TEST SCORES

The test included in this book is designed to provide practice answering exam-style questions along with a review of nursing content. Your results on this test indicate where you are NOW. It is NOT designed to predict your ability to pass the NCLEX-PN® exam.

- If you scored 70% or better, you have a good understanding of essential nursing content and you are able to utilize the critical thinking skills required to answer exam-style questions.
- If you scored 60 to 69%, you have areas of essential nursing content that need further review, or you may need continued work to master the critical thinking skills needed to correctly answer exam-style questions.
- If you scored 59% or less, you need concentrated study of nursing content and continued practice utilizing the critical thinking skills required to be successful on the NCLEX-PN® exam.

If you are looking for additional preparation materials for the NCLEX-PN® exam, Kaplan's NCLEX-PN® Question Bank provides access to 1,000 practice questions. See the instructions in this book for how to sample the Question Bank for free. This resource is designed to develop both your knowledge of the nursing content as well as your critical thinking skills. Learn more at: *kaplannursing.com* or call 213-452-5700 (in Canada call 800-533-8850).

ANSWER KEY

1.	**3**	38.	**3**	75.	**3**	111.	**4**
2.	**1**	39.	**3**	76.	**3**	112.	**4**
3.	**4**	40.	**2**	77.	**1**	113.	**3**
4.	**2**	41.	**3**	78.	**3**	114.	**See explanation**
5.	**1**	42.	**1**	79.	**3**		
6.	**1**	43.	**1**	80.	**3**	115.	**4**
7.	**3**	44.	**2**	81.	**125**	116.	**1**
8.	**2**	45.	**2**	82.	**1**	117.	**3**
9.	**2**	46.	**2**	83.	**3**	118.	**2**
10.	**1**	47.	**3**	84.	**3**	119.	**1**
11.	**3**	48.	**2**	85.	**3**	120.	**3**
12.	**2**	49.	**1**	86.	**4**	121.	**2**
13.	**4**	50.	**4**	87.	**4**	122.	**4**
14.	**3**	51.	**4**	88.	**2**	123.	**1**
15.	**2**	52.	**2**	89.	**2**	124.	**2**
16.	**4**	53.	**4**	90.	**3**	125.	**3**
17.	**2**	54.	**3**	91.	**1**	126.	**4**
18.	**2**	55.	**2**	92.	**2**	127.	**1**
19.	**2**	56.	**1**	93.	**3**	128.	**1**
20.	**4**	57.	**2**	94.	**3**	129.	**4**
21.	**3**	58.	**4**	95.	**2**	130.	**465**
22.	**3**	59.	**4**	96.	**4**	131.	**2**
23.	**2**	60.	**2**	97.	**4**	132.	**4**
24.	**3**	61.	**2**	98.	**3**	133.	**4**
25.	**2**	62.	**3**	99.	**1**	134.	**4**
26.	**4**	63.	**2**	100.	**2**	135.	**2**
27.	**1**	64.	**2**	101.	**2**	136.	**2**
28.	**1**	65.	**2**	102.	**See explanation**	137.	**2**
29.	**4**	66.	**3**			138.	**2**
30.	**1**	67.	**2**	103.	**2**	139.	**3**
31.	**3**	68.	**3**	104.	**725**	140.	**3**
32.	**4**	69.	**4**	105.	**1**	141.	**3**
33.	**3**	70.	**4**	106.	**3**	142.	**4**
34.	**3**	71.	**1**	107.	**1**	143.	**3**
35.	**4**	72.	**1**	108.	**3**	144.	**4**
36.	**2**	73.	**4**	109.	**2, 3, 5, 6**	145.	**2, 3, 4**
37.	**1**	74.	**4**	110.	**2**		

PRACTICE TEST ANSWERS AND EXPLANATIONS

1. The Answer is 3

The LPN/LVN is gathering data from a client who is being treated for obsessive-compulsive disorder. Which of the following is the *MOST* important question the LPN/LVN should ask this client?

Reworded Question: What are the signs and symptoms of obsessive-compulsive disorder?

Strategy: "*MOST* important" indicates there may be more than one correct response.

Needed Info: Obsessive-compulsive disorder is characterized by a history of obsessions and compulsions. Obsessions are recurrent and persistent thoughts, ideas, impulses, or images that are experienced as intrusive and senseless. The client knows that the thoughts are ridiculous or morbid but cannot stop, forget, or control them. Compulsions are repetitive behaviors performed in a certain way to prevent discomfort and neutralize anxiety.

Category: Data Collection/Psychosocial Integrity

(1) "Do you find yourself forgetting simple things?"—should be used to assess client with suspected cognitive disorder

(2) "Do you find it hard to stay on a task?"—assesses for disorders that disrupt the ability to concentrate, such as depression

(3) "Do you have trouble controlling upsetting thoughts?"—CORRECT: one feature of obsessive-compulsive disorder is the client's inability to control intrusive thoughts that repeat over and over

(4) "Do you experience feelings of panic in a closed area?"—appropriate for client with suspected panic disorder related to closed spaces or claustrophobia

2. The Answer is 1

The LPN/LVN is caring for a client who states, "I just want to die." The LPN/LVN should examine the client's medical record for which of the following documents?

Reworded Question: What data does the LPN/LVN need to know?

Strategy: Determine the document that would address a client's choice to die.

Needed Info: Advance directives: specific instructions by the client that are legally binding. Clients with advance directives must provide them in written form to the healthcare provider. Advance directives include: "do not resuscitate," living will, durable power of attorney/healthcare surrogate.

Category: Data Collection/Safe and Effective Care Environment/Coordinated Care

(1) Advance directives—CORRECT: advance directives specify the client's wishes regarding healthcare decisions

(2) Power of attorney—surrogate or proxy if the client is incompetent

(3) "Do not resuscitate order"—only one part of advance directives

(4) Living will—only one part of advance directives

3. The Answer is 4

A newly admitted client with a history of convulsions suddenly says to the LPN/LVN, "I hear drums." Which of the following should the LPN/LVN do *FIRST*?

Reworded Question: What does a sudden visual, olfactory, or auditory sensation often signal in a client with a history of convulsions?

Strategy: Quickly review the most likely causes of the client's unusual perception.

Needed Info: Aura: brief sensory alteration often preceding seizure or migraine, likely for client with history of convulsions. Petit mal seizures: usually occur in children, not associated with an aura. Grand mal seizures: involve loss of consciousness and convulsions.

Category: Evaluation/Physiological Integrity/Physiological Adaptation

(1) Tell the client to ignore the drums—client is experiencing an auditory sensation that may signal the start of a convulsion

(2) Place the client in a darkened room away from the nurses' station—needs continued observation

(3) Continue to question the client—many adults experience unusual sensory perceptions (an aura) before the onset of a seizure; this client has a history of seizures

(4) Insert an oral airway in the client—CORRECT: airway prevents client from biting cheek or tongue during a seizure

---

4. The Answer is 2

A client diagnosed with multiple myeloma is admitted to the unit after developing pneumonia. When the LPN/LVN enters the client's room wearing a mask, the client says in an irritated tone of voice, "Why are you wearing that mask?" Which of the following responses by the LPN/LVN is *BEST*?

Reworded Question: What is the most therapeutic response?

Strategy: Remember therapeutic communication.

Needed Info: Multiple myeloma: a neoplastic disease that infiltrates bone and bone marrow, causes anemia, renal lesions, and high globulin levels in blood; pneumonia is inflammatory process resulting in edema of lung tissue and extravasation of fluid into alveoli, causing hypoxia.

Category: Data Collection/Safe and Effective Care Environment/Safety and Infection Control

(1) "The chest X-ray taken this morning indicates you have pneumonia."—does not assess what

client knows; physician responsible for telling client the medical diagnosis

(2) "What have you been told about the X-rays that were taken this morning?"—CORRECT: data collection; determines what client knows before responding; allows client to verbalize

(3) "You have been placed on contact precautions due to your infection."—pneumonia requires droplet precautions

(4) "I am trying to protect you from the germs in the hospital."—pneumonia requires droplet precautions

---

5. The Answer is 1

A nursing team consists of an RN, an LPN/LVN, and a nursing assistant. The LPN/LVN should be assigned to which of the following clients?

Reworded Question: Which client is an appropriate assignment for the LPN/LVN?

Strategy: Think about the skill level involved in each client's care.

Needed Info: LPN/LVN: assists with implementation of care; performs procedures; differentiates normal from abnormal; cares for stable clients with predictable conditions; has knowledge of asepsis and dressing changes; administers medications (varies with educational background and state nurse practice act).

Category: Planning/Safe and Effective Care Environment/Coordinated Care

(1) A 72-year-old client with diabetes who requires a dressing change for a stasis ulcer—CORRECT: stable client with an expected outcome

(2) A 42-year-old client who has cancer of the bone and is complaining of pain—requires assessment; RN is the appropriate caregiver

(3) A 55-year-old client with terminal cancer who is being transferred to hospice home care—requires nursing judgment; RN is the appropriate caregiver

(4) A 23-year-old client who has a fracture of the right leg and asks to use the urinal—standard unchanging procedure; would be assigned to the nursing assistant

6. The Answer is 1

To determine the structural relationship of one hospital department with another, the LPN/LVN should consult which of the following?

Reworded Question: How does the LPN/LVN determine the relationship of one hospital department to another?

Strategy: Think about each answer.

Needed Info: The lateral lines on an organizational chart define the division and specializations of labor; the vertical lines explain the lines of authority and responsibility.

Category: Implementation/Safe and Effective Care/Coordinated Care

(1) Organizational chart—CORRECT: delineates the overall organization structure, showing which departments exist and their relationships with one another both laterally and vertically

(2) Job descriptions—focus is not on departmental relationships

(3) Personnel policies—defines policies for the organization's employees

(4) Policies and Procedures Manual—defines standards of care for an institution

7. The Answer is 3

A client complains of pain in his right lower extremity. The physician orders codeine 60 mg and aspirin grains X PO every 4 hours, as needed for pain. Each codeine tablet contains 15 mg of codeine. Each aspirin tablet contains 325 mg of aspirin. Which of the following should the LPN/LVN administer?

Reworded Question: What amount of medication should you give?

Strategy: Remember how to calculate dosages.

Needed Info: 60 mg = 1 grain.

Category: Implementation/Physiological Integrity/Pharmacological Therapies

(1) 2 codeine tablets and 4 aspirin tablets—inaccurate

(2) 4 codeine tablets and 3 aspirin tablets—inaccurate

(3) 4 codeine tablets and 2 aspirin tablets—CORRECT: $60/x = 15/1$, $x = 4$; 10 grains = 600 mg; $325/1 = 600/x$, $x = 1.8$ (round to 2)

(4) 3 codeine tablets and 3 aspirin tablets—inaccurate

8. The Answer is 2

The LPN/LVN cares for a client receiving paroxetine (Paxil). It is *MOST* important for the LPN/LVN to report which of the following to the physician?

Reworded Question: What is a potential drug interaction?

Strategy: "*MOST* important" indicates priority.

Needed Info: Paxil is a selective serotonin reuptake inhibitor (SSRI) used to treat depression, panic disorder, obsessive-compulsive disorder; side effects include palpitations, bradycardia, nausea and vomiting, and decreased appetite.

Category: Evaluation/Physiological Integrity/Pharmacological Therapies

(1) The client states there is no change in her appetite—causes anorexia; monitor weight and nutritional intake; report continued weight loss

(2) The client states she has started taking digoxin (Lanoxin)—CORRECT: may decrease effectiveness of digoxin

(3) The client states she applies sunscreen before going outside—appropriate action; prevents photosensitivity reactions

(4) The client states she drives her car to work—driving is acceptable after determining client's response to drug

9. The Answer is 2

A client with a DNR (do not resuscitate) physician's order experiences a cardiac arrest. Which of the following is the *FIRST* action the LPN/LVN should take?

Reworded Question: What actions are appropriate for a client with a DNR order who has no heartbeat?

Strategy: Determine which actions meet DNR standards.

Needed Info: DNR requires a written physician's order in the medical record, no extraordinary care given in the event of the client's death. Extraordinary care after cardiac or pulmonary cessation: cardiopulmonary resuscitation (CPR), medications, ventilators, defibrillation.

Category: Data Collection/Safe and Effective Care Environment/Coordinated Care

(1) Administer lifesaving medications—DNR means these medications are not given

(2) Assess the client for signs of death—CORRECT: client has signs of death and requires further assessment to confirm that the client is indeed dead

(3) Open the airway and give 2 breaths—CPR should not be initiated for clients with DNR orders

(4) Summon the emergency code team—CPR should not be initiated for clients with DNR orders

---

10. The Answer is 1

An LPN/LVN is working in the newborn nursery. Which of the following client-care assignments should the LPN/LVN question?

Reworded Question: Which infant is outside the scope of practice for an LPN/LVN?

Strategy: Remember the ABCs (airway, breathing, circulation).

Needed Info: Need to meet client's needs. Physical stability of client is LPN/LVN's first concern. Most unstable client should be cared for by RN.

Category: Evaluation/Safe and Effective Care Environment/Coordinated Care

(1) A 2-day-old infant lying quietly alert with a heart rate of 185—CORRECT: infant has tachycardia; normal resting rate is 120–160; requires further investigation

(2) A 1-day-old infant crying with the anterior fontanel bulging—crying causes increased intracranial pressure, which causes fontanel to bulge

(3) A 12-hour-old infant being held; respirations 45 breaths per minute and irregular—normal

respiratory rate is 30–60 breaths per minute with apneic episodes

(4) A 5-hour-old infant sleeping with hands and feet blue bilaterally—acrocyanosis is normal for 2–6 hours postdelivery due to poor peripheral circulation

---

11. The Answer is 3

While inserting a nasogastric tube, the LPN/LVN should use which of the following protective measures?s

Reworded Question: What is the correct standard precaution?

Strategy: Think about each answer choice. How is each measure protecting the LPN/LVN?

Needed Info: Mask, eye protection, face shield protect mucous membrane exposure; used if activities are likely to generate splash or sprays. Gowns used if activities are likely to generate splashes or sprays.

Category: Planning/Safe and Effective Care Environment/Safety and Infection Control

(1) Gloves, gown, goggles, and surgical cap—surgical caps offer protection to hair but aren't required

(2) Sterile gloves, mask, plastic bags, and gown—plastic bags provide no direct protection and aren't part of standard precautions

(3) Gloves, gown, mask, and goggles—CORRECT: must use standard precautions on all clients; prevent skin and mucous membrane exposure when contact with blood or other body fluids is anticipated

(4) Double gloves, goggles, mask, and surgical cap—surgical cap not required; unnecessary to double glove

---

12. The Answer is 2

The LPN/LVN is caring for clients in the outpatient clinic. Which of the following clients should the LPN/LVN see *FIRST*?

Reworded Question: Which client should the LPN/LVN see first?

Strategy: Think ABCs.

Needed Info: Need to meet client's needs. Physical stability is LPN/LVN's first concern. Client with most serious problem should be seen first.

Category: Planning/Safe and Effective Care Environment/Coordinated Care

(1) A client with hepatitis A who states, "My arms and legs are itching."—caused by accumulation of bile salts under the skin; treat with calamine lotion and antihistamines

(2) A client with a cast on the right leg who states, "I have a funny feeling in my right leg."—CORRECT: may indicate neurovascular compromise; requires immediate data collection

(3) A client with osteomyelitis of the spine who states, "I am so nauseous that I can't eat."—requires follow-up, but not highest priority

(4) A client with rheumatoid arthritis who states, "I am having trouble sleeping."—requires data collection, but not a priority

13. The Answer is 4

Which of the following client assignments should an LPN/LVN question?

Reworded Question: Which client is an inappropriate assignment for an LPN/LVN?

Strategy: Think about the skill level involved in each client's care.

Needed Info: Determine nursing care required to meet clients' needs; take into account time required, complexity of activities, acuity of client, infection control issues. Consider knowledge and abilities of staff members and decide which staff person is best able to provide care.

Category: Planning/Safe and Effective Care Environment/Coordinated Care

(1) A client with a chest tube who is ambulating in the hall—LPN/LVN can care for client

(2) A client with a colostomy who requires assistance with a colostomy irrigation—LPN/LVN can care for client

(3) A client with a right-sided cerebrovascular accident (CVA) who requires assistance with bathing—LPN/LVN can care for client

(4) A client who is refusing medication to treat cancer of the colon—CORRECT: requires the assessment skills of the RN

14. The Answer is 3

The LPN/LVN is caring for a client with hepatitis B. The client is to be discharged the next day. The LPN/LVN would be *MOST* concerned if the client made which of the following statements?

Reworded Question: What is an incorrect statement about care with hepatitis B?

Strategy: "*MOST* concerned" indicates you are looking for an incorrect statement.

Needed Info: Hepatitis A (HAV): high risk groups include young children, institutions for custodial care, international travelers; fecal/oral transmission, poor sanitation; nursing considerations include prevention, improved sanitation, treat with gammaglobulin early post-exposure, no preparation of food. Hepatitis B (HBV): high risk groups include drug addicts, fetuses from infected mothers, homosexually active men, transfusions, healthcare workers; transmission by parenteral, sexual contact, blood/body fluids; nursing considerations include vaccine (Heptavax-B, Recombivax HB), immune globulin (HBLg) postexposure, chronic carriers (potential for chronicity 5–10%). Hepatitis C (HVC): high risk groups include transfusions, international travelers; transmission by blood/body fluids; nursing considerations include great potential for chronicity. Delta hepatitis: high risk groups same as for HBV; transmission coinfects with HBV, close personal contact.

Category: Evaluation/Safe and Effective Care Environment/Coordinated Care

(1) "I must not share eating utensils with my family."—prevents transmission; handwashing before eating and after toileting very important

(2) "I must use my own bath towel."—prevents transmission; don't share bed linens

(3) "I'm glad that my husband and I can continue to have intimate relations."—CORRECT: avoid sexual contact until serologic indicators return to normal

(4) "I must eat small, frequent feedings."—easier to tolerate than three standard meals; diet should be high in carbohydrates and calories

15. The Answer is 2

The LPN/LVN carries out the plan for care of a client with anemia who is complaining of weakness. Which of the following tasks could be assigned to the nursing assistant?

Reworded Question: What is an appropriate assignment for the nursing assistant?

Strategy: Think about the skill level involved in each task.

Needed Info: Unlicensed assistive personnel (UAPs): assist with direct client care activities (bathing, transferring, ambulating, feeding, toileting, obtaining vital signs/height/weight/intake/output, housekeeping, transporting, stocking supplies); includes nurse aides, assistants, technicians, orderlies, nurse extenders; scope of nursing practice is limited.

Category: Evaluation/Safe and Effective Care Environment/Coordinated Care

(1) Listen to the client's breath sounds—requires head-to-toe assessment; could be performed by LPN/LVN and reported to RN

(2) Set up the client's lunch tray—CORRECT: standard, unchanging procedure; decreases cardiac workload

(3) Obtain a diet history—involves data collection; could be performed by LPN/LVN and reported to RN

(4) Instruct the client on how to balance rest and activity—teaching required; could be performed by LPN/LVN following established plan of care

16. The Answer is 4

The LPN/LVN is caring for clients on the surgical floor and has just received report from the RN. Which of the following clients should the LPN/LVN see *FIRST*?

Reworded Question: Which client is the least stable?

Strategy: Think ABCs.

Needed Info: Need to meet the client's needs. Physical stability is the LPN/LVN's first concern. Most unstable client should be seen first.

Category: Planning/Safe and Effective Care Environment/Coordinated Care

(1) A 35-year-old admitted 3 days ago with a gunshot wound; 1.5-cm area of dark drainage noted on the dressing—does not indicate acute bleeding; small amount of blood

(2) A 43-year-old who had a mastectomy 2 days ago; 23 mL of serosanguinous fluid noted in the Jackson-Pratt drain—expected outcome

(3) A 59-year-old with a collapsed lung due to an accident; no drainage noted in the previous 8 hours—indicates resolution

(4) A 62-year-old who had an abdominal-perineal resection 3 days ago; client complains of chills—CORRECT: at risk for peritonitis; should be assessed by the RN for further symptoms of infection

17. The Answer is 2

A client scheduled for a cardiac catheterization says to the LPN/LVN, "I know you were in here when the doctor had me sign the consent form for the test. I thought I understood everything, but now I'm not so sure." Which of the following responses by the LPN/LVN is *BEST*?

Reworded Question: Which response is most therapeutic?

Strategy: "*BEST*" indicates that discrimination is required to answer the question.

Needed Info: Informed consent is obtained by the individual who will perform the test; explanation of the test and expected results, anticipated risks and discomforts, potential benefits, possible alternatives are discussed; consent can be withdrawn at any time.

Category: Evaluation/Safe and Effective Care Environment/Coordinated Care

(1) "Why didn't you listen more closely?"—"why" questions are nontherapeutic; does not respond to the client's feelings or concerns

(2) "You sound as if you would like to ask more questions."—CORRECT: directly responds

to client's statement by paraphrasing; implies encouragement of expression of client's concern

(3) "I'll get you a pamphlet about cardiac catheterization."—may be helpful, but first the nurse needs to clarify the client's concerns by discussion

(4) "That often happens when this procedure is explained to clients."—does convey acceptance and lets the client know that his response is not abnormal; response is closed and does not allow client to express feelings or concerns

18. The Answer is 2

A 1-day-old newborn diagnosed with intrauterine growth retardation is observed by the LPN/LVN to be restless, irritable, and fist-sucking, and has a high-pitched, shrill cry. Based on this data, which of the following actions should the LPN/LVN take *FIRST*?

Reworded Question: What do you do for a newborn experiencing withdrawal?

Strategy: Determine the outcome of each answer.

Needed Info: Drug withdrawal may manifest from as early as 12 hours after birth up to 10 days after delivery. Symptoms: high-pitched cry, hyperreflexia, decreased sleep, diaphoresis, tachypnea, excessive mucus, vomiting, uncoordinated sucking. Nursing care: assess muscle tone, irritability, vital signs; administer phenobarbital as ordered; report symptoms of respiratory distress; reduce stimulation; provide adequate nutrition/fluids; monitor mother/child interactions.

Category: Implementation/Health Promotion and Maintenance

(1) Massage the infant's back—may result in overstimulation of the infant

(2) Tightly swaddle the infant in a flexed position—CORRECT: promotes infant's comfort and security

(3) Schedule feeding times every 3–4 hours—small, frequent feedings are preferable

(4) Encourage eye contact with the infant during feedings—may result in overstimulation of infant

19. The Answer is 2

The LPN/LVN visits a neighbor who is at 20 weeks' gestation. The neighbor complains of nausea, headache, and blurred vision. The LPN/LVN notes that the neighbor appears nervous, is diaphoretic, and is experiencing tremors. It would be *MOST* important for the LPN/LVN to ask which of the following questions?

Reworded Question: What is the priority data collection question?

Strategy: "*MOST* important" indicates there may be more than one correct response.

Needed Info: Data collection: irritability, confusion, tremors, blurring of vision, coma, seizures, hypotension, tachycardia, skin cool and clammy, diaphoresis. Plan/implementation: liquids containing sugar if conscious, skim milk is ideal if tolerated; dextrose 50% IV if unconscious, glucagon; follow with additional carbohydrate in 15 minutes; determine and treat cause; client education; exercise regimen.

Category: Data Collection/Health Promotion and Maintenance

(1) "Are you having menstrual-like cramps?"—symptoms of preterm labor

(2) "When did you last eat or drink?"—CORRECT: classic symptoms of hypoglycemia; offer carbohydrate

(3) "Have you been diagnosed with diabetes?"—need to determine if she is hypoglycemic

(4) "Have you been lying on the couch?"—not relevant to hypoglycemia

20. The Answer is 4

The LPN/LVN notes that a child newly admitted to the pediatric unit is scratching her head almost constantly. It would be *MOST* important for the LPN/LVN to take which of the following actions?

Reworded Question: What might head scratching indicate?

Strategy: Determine if data collection or implementation is appropriate.

Needed Info: Pediculosis (lice). Data collection: scalp—white eggs (nits) on hair shafts, itchy; body—macules and papules; pubis—red macules.

Category: Data Collection/Health Promotion and Maintenance

(1) Discuss basic hygiene with the parents—makes an assumption; must collect data first

(2) Instruct the child not to sleep with her dog—must first collect data to determine the problem

(3) Inform the parents that they must contact an exterminator—not enough information to make this determination

(4) Observe the scalp for small white specks—CORRECT: nits (eggs) appear as small, white, oval flakes attached to hair shaft

21. The Answer is 3

A suicidal client who was admitted to the psychiatric unit for treatment and observation a week ago suddenly appears cheerful and motivated. The LPN/LVN should be aware of which of the following?

Reworded Question: What is the significance of sudden mood changes in a depressed client?

Strategy: Know the signs of impending suicide.

Needed Info: Data collection for suicidal ideation, suicidal gestures, suicidal threats, and actual suicidal attempt. Clients who have developed a suicide plan are more serious about following through, and are at grave risk. Clients emerging from severe depression have more energy with which to formulate and carry out a suicide plan (for which they had no energy before treatment). The LPN/LVN should determine risk for suicide; suspect suicidal ideation in depressed client; ask the client if he is thinking about suicide; ask the client about the advantages and disadvantages of suicide to determine how client sees his situation; evaluate client's access to a method of suicide; develop a formal "no suicide" contract with client; and support the client's reason to live.

Category: Planning/Psychosocial Integrity

(1) The client is probably sleeping well because of the medication—improved sleep patterns would not explain the client's sudden mood change

(2) The client has made new friends and has a support group—support on the nursing unit would not explain the mood change

(3) The client may have finalized a suicide plan—CORRECT: as depressed clients improve, their risk for suicide is greater because they are able to mobilize more energy to plan and execute suicide

(4) The client is responding to treatment and is no longer depressed—sudden cheerful and energetic mood does not indicate resolution of depression

22. The Answer is 3

The LPN/LVN is caring for clients in the GYN clinic. A client complains of an off-white vaginal discharge with a curdlike appearance and vulvar itching. It would be *MOST* important for the LPN/LVN to ask which of the following questions?

Reworded Question: What is a predisposing factor to developing candidiasis?

Strategy: "*MOST* important" indicates there may be more than one correct response.

Needed Info: Candida albicans. Symptoms: odorless, cheesy white discharge; itching, inflames vagina and perineum. Treatment: topical clotrimazole (Gyne-Lotrimin), nystatin (Mycostatin).

Category: Data Collection/Health Promotion and Maintenance

(1) "Do you douche?"—not a factor in the development of candidiasis

(2) "Are you sexually active?"—candidiasis not usually sexually transmitted; predisposing factors include glycosuria, pregnancy, and oral contraceptives

(3) "What kind of birth control do you use?"—CORRECT: oral contraceptives predispose individuals to candidiasis

(4) "Have you taken any cough medicine?"—no relationship between cough medicine and candidiasis

23. The Answer is 2

The physician orders an Ace bandage wrap for a client's left leg from toes to mid-thigh. The LPN/LVN should do which of the following?

Reworded Question: What should an LPN/LVN do for a bandaged extremity?

Strategy: Think of what is most important for a bandaged extremity.

Needed Info: Quality of circulation: determined by observing the color, motion, and sensitivity (CMS) of an affected body part, particularly distal to the bandage.

Category: Data Collection/Safe and Effective Care Environment/Safety and Infection Control

(1) Increase friction between the skin and bandage surfaces—would cause skin breakdown

(2) Leave a small distal part of the extremity exposed—CORRECT: enables the LPN/LVN to determine the CMS of a distal body part

(3) Use multiple pins to secure the bandage—unnecessary

(4) Position the left leg in abduction—unnecessary

24. The Answer is 3

A client recovering from a laparoscopic laser cholecystectomy says to the LPN/LVN, "I hate the thought of eating a low-fat diet for the rest of my life." Which of the following responses by the LPN/LVN is *MOST* appropriate?

Reworded Question: Is a low-fat diet required indefinitely?

Strategy: "*MOST* appropriate" indicates discrimination may be required to answer the question.

Needed Info: Laparoscopic laser cholecystectomy is removal of the gallbladder by laser through a laparoscope; monitor T-tube if present; observe for jaundice; monitor intake and output; monitor for pain and encourage early ambulation to rid the body of carbon dioxide.

Category: Implementation/Physiological Integrity/Physiological Adaptation

(1) "I will ask the dietician to come talk to you."—passing the buck; nurse should respond to the client

(2) "What do you think is so bad about following a low-fat diet?"—does not respond directly to the client's statement

(3) "It may not be necessary for you to follow a low-fat diet for that long."—CORRECT: fat restriction is usually lifted as the client tolerates fat;

biliary ducts dilate sufficiently to accommodate bile volume that was held by the gallbladder

(4) "At least you will be alive and not suffering that pain."—nontherapeutic and judgmental

25. The Answer is 2

The LPN/LVN is caring for clients in a pediatric clinic. The mother of a 14-year-old male privately tells the LPN/LVN that she is worried about her son because she unexpectedly walked into his room and discovered him masturbating. Which of the following responses by the LPN/LVN is *MOST* appropriate?

Reworded Question: What is the most therapeutic response?

Strategy: Remember therapeutic communication.

Needed Info: Male changes in puberty: increase in genital size; breast swelling; pubic, facial, axillary, and chest hair; deepening voice; production of functional sperm; nocturnal emissions. Psychosexual development: masturbation as expression of sexual tension; sexual fantasies; experimental sexual intercourse.

Category: Implementation/Health Promotion and Maintenance

(1) "Tell your son he could go blind doing that."—false information

(2) "Masturbation is a normal part of sexual development."—CORRECT: true statement provides opportunity for sexual self-exploration

(3) "He's really too young to be masturbating."—boys typically begin masturbating in early adolescence

(4) "Why don't you give him more privacy?"—judgmental; doesn't take advantage of opportunity to teach

26. The Answer is 4

A client begins to breathe very rapidly. Which of the following actions by the LPN/LVN would be the *MOST* appropriate?

Reworded Question: What is the most appropriate action for a client experiencing tachypnea?

Strategy: "*MOST* appropriate" indicates priority.

Needed Info: Tachypnea: rapid respirations, respirations greater than 20/minute. Changes in respiratory rate: gather additional data in order to provide complete information to the RN and physician.

Category: Data Collection/Safe and Effective Care Environment/Coordinated Care

(1) Assess the apical pulse—initial data collection should be directed at respiratory data

(2) Measure blood pressure and pulse—initial data collection should be directed at respiratory data

(3) Notify the physician—the physician will need more data in order to respond to client condition changes

(4) Obtain an oxygen saturation—CORRECT: provides the LPN/LVN with data about the client's oxygen saturation

27. The Answer is 1

The LPN/LVN plans morning care for a client hospitalized after a cerebrovascular accident (CVA) resulting in left-sided paralysis and homonymous hemianopia. During morning care, the LPN/LVN should do which of the following?

Reworded Question: What should you do for morning care for this client?

Strategy: Think about the consequences of each answer choice.

Needed Info: Homonymous hemianopia: blindness in half of each visual field caused by damage to brain. Client cannot see past midline toward the side opposite the lesion without turning the head toward that side. Approach client from side that is not visually impaired. Reduce noise and complexity of decision making.

Category: Implementation/Physiological Integrity/Physiological Adaptation

(1) Provide care from the client's right side—CORRECT: approach from side with intact vision

(2) Speak loudly and distinctly when talking with the client—no hearing loss

(3) Reduce the level of lighting in the client's room to prevent glare—increase light to assist with vision

(4) Provide all of the client's care to reduce his energy expenditure—encourage independence

28. The Answer is 1

A primigravid woman comes to the clinic for her initial prenatal visit. She is at 32 weeks' gestation and says that she has just moved from out of state. The client says that she has had periodic headaches during her pregnancy, and that she is continually bumping into things. The LPN/LVN notes numerous bruises in various stages of healing around the client's breasts and abdomen. Vital signs are: BP 120/80, pulse 72, resp 18, and FHT 142. Which of the following responses by the LPN/LVN is *BEST*?

Reworded Question: What might bruising indicate?

Strategy: Determine if it is appropriate to collect data or implement.

Needed Info: Symptoms of domestic abuse: frequent visits to physician's office or emergency room for unexplained trauma; client being cued, silenced, or threatened by an accompanying family member; evidence of multiple old injuries, scars, healed fractures seen on X-ray; fearful, evasive, or inconsistent replies, or nonverbal behaviors such as flinching when approached or touched. Nursing care: provide privacy during initial interview to ensure perpetrator of violence does not remain with client; carefully document all injuries (with consent); determine safety of client by asking specific questions about weapons, substance abuse, extreme jealousy; develop with client a safety or escape plan; refer client to community resources.

Category: Data Collection/Health Promotion and Maintenance

(1) "Are you battered by your partner?"—CORRECT: evidence of injury should be investigated; assess head, neck, chest, abdomen, breasts, upper extremities

(2) "How do you feel about being pregnant?"—injuries take priority

(3) "Tell me about your headaches."—injuries take priority

(4) "You may be more clumsy due to your size."—assumption; need to collect data

29. The Answer is 4

The LPN/LVN is providing care for a client with chronic lung disease who is receiving oxygen through a nasal cannula. The LPN/LVN should expect which of the following to occur?

Reworded Question: What physiological changes occur with chronic obstructive pulmonary disease (COPD) that affect oxygen usage?

Strategy: Note the guidelines for oxygen use for clients with COPD.

Needed Info: Clients with COPD retain high amounts of carbon dioxide. Client's respiratory drive may be controlled by the level of oxygen present in the arterial blood. Administration of oxygen at high-liter flows can suppress the respiratory drive. Humidification effective only for flow rates above 5 liters.

Category: Planning/Physiological Integrity/Physiological Adaptation

(1) Arterial blood gases will be drawn q 2 hours—blood gases are not drawn that often unless the client is in acute distress

(2) The client's oral intake will be restricted—fluids should be encouraged, not restricted

(3) The client will be on strict bed rest—client should rest as needed: strict bed rest is unnecessary

(4) The oxygen flow rate will be set at 3 L/min or less—CORRECT: the respiratory drive for clients with COPD can be suppressed by high levels of oxygen

30. The Answer is 1

The LPN/LVN cares for a child who is in a leg cast for treatment of a fractured right ankle. It is *MOST* important for the LPN/LVN to reinforce which of the following activities after discharge?

Reworded Question: What is the priority action for a client in a cast?

Strategy: Determine the outcome of each answer choice.

Needed Info: Immediate nursing care for plaster cast: don't cover cast until dry (48 hours), handle with palms not fingertips; don't rest on hard surfaces; elevate affected limb above heart on soft surface until dry; don't use head lamp; check for blueness or paleness, pain, numbness, tingling (if present, elevate area; if it persists, contact physician); child should remain inactive while cast is drying. Intermediate nursing care: mobilize client, isometric exercises; check for break in cast or foul odor; tell client not to scratch skin under cast and not to put anything underneath cast; if fiberglass cast gets wet, dry with hair dryer on cool setting. After-cast nursing care: wash skin gently, apply baby powder/cornstarch/baby oil; have client gradually adjust to movement without support of cast; swelling is common, elevate limb and apply elastic bandage.

Category: Implementation/ Physiological Integrity/ Reduction of Risk Potential

(1) The child performs isometric exercises of the right leg—CORRECT: contraction of muscle without moving joint; promotes venous return and circulation, prevents thrombi; quadriceps setting (push back knees into bed) and gluteal setting (push heels into bed)

(2) The mother gently massages the child's right foot with emollient cream—will help prevent dryness of foot but does not address skin under cast

(3) The mother cleans the leg cast with mild soap and water—unnecessary to clean cast

(4) The mother elevates the right leg on several pillows—unnecessary

31. The Answer is 3

The LPN/LVN is caring for a client who had a thyroidectomy 12 hours ago for treatment of Graves' disease. The LPN/LVN would be *MOST* concerned if which of the following were observed?

Reworded Question: What is a complication after a thyroidectomy?

Strategy: "*MOST* concerned" indicates a complication.

Needed Info: Nursing care for Graves' disease/hyperthyroidism: limit activities to quiet and provide frequent rest periods; advise light, cool clothing; avoid stimulants; use calm, unhurried approach; administer antithyroid medication, irradiation with I^{131} PO. Post-thyroidectomy care: low or semi-Fowler's position; support head, neck, and shoulders to prevent flexion or hyperextension of suture line;

tracheostomy set at bedside; observe for complications—laryngeal nerve injury, thyroid storm, hemorrhage, respiratory obstruction, tetany (decreased calcium from parathyroid involvement), check Chvostek's and Trousseau's signs.

Category: Data Collection/Physiological Integrity/Reduction of Risk Potential

(1) The client's blood pressure is 138/82, pulse 84, respirations 16, oral temp 99° F (37.2° C)—vital signs within normal limits

(2) The client supports his head and neck when turning his head to the right—prevents stress on the incision

(3) The client spontaneously flexes his wrist when the blood pressure is obtained—CORRECT: carpal spasms indicate hypocalcemia

(4) The client is drowsy and complains of a sore throat—expected outcome after surgery

32. The Answer is 4

A client is admitted with complaints of severe pain in the right lower quadrant of the abdomen. To assist with pain relief, the LPN/LVN should take which of the following actions?

Reworded Question: What is an appropriate nonpharmacological method for pain relief?

Strategy: Determine the outcome of each answer choice.

Needed Info: Establish a 24-hour pain profile. Teach client about pain and its relief: explain quality and location of impending pain; slow, rhythmic breathing to promote relaxation; effects of analgesics and benefits of preventative approach; splinting techniques to reduce pain. Reduce anxiety and fears. Provide comfort measures: proper positioning; cool, well-ventilated, quiet room; back rub; allow for rest.

Category: Implementation/Physiological Integrity/Basic Care and Comfort

(1) Encourage the client to change positions frequently in bed—unnecessary movement will increase pain, should be avoided

(2) Massage the right lower quadrant of the abdomen—if appendicitis is suspected, massage or palpation should never be performed as these actions may cause the appendix to rupture

(3) Apply warmth to the abdomen with a heating pad—if pain is caused by appendicitis, increased circulation from heat may cause appendix to rupture

(4) Use comfort measures and pillows to position the client—CORRECT: nonpharmacological methods of pain relief

33. The Answer is 3

Which of the following actions by the LPN/LVN would be considered negligence?

Reworded Question: What is incorrect behavior?

Strategy: Think about the consequences of each action.

Needed Info: Negligence is the unintentional action or failure to act of an LPN/LVN that a reasonable person would or would not perform in similar circumstances; can be an act of commission or omission. Standards of care: the actions that other LPN/LVNs would take in the same or similar circumstances that provide for quality care. Nurse practice acts: state laws that determine the scope of the practice of nursing.

Category: Implementation/Safe and Effective Care Environment/Safety and Infection Control

(1) Administering subQ (subcutaneous) heparin into a client's abdomen without first aspirating for blood—correct procedure

(2) Crushing furosemide (Lasix) and adding to a teaspoon of applesauce for an elderly client—correct procedure

(3) Lowering the bed side rails after administering meperidine (Demerol) and hydroxyzine (Vistaril) to a client preoperatively—CORRECT: bed side rails should be raised after administering preoperative medication

(4) Placing a used syringe and needle in a sharps container in a client's room—correct procedure

34. The Answer is 3

The LPN/LVN teaches an elderly client with right-sided weakness how to use a cane. Which of the following behaviors by the client indicates that the teaching was effective?

Reworded Question: What is the appropriate technique used to ambulate with a cane?

Strategy: Determine the outcome of each answer choice.

Needed Info: Cane tip should have concentric rings (shock absorber for stability). Flex elbow 30 degrees and hold handle up; tip of cane should be 15 cm lateral to base of the fifth toe. Hold cane in hand opposite affected extremity; advance cane and affected leg; lean on cane when moving good leg. To manage stairs, step up on good leg, place the cane and affected leg on step; reverse when going down ("up with the good, down with the bad"); same sequence used with crutches.

Category: Evaluation/Physiological Integrity/Basic Care and Comfort

(1) The man holds the cane with his right hand, moves the cane forward followed by the right leg, and then moves the left leg—should hold cane with the stronger (left) hand

(2) The man holds the cane with his right hand, moves the cane forward followed by his left leg, and then moves the right leg—should hold cane with the stronger (left) hand

(3) The man holds the cane with his left hand, moves the cane forward followed by the right leg, and then moves the left leg—CORRECT: the cane acts as a support and aids in weight-bearing for the weaker right leg

(4) The man holds the cane with his left hand, moves the cane forward followed by his left leg, and then moves the right leg—cane needs to be a support and aid in weight-bearing for the weaker right leg

35. The Answer is 4

The LPN/LVN has been caring for a 72-year-old client for the past 2 days. The client's vital signs have been within normal limits. This morning her vital signs are: tympanic temperature 103.6° F (39.77° C), pulse 82 regular and strong, respirations 14

shallow and unlabored, BP 134/88. What should the LPN/LVN's next action be?

Reworded Question: What do you do first when you obtain a vital sign that represents a significant change in the client's status and conflicts with other data?

Strategy: Think about what other vital sign changes occur with a significant temperature elevation.

Needed Info: Vitals in normal range: pulse 82, respirations 14, BP 134/88 (slightly elevated likely due to age). Temperature significantly elevated: should result in a more rapid pulse rate and an increased respiratory rate due to increased cellular metabolism. Validation of the temperature reading with another thermometer is required to determine the accuracy of the initial temperature reading.

Category: Planning/Physiological Integrity/Physiological Adaptation

(1) Call the physician immediately to report the vital signs—the LPN/LVN should take responsibility for gathering additional data before calling the physician

(2) Proceed with the client's care—a temperature elevation to 103.6° F (39.77° C) is not normal

(3) Record the vital signs on the graphic record in the chart—the LPN/LVN should insure that the readings obtained are accurate before recording them in a legal document

(4) Retake the temperature with a different thermometer—CORRECT: a temperature of 103.6° F (39.77° C) is abnormal without a corresponding increase in pulse and respiratory rate, the thermometer is likely defective

36. The Answer is 2

A 46-year-old man is admitted to the hospital with a fractured right femur. He is placed in balanced suspension traction with a Thomas splint and Pearson attachment. During the first 48 hours, the LPN/LVN should gather data related to which of the following complications?

Reworded Question: What complication of a fracture is seen in the first 48 hours?

Strategy: Be careful! They are asking for the complication that occurs during the first 48 hours. Later complications may be included.

Needed Info: Complications of fractures: 1) compartment syndrome (increased pressure externally [casts, dressings] or internally [bleeding, edema] resulting in compromised circulation); signs/symptoms (S/S): pallor, weak pulse, numbness, pain, 2) shock: bone is vascular, 3) fat embolism, 4) deep vein thrombosis, 5) infection, avascular necrosis, 6) delayed union, nonunion, malunion.

Category: Data Collection/Physiological Integrity/ Physiological Adaptation

(1) Pulmonary embolism—obstruction of pulmonary system by thrombus from venous system or right side of heart; seen 2–3 days to several weeks after fracture

(2) Fat embolism—CORRECT: fat moves into bloodstream from fracture; formed by alteration in lipids in blood; fat combines with platelets to form emboli; S/S: abnormal behavior due to cerebral anoxia (confusion, agitation, delirium, coma), abnormal arterial blood gases (ABGs) (pO_2 below 60 mmHg), increased respiration; chest pain, dyspnea, pallor, hypertension, petechiae on chest, upper arms, abdomen; treatment: high Fowler's, high O_2 concentration, ventilation with positive end expiratory pressure (PEEP) to decrease pulmonary edema, IVs, steroids, Dextran to prevent shock

(3) Avascular necrosis—(seen later than 48 hrs) bone loses blood supply and dies; seen with chronic renal disease or prolonged steroid use; treatment: bone graph, joint fusion, prosthetic replacement

(4) Malunion—bone fragments heal in deformed position as a result of inadequate reduction and immobilization; treatment: surgical or manual manipulation to realign

37. The Answer is 1

The LPN/LVN is helping a nursing assistant provide a bed bath to a comatose client who is incontinent. The LPN/LVN should intervene if which of the following actions is noted?

Reworded Question: What is an incorrect action?

Strategy: "Should intervene" indicates that you are looking for something wrong.

Needed Info: Standard precautions (barrier) used with all clients: primary strategy for nosocomial infection control. Most important way to reduce transmission of pathogens. Gloves: use clean, non-sterile when touching blood, body fluids, secretions, excretions, contaminated articles; remove promptly after use, before touching items and environmental surfaces.

Category: Evaluation/Safe and Effective Care Environment/Safety and Infection Control

(1) The nursing assistant answers the phone while wearing gloves—CORRECT: contaminated gloves should be removed before the phone is answered

(2) The nursing assistant log-rolls the client to provide back care—correct way to roll a client to maintain proper alignment

(3) The nursing assistant places an incontinence diaper under the client—appropriate to use incontinence diapers for this client

(4) The nursing assistant positions the client on the left side, head elevated—appropriate position to prevent aspiration and protect the airway

38. The Answer is 3

A 70-year-old woman is transferred to the orthopedic unit from the emergency room after being found on the floor by her daughter. X-rays reveal a displaced subcapital fracture of the left hip and osteoarthritis. When comparing the legs, the LPN/LVN would most likely make which of the following observations?

Reworded Question: What is a symptom of a hip fracture?

Strategy: Think about each answer choice.

Needed Info: Symptoms of fracture: swelling, pallor, ecchymosis; loss of sensation to other body parts; deformity; pain/acute tenderness; muscle spasms; loss of function, abnormal mobility; crepitus (grating sound on movement); shortening of affected limb; decreased or absent pulses distal to injury; affected extremity colder than contralateral part. Emergency nursing care: immobilize joint above and below fracture by use of splints before client is moved; in open fracture, cover the wound with sterile dressings or cleanest material available, control bleeding by direct pressure; check temp, color, sensation, capillary refill distal to fracture; in emergency room, give narcotic adequate to relieve pain (except in presence of head injury).

Category: Data Collection/Physiological Integrity/Physiological Adaptation

(1) The client's left leg is longer than the right leg and externally rotated—leg is shorter due to contraction of muscles attached above and below fracture site

(2) The client's left leg is shorter than the right leg and internally rotated—leg is usually externally rotated

(3) The client's left leg is shorter than the right leg and adducted—CORRECT: extremity shortens due to contraction of muscles attached above and below fracture site, fragments overlap by 1–2 inches

(4) The client's left leg is longer than the right leg and is abducted—extremity shortens and externally rotates

39. The Answer is 3

The LPN/LVN is caring for a client with a cast on the left leg. The LPN/LVN would be *MOST* concerned if which of the following is observed?

Reworded Question: What is a complication of a cast?

Strategy: "*MOST* concerned" indicates a complication.

Needed Info: Immediate nursing care for plaster cast: Don't cover cast until dry (48 hours), handle with palms not fingertips; don't rest on hard surfaces; elevate affected limb above heart on soft surface until dry; don't use head lamp; check for blueness or paleness, pain, numbness, tingling (if present, elevate area; if it persists, contact physician); client should remain inactive while cast is drying. Intermediate nursing care: Mobilize client, isometric exercises; check for break in cast or foul odor; tell client not to scratch skin under cast and not to put anything underneath cast; if fiberglass cast gets wet, dry with hair dryer on cool setting. After-cast nursing care: Wash skin gently, apply baby

powder/cornstarch/baby oil; have client gradually adjust to movement without support of cast; swelling is common, elevate limb and apply elastic bandage.

Category: Data Collection/Physiological Integrity/Physiological Adaptation

(1) Capillary refill time is less than 3 seconds—capillary refill time is within normal limits

(2) Client complains of discomfort and itching—a casted extremity may itch or feel uncomfortable due to prolonged immobility

(3) Client complains of tightness and pain—CORRECT: client with a pressure ulcer usually reports pain and tightness in the area; infection or necrosis will result in feeling of warmth and a foul odor

(4) Client's foot is elevated on a pillow—newly casted extremity may be slightly elevated to help relieve edema; should remain in correct anatomical position and below heart level to allow sufficient arterial perfusion

40. The Answer is 2

The LPN/LVN is assisting with discharging a client from an inpatient alcohol treatment unit. Which of the following statements by the client's wife indicates that the family is coping adaptively?

Reworded Question: What indicates that the client's family is coping with the client's alcoholism?

Strategy: Think about what each statement means.

Needed Info: Nursing care for chronic alcohol dependence: safety; monitor for withdrawal; reality orientation; increase self-esteem and coping skills; balanced diet; abstinence from alcohol; identify problems related to drinking in family relationships, work, etc.; help client to see/admit problem; confront denial with slow persistence; maintain relationship with client; establish control of problem drinking; provide support; Alcoholics Anonymous; disulfiram (Antabuse): drug used to maintain sobriety, based on behavioral therapy.

Category: Evaluation/Psychosocial Integrity

(1) "My husband will do well as long as I keep him engaged in activities that he likes."—wife is accepting responsibility; codependent behavior

(2) "My focus is learning how to live my life."—CORRECT: wife is working to change codependent patterns

(3) "I am so glad that our problems are behind us."—unrealistic; discharge is not the final step of treatment

(4) "I'll make sure that the children don't give my husband any problems."—wife is accepting responsibility; codependent behavior

41. The Answer is 3

An LPN/LVN is caring for clients in the mental health clinic. A woman comes to the clinic complaining of insomnia and anorexia. The client tearfully tells the LPN/LVN that she was laid off from a job that she had held for 15 years. Which of the following responses by the LPN/LVN is *MOST* appropriate?

Reworded Question: What is the most therapeutic response?

Strategy: Remember therapeutic communication.

Needed Info: Nursing considerations, explore client's understanding of the problem: focus on the present; emphasize client's strengths; avoid blaming; determine how client handled similar situations; provide support; mobilize client's coping strategies.

Category: Implementation/Psychosocial Integrity

(1) "Did your company give you a severance package?"—yes/no question, nontherapeutic

(2) "Focus on the fact that you have a healthy, happy family."—gives advice, false assurance

(3) "Tell me what happened."—CORRECT: explores situation; allows client to verbalize

(4) "Losing a job is common nowadays."—dismisses the client's concern

42. The Answer is 1

A client with a history of alcoholism is transferred to the unit in an agitated state. He is vomiting and diaphoretic. He says he had his last drink 5 hours ago. The LPN/LVN would expect to administer which of the following medications?

Reworded Question: What is the best medication to treat acute alcohol withdrawal?

Strategy: Think about the action of each drug.

Needed Info: Alcohol sedates the central nervous system (CNS); rebound during withdrawal. Early symptoms occur 4–6 hours after last drink. Symptoms: tremors; easily startled; insomnia; anxiety; anorexia; alcoholic hallucinosis (48 hours after last drink). Nursing care: administer sedation as needed, usually benzodiazepines; monitor vital signs, particularly pulse; take seizure precautions; provide quiet, well-lit environment; orient client frequently; don't leave hallucinating, confused client alone; administer anticonvulsants as needed, thiamine IV or IM, and IV glucose.

Category: Planning/Psychosocial Integrity

(1) Chlordiazepoxide hydrochloride (Librium)—CORRECT: antianxiety; used to treat symptoms of acute alcohol withdrawal; side effects (S/E): lethargy, hangover, agranulocytosis

(2) Disulfiram (Antabuse)—used as a deterrent to compulsive drinking; contraindicated if client drank alcohol in previous 12 hours

(3) Methadone hydrochloride (Dolophine)—opioid analgesic; used to treat narcotic withdrawal syndrome; S/E: seizures, respiratory depression

(4) Naloxone hydrochloride (Narcan)—narcotic antagonist used to reverse narcotic-induced respiratory depression; S/E: ventricular fibrillation, seizures, pulmonary edema

43. The Answer is 1

An elderly client is admitted to a long-term care setting. The client is occasionally confused and her gait is often unsteady. Which of the following actions by the LPN/LVN is *MOST* appropriate?

Reworded Question: What are visual cues for a client who is confused?

Strategy: Determine the outcome of each answer choice.

Needed Info: Nursing care for Alzheimer's disease: provide calm, predictable environment with regular routine; give clear and simple explanations; display clock and calendar; color-code objects and areas; monitor medications and food intake; secure doors leading from house/unit; gently distract and redirect during wandering behavior; avoid restraints (increases combativeness); organize daily activities into short, achievable steps; discourage long naps during the day. If client experiences catastrophic reaction, remain calm and stay with client; provide distraction such as music, rocking, stroking.

Category: Implementation/Psychosocial Integrity

(1) Ask the client's family to provide personal items such as photos or mementos—CORRECT: provides visual stimulation to reduce sensory deprivation

(2) Select a room with a bed by the door so the client can look down the hall—provides only occasional stimulation

(3) Suggest the client eat her meals in the room with her roommate—needs to eat in the dining hall with others for stimulation

(4) Encourage the client to ambulate in the halls twice a day—unsafe due to unsteady gait and confusion

44. The Answer is 2

The LPN/LVN reinforces how to use a standard aluminum walker with an elderly client. Which of the following behaviors by the client indicates that the teaching was effective?

Reworded Question: What is the correct technique when ambulating with a walker?

Strategy: Determine the outcome of each answer choice.

Needed Info: Elbows flexed at 20–30-degree angle when standing with hands on grips. Lift and move walker forward 8–10 inches. With partial or non-weight-bearing, put weight on wrists and arms and step forward with affected leg, supporting self on arms, and follow with good leg. Nurse should stand behind client, hold onto gait belt at waist as needed for balance. Sit down by grasping armrest on affected side, shift weight to good leg and hand, lower self into chair. Client should wear sturdy shoes.

Category: Evaluation/Physiological Integrity/Basic Care and Comfort

(1) The client slowly pushes the walker forward 12 inches, then takes small steps forward while leaning on the walker—should not push the walker

(2) The client lifts the walker, moves it forward 10 inches, and then takes several small steps forward—CORRECT: walker needs to be picked up, placed down on all legs

(3) The client supports his weight on the walker while advancing it forward, then takes small steps while balancing on the walker—should not support weight on walker while trying to move it

(4) The client slides the walker 18 inches forward, then takes small steps while holding onto the walker for balance—walker should be picked up, not slid forward

45. The Answer is 2

An LPN/LVN is providing care for a group of elderly clients in a residential home setting. The LPN/LVN knows that the elderly are at greater risk of developing sensory deprivation for which of the following reasons?

Reworded Question: Why do the elderly have sensory deprivation?

Strategy: Think about each answer choice.

Needed Info: Plan/implementation: assist client with adjusting to lifestyle changes; allow client to verbalize concerns; prevent isolation; provide assistance as required.

Category: Implementation/Psychosocial Integrity

(1) Increased sensitivity to the side effects of medications—many medications alter GI functioning but do not cause decreased vision, hearing, or taste

(2) Decreased visual, auditory, and gustatory abilities—CORRECT: gradual loss of sight, hearing, and taste interferes with normal functioning

(3) Isolation from their families and familiar surroundings—clients are in contact with other residents and staff who provide stimulation

(4) Decreased musculoskeletal function and mobility—clients can be placed in wheelchairs and moved

46. The Answer is 2

The LPN/LVN would expect which of the following clients to be able to sign a consent form for nonemergent medical treatment?

Reworded Question: Which of these clients can give consent for his or her own medical treatment?

Strategy: Think about the requirements for informed consent in nonemergent medical situations.

Needed Info: Clients requiring consent by an agent: under 18 years of age unless emancipated, declared legally incompetent, under the influence of drugs or alcohol, unable to understand or respond to information. In emergency situations: assumption that clients would want to be treated.

Category: Planning/Safe and Effective Care Environment/Coordinated Care

(1) A 10-year-old with a right tibia and fibula fracture—this child requires the consent of the legal guardian in this nonemergent situation

(2) A 21-year-old requiring surgery for acute appendicitis—CORRECT: this client can provide her own informed consent

(3) A 35-year-old who is confused after an automobile accident—informed consent would be required from a spouse or family member in this nonemergent situation

(4) A 73-year-old who has been legally declared incompetent—consent is required from the legal guardian in this nonemergent situation

47. The Answer is 3

An LPN/LVN is assisting with the discharge of a client with a diagnosis of hepatitis of unknown etiology. The LPN/LVN knows that teaching has been successful if the client makes which of the following statements?

Reworded Question: What is a correct statement about hepatitis?

Strategy: Determine the outcome of each statement.

Needed Info: Hepatitis A (HAV): high risk groups include young children, institutions for custodial care, international travelers; by fecal/oral transmission, poor sanitation; nursing considerations include prevention, improved sanitation, treat with gammaglobulin early postexposure, no preparation of food. Hepatitis B (HBV): high risk groups include drug addicts, fetuses from infected mothers, homosexually active men, transfusions, health care workers; transmission by parenteral, sexual contact, blood/body fluids; nursing considerations include vaccine (Heptavax-B, Recombivax HB), immune globulin (HBLg) postexposure, chronic carriers (potential for chronicity 5–10%). Hepatitis C (HVC): high risk groups include transfusions, international travelers; transmission by blood/body fluids; nursing considerations include great potential for chronicity. Delta hepatitis: high risk groups same as for HBV; transmission coinfects with HBV, close personal contact.

Category: Evaluation/Physiological Integrity/Reduction of Risk Potential

(1) "I am so sad that I am not able to hold my baby."—hepatitis not spread by casual contact

(2) "I will eat after my family eats."—can eat with family; cannot share eating utensils

(3) "I will make sure that my children don't eat or drink from my dishware."—CORRECT: to prevent transmission, families should not share eating utensils or drinking glasses; wash hands before eating and after using toilet

(4) "I'm glad that I don't have to get help taking care of my children."—need to alternate rest and activity to promote hepatic healing; mothers of young children will need help

48. The Answer is 2

The LPN/LVN checks the IV flow rate for a postoperative client. The client is to receive 3,000 mL of Ringer's lactate solution IV to run over 24 hours. The IV infusion set has a drop factor of 10 drops per milliliter. The LPN/LVN would expect the client's IV to be running at how many drops per minute?

Reworded Question: What is the IV flow rate?

Strategy: Remember the formula to calculate IV flow rate: total volume × drop factor divided by the time in minutes.

Needed Info: Ringer's lactate: electrolyte solution used to expand extracellular fluid volume, and reduce blood viscosity.

Category: Implementation/Physiological Integrity/ Pharmacological Therapies

(1) 18—incorrect

(2) 21—CORRECT: (3,000 × 10) divided by (24 × 60) = 30,000 divided by 1,440 = 20.8 = 21

(3) 35—incorrect

(4) 40—incorrect

49. The Answer is 1

A client with emphysema becomes restless and confused. Which of the following actions should the LPN/LVN take next?

Reworded Question: What should the LPN/LVN do to raise the oxygen levels of a client with emphysema?

Strategy: Determine the outcome of each answer choice.

Needed Info: Emphysema: overinflation of alveoli resulting in destruction of alveoli walls; predisposing factors include smoking, chronic infections, environmental pollution. Teaching includes breathing exercises; stop smoking; avoid hot/cold air or allergens; instructions regarding medications; avoid crowds or close contact with persons who have colds or flu; adequate rest and nutrition; oral hygiene; prophylactic flu vaccines; observe sputum for indications of infection.

Category: Implementation/Physiological Integrity/ Reduction of Risk Potential

(1) Encourage the client to perform pursed-lip breathing—CORRECT: prevents collapse of lung unit and helps client control rate and depth of breathing

(2) Check the client's temperature—confusion is probably due to decreased oxygenation

(3) Assess the client's potassium level—confusion is probably due to decreased oxygenation, not electrolyte imbalance

(4) Increase the client's oxygen flow rate to 5 L/min—should receive low flow oxygen to prevent carbon dioxide narcosis

50. The Answer is 4

The LPN/LVN cares for a client following surgery for removal of a cataract in the right eye. The client complains of severe eye pain in her right eye. Which of the following activities should the LPN/LVN do *FIRST*?

Reworded Question: Is pain after cataract surgery normal?

Strategy: Remember what you know about cataract removal.

Needed Info: Cataract: change in the transparency of crystalline lens of eye. Causes: aging, trauma, congenital, systemic disease. S/S: blurred vision, decrease in color perception, photophobia. Treated by removal of lens under local anesthesia with sedation. Intraocular lens implantation, eyeglasses, or contact lenses after surgery. Complications: glaucoma, infection, bleeding, retinal detachment.

Category: Planning/Physiological Integrity/Reduction of Risk Potential

(1) Administer an analgesic to the client—mild discomfort treated with analgesics

(2) Recheck the client in 30 minutes—action should be taken immediately

(3) Document the finding in the client's chart— action should be taken immediately

(4) Report the finding to the RN—CORRECT: ruptured blood vessel or suture causing hemorrhage or increased intraocular pressure; notify physician if restless, increased pulse, drainage on dressing

51. The Answer is 4

The LPN/LVN is caring for a client 4 hours after intracranial surgery. Which of the following actions should the LPN/LVN take immediately?

Reworded Question: What is a priority after intracranial surgery?

Strategy: Determine the outcome of each answer choice.

Needed Info: Monitor vital signs hourly. Elevate head 15–30 degrees to promote venous drainage from brain. Avoid neck flexion and head rotation (support in cervical collar or neck rolls). Reduce environmental stimuli. Prevent the Valsalva maneuver; teach client to exhale while turning or moving in bed. Administer stool softeners. Restrict fluids to 1,200–1,500 mL/day. Administer medications: osmotic diuretics, corticosteroid therapy, anticonvulsant meds.

Category: Implementation/Physiological Integrity/Reduction of Risk Potential

(1) Turn, cough, and deep-breathe the client—coughing is discouraged, can increase intracranial pressure

(2) Place the client with the neck flexed and head turned to the side—will increase intracranial pressure (ICP); keep head in a neutral position

(3) Perform passive range-of-motion exercises—changes in client's position can increase intracranial pressure

(4) Move client to the head of the bed using a turning sheet—CORRECT: client's body should be moved as a unit to prevent increased ICP; prevent disruption of the ICP monitoring system

52. The Answer is 2

A 6-year-old child with a congenital heart disorder is admitted with congestive heart failure. Digoxin (Lanoxin) 0.12 mg is ordered for the child. The bottle of Lanoxin contains 0.05 mg of Lanoxin in 1 mL of solution. Which of the following amounts should the LPN/LVN administer to the child after validating the dose with the RN?

Reworded Question: How much of the medication should you give?

Strategy: Remember how to calculate dosages. Be careful and don't make math errors.

Needed Info: Formula: dose on hand over 1 mL = dose desired.

Category: Implementation/Physiological Integrity/Pharmacological Therapies

(1) 1.2 mL—inaccurate

(2) 2.4 mL—CORRECT: $0.05 \text{ mg}/1 \text{ mL} = 0.12 \text{ mg}/x$ mL, $0.05x = 0.12$, $x = 2.4$ mL

(3) 3.5 mL—inaccurate

(4) 4.2 mL—inaccurate

53. The Answer is 4

The LPN/LVN is caring for a client diagnosed with chronic lymphocytic leukemia, hospitalized for treatment of hemolytic anemia. The LPN/LVN should expect to implement which of the following actions?

Reworded Question: What should you do for a client with anemia?

Strategy: Although the client has leukemia, he is admitted with anemia. You must focus on the anemia.

Needed Info: Lymphocytic leukemia: characterized by proliferation of lymphocytes. S/S: fatigue, weakness, HA, easy bruising, bleeding gums, epistaxis, fever, generalized pain. Diagnostic tests: CBC, bone marrow aspiration, lumbar puncture, X-rays, lymph node biopsy. Treatment: total body irradiation or radiation to spleen, chemotherapy. Nursing responsibilities: low-bacteria diet (no raw fruits or vegetables), institute bleeding precautions (soft toothbrush, don't floss, no injections, no aspirin, pad bed rails, use air mattress, use paper tape), antiemetics, comfort measures. Hemolytic anemia S/S: jaundice, splenomegaly, hepatomegaly, fatigue, weakness. Treatment: O_2, blood transfusions, corticosteroids.

Category: Planning/Physiological Integrity/Physiological Adaptation

(1) Encourage activities with other clients in the day room—does not meet need for rest

(2) Isolate the client from visitors—no info given about white blood cell count or reverse isolation; on reverse isolation if neutrophil count is less than 500/mm^3

(3) Provide a diet high in vitamin C—needed for wound healing and resistance to infection; not best choice

(4) Maintain a quiet environment—CORRECT: primary problem activity intolerance due to fatigue

54. The Answer is 3

The LPN/LVN is caring for a client with cervical cancer. The LPN/LVN notes that the radium implant has become dislodged. Which of the following actions should the LPN/LVN take *FIRST*?

Reworded Question: What is the best action when a radium implant becomes dislodged?

Strategy: Think about the outcome of each answer choice.

Needed Info: Limit radioactive exposure: assign client to private room; place "Caution: Radioactive Material" sign on door; wear dosimeter film badge at all times when interacting with client (measures amount of exposure); do not assign pregnant nurse to client; rotate staff caring for client; organize tasks so limited time is spent in client's room; limit visitors; encourage client to do own care; provide shield in room. Client care: use antiemetics for nausea; consider body image; provide comfort measures; provide good nutrition.

Category: Implementation/Physiological Integrity/ Reduction of Risk Potential

(1) Stay with the client and contact radiology—need to secure the implant in a lead container kept in the client's room

(2) Wrap the implant in a blanket and place it behind a lead shield—pick up implant with long-handled forceps

(3) Pick up the implant with long-handled forceps and place it in a lead container—CORRECT: never touch implant with bare hands; forceps and container should be placed in client's room

(4) Obtain a dosimeter reading on the client and report it to the physician—need to place implant in lead container

55.　The Answer is 2

The LPN/LVN comes to the home of a client with cellulitis of the left leg to perform a daily dressing change. The client tells the LPN/LVN that the nursing assistant changed the dressing earlier that morning. Which of the following actions by the LPN/LVN is *BEST*?

Reworded Question: What is the correct chain of command for reporting a problem?

Strategy: Think about the chain of command.

Category: Implementation/Safe and Effective Care Environment/Coordinated Care

(1) Tell the client that the nursing assistant did a good job with the dressing change—does not address the problem of the nursing assistant performing the dressing change

(2) Notify the RN supervisor of the situation— CORRECT: correct chain of command for reporting this problem

(3) Ask the client to describe the dressing change— does not address the problem of the nursing assistant performing the dressing change

(4) Report the nursing assistant to the home care agency—incorrect chain of command; should report problem to next person in direct line of authority in same area

56.　The Answer is 1

The LPN/LVN is caring for a client with pernicious anemia. The LPN/LVN reinforces teaching about the plan of care. The LPN/LVN should report which of the following statements to the RN?

Reworded Question: What is true about pernicious anemia?

Strategy: Determine the outcome of each answer choice.

Needed Info: Pernicious anemia is caused by failure to absorb vitamin B_{12} because of a deficiency of intrinsic factor from the gastric mucosa. Symptoms: pallor, slight jaundice, glossitis, fatigue, weight loss, paresthesias of hands and feet, disturbances of balance and gait. Treatment: vitamin B_{12} IM monthly.

Category: Evaluation/Physiological Integrity/Physiological Adaptation

(1) "In order to get better, I will need to take iron pills."—CORRECT: pernicious anemia is due to vitamin B deficiency, not iron deficiency

(2) "I am going to attend smoking cessation classes."—no reason to report

(3) "I will learn how to perform IM injections."— many clients instructed how to give monthly IM B_{12} injection

(4) "I need to eat a balanced diet."—no reason to report

57. The Answer is 2

The LPN/LVN is caring for clients on a general medical/surgical unit of an acute care facility. Four clients have been admitted in the last 20 minutes. Which of the admissions should the LPN/LVN see *FIRST*?

Reworded Question: Who is the priority client?

Strategy: Think ABCs.

Needed Info: Factors to consider: chief complaint; age of client; medical history; potential for life-threatening event.

Category: Planning/Physiological Integrity/Reduction of Risk Potential

(1) A client complaining of vomiting and diarrhea—airway issue takes priority

(2) A client with third-degree burns to the face—CORRECT: face, neck, chest, or abdominal burns result in severe edema, causing airway restriction

(3) A client with a fractured left hip—airway issue takes priority

(4) A client complaining of epigastric pain—airway issue takes priority

58. The Answer is 4

The LPN/LVN is caring for a client with a diagnosis of COPD, bronchitis-type, in the long-term care facility. The client is wheezing, and his oxygen saturation is 85%. Four hours ago, the oxygen saturation was 88%. It is *MOST* important for the LPN/LVN to take which of the following actions?

Reworded Question: What is the best action for a client with COPD?

Strategy: Determine the outcome of each answer choice.

Needed Info: Emphysema: overinflation of alveoli resulting in destruction of alveoli walls; predisposing factors include smoking, chronic infections, environmental pollution. Teaching includes breathing exercises; stop smoking; avoid hot/cold air or allergens; instructions regarding medications; avoid crowds or close contact with persons who have colds or flu; adequate rest and nutrition; oral hygiene; prophy-

lactic flu vaccines; observe sputum for indications of infection.

Category: Implementation/Physiological Integrity/Pharmacological Therapies

(1) Administer beclomethasone (Vanceril), 2 puffs per metered-dose inhaler—administer brochodilator first to open passageways

(2) Listen to breath sounds—situation does not require further data collection

(3) Increase oxygen to 4 L per mask—increased oxygen levels in client's blood may lead to respiratory depression

(4) Administer albuterol (Proventil), 2 puffs per metered-dose inhaler—CORRECT: brochodilator, relaxes bronchial smooth muscles

59. The Answer is 4

The LPN/LVN is caring for a client hospitalized for observation following a fall. The client states, "My friend fell last year, and no one thought anything was wrong. She died 2 days later!" Which of the following responses by the LPN/LVN is *BEST*?

Reworded Question: What is the most therapeutic response?

Strategy: Remember therapeutic communication.

Needed Info: Therapeutic communication: using silence (allows client time to think and reflect; conveys acceptance; allows client to take lead in conversation); using general leads or broad openings (encourages client to talk, indicates interest in client); clarification (encourages description of feelings and details of particular experience; makes sure LPN/LVN understands client); reflecting (paraphrases what client says; reflects what client says, especially feelings conveyed).

Category: Implementation/Psychosocial Integrity

(1) "This happens to quite a few people."—nontherapeutic; doesn't address client's concerns

(2) 'We are monitoring you, so you'll be okay."—nontherapeutic; "don't worry" response

(3) "Don't you think I'm taking good care of you?"—nontherapeutic; focus is on the LPN/LVN

(4) "You're concerned that it might happen to you?"—CORRECT: reflects client's feelings

60. The Answer is 2

The LPN/LVN is caring for clients on the pediatric unit. An 8-year-old client with second- and third-degree burns on the right thigh is being admitted. The LPN/LVN should expect the new client to be placed with which one of the following roommates?

Reworded Question: Who is the appropriate roommate for a client with burns?

Strategy: Think about the transmission of diseases.

Needed Info: Droplet precautions: used with pathogens transmitted by infectious droplets; involves contact of conjunctivae or mucous membranes of nose or mouth, or during coughing, sneezing, talking, or procedures such as suctioning or bronchoscopy; private room or with client with same infection; spatial separation of 3 feet between infected client and visitors or other clients; door may remain open; place mask on client during transportation.

Category: Implementation/Physiological Integrity/Physiological Adaptation

(1) A 2-year-old with chickenpox—infectious disease

(2) A 4-year-old with asthma—CORRECT: client not infectious; lowest risk of cross-contamination

(3) A 9-year-old with acute diarrhea—requires contact precautions

(4) A 10-year-old with methicillin-resistant *Staphylococcus aureus* (MRSA)—requires contact isolation

61. The Answer is 2

In order to evaluate the effectiveness of a client's heparin therapy, the LPN/LVN should monitor which of the following laboratory values?

Reworded Question: What blood work is done to monitor heparin therapy?

Strategy: Remember what information is most important for a client receiving heparin therapy.

Needed Info: Heparin: anticoagulant. Side effects: hemorrhage, thrombocytopenia. Antidote: protamine sulfate. When given subQ, inject slowly; leave needle in place 10 seconds, then withdraw; don't massage site; rotate sites. Nursing responsibilities: check for bleeding gums, bruises, nosebleeds, petechiae, melena, tarry stools, hematuria; use electric razor and soft toothbrush.

Category: Data Collection/Physiological Integrity/Reduction of Risk Potential

(1) Platelet count—evaluates platelet production; not altered

(2) Partial thromboplastin time—CORRECT: or clotting time; 1.5–2 × control, clotting time 2–3 × control

(3) Bleeding time—duration of bleeding after small puncture wound; detects platelet and vascular problems; not altered

(4) Prothrombin time—used to monitor Coumadin therapy

62. The Answer is 3

The LPN/LVN is reinforcing teaching with a client who is scheduled for a paracentesis. Which of the following statements by the client indicates that teaching has been successful?

Reworded Question: What is a correct statement about paracentesis?

Strategy: Determine the outcome of each answer choice.

Needed Info: Paracentesis: removal of fluid from the peritoneal cavity; 2–3 liters may be removed. Prep: informed consent; void, take vital signs; measure abdominal girth; weigh client. During procedure: take vital signs q 15 minutes. After procedure: document amount, color, characteristics of drainage obtained; assess pressure dressing for drainage; position in bed until vital signs are stable.

Category: Evaluation/Physiological Integrity/Reduction of Risk Potential

(1) "I will be in surgery for less than 1 hour."—not a surgical procedure

(2) "I must not void prior to the procedure."—bladder is emptied prior to the procedure to prevent puncture

(3) "The physician will remove 2–3 liters of fluid."—CORRECT: fluid removed slowly to decrease ascites; can remove 4–6 liters in severe cases

(4) "I will lie on my back and breathe slowly."—positioned in an upright position with feet supported

63. The Answer is 2

The LPN/LVN is performing chest physiotherapy on an elderly client with chronic airflow limitations (CAL). Which of the following actions should the LPN/LVN take *FIRST*?

Reworded Question: What should the nurse do prior to beginning chest physiotherapy?

Strategy: Determine whether to collect data or implement.

Needed Info: Postural drainage: uses gravity to facilitate removal of bronchial secretions; client is placed in a variety of positions to facilitate drainage into larger airways; secretions may be removed by coughing or suctioning. Percussion and vibration: usually performed during postural drainage to augment the effect of gravity drainage; percussion: rhythmic striking of chest wall with cupped hands over areas where secretions are retained; vibration: hand and arm muscles of person doing vibration are tensed, and a vibrating pressure is applied to chest as client exhales.

Category: Data Collection/Physiological Integrity/ Reduction of Risk Potential

(1) Perform chest physiotherapy prior to meals—prevents nausea, vomiting, aspiration

(2) Auscultate the chest prior to beginning the procedure—CORRECT: identify areas of the lung that require drainage; auscultate chest at end of procedure to determine effectiveness

(3) Administer bronchodilators after the procedure—given before chest physiotherapy to dilate the bronchioles and to liquify secretions

(4) Percuss each lobe prior to asking the client to cough—may cause fractures of the ribs; percussion helps loosen thick secretions

64. The Answer is 2

In which of the following situations would it be *MOST* appropriate for the LPN/LVN to wear a protective gown and clean gloves?

Reworded Question: Which of these clients poses the greatest risk for spreading disease requiring both gloves and a gown?

Strategy: Note how microorganisms are most frequently spread.

Needed Info: Spread of microorganisms: contact directly with a source of infection, contact with surfaces contaminated with microorganisms, some airborne diseases, includes all bodily waste and fluids except sweat. Standard precautions: Centers for Disease Control and Prevention (CDC) recommends barrier techniques to prevent spread of microorganisms; common barriers include gloves, masks, goggles, and gowns; choose appropriate barrier for the situation.

Category: Implementation/Safe and Effective Care Environment/ Safety and Infection Control

(1) Administering oral medications to a client with AIDS—there is no contact with body fluids

(2) Assisting in the care of a car-accident victim who is bleeding—CORRECT: blood from this client may contact the nurse's skin when performing care or gathering data; gloves protect hands and gowns protect the skin of the arms as well as skin under clothing

(3) Bathing a client with an abdominal wound infection—gloves are adequate protection

(4) Changing the linen of a client with sickle-cell anemia—if bed is soiled, gloves should be adequate protection; linen should not be in contact with the nurse's uniform

65. The Answer is 2

A client is to receive 1,000 mL of 5% dextrose in 0.45 NaCl intravenous solution in an 8-hour period. The intravenous set delivers 15 drops per milliliter. The LPN/LVN should expect the flow rate to be how many drops per minute?

Reworded Question: What is the correct IV flow rate?

Strategy: Use the correct formula and be careful not to make math errors.

Needed Info: Formula: total volume × drip factor divided by the total time in minutes.

Category: Planning/Physiological Integrity/Pharmacological Therapies

(1) 15—incorrect

(2) 31—CORRECT: (1,000 × 15) divided by (8 × 60)

(3) 45—incorrect

(4) 60—incorrect

66. The Answer is 3

A client is admitted to the hospital with complaints of seizures and a high fever. A brain scan is ordered. Before the scan, the client asks the LPN/LVN what position he will be in while the procedure is being done. Which of the following statements by the LPN/LVN is *MOST* accurate?

Reworded Question: What is the proper position for a brain scan?

Strategy: Visualize the procedure.

Needed Info: Brain scan: measures amount of uptake by the brain of radioactive isotopes. Damaged tissue absorbs more than normal tissue. Nursing care before: withhold meds (antihypertensives, vasoconstrictors, vasodilators for 24 hours). During the test, client will need to change position while pictures of the brain are taken. Test is painless. After test, force fluids to promote excretion of isotopes. Urine doesn't need special handling.

Category: Implementation/Physiological Integrity/Reduction of Risk Potential

(1) "You will be in a side-lying position, with the foot of the bed elevated."—incorrect

(2) "You will be in a semi-upright sitting position, with your knees flexed."—incorrect

(3) "You will be lying on your back with a small pillow under your head."—CORRECT

(4) "You will be flat on your back, with your feet higher than your head"—incorrect

67. The Answer is 2

A client with a diagnosis of delirium is admitted to the hospital. To evaluate the cause of the client's delirium, blood is sent to the laboratory for analysis. The results are as follows: Na^+ 156, Cl^- 100, K^+ 4.0, HCO_3 21, BUN 86, glucose 100. Based on these laboratory results, the LPN/LVN would expect to see which of the following nursing diagnoses on the client's care plan?

Reworded Question: What nursing diagnosis is appropriate?

Strategy: Determine if each lab value is normal or abnormal. Decide what the abnormal lab values indicate about the client and how it would influence the appropriate nursing diagnosis for that client.

Needed Info: Normal Na^+: 135–145 mEq/L. Hypernatremia: dehydration and insufficient water intake. Normal Cl^-: 95–105 mEq/L. Normal K^+: 3.5–5.0 mEq/L. Normal HCO_3: 22–26 mEq/L. Decreased levels seen with starvation, renal failure, diarrhea. Normal blood, urea, nitrogen (BUN): 6–20 mg/100 mL. Elevated levels indicate rapid protein catabolism, kidney dysfunction, dehydration. Normal glucose: 70–100 mg/dL.

Category: Planning/Physiological Integrity/Reduction of Risk Potential

(1) Alteration in patterns of urinary elimination—would have altered K^+

(2) Fluid volume deficit—CORRECT: elevated Na^+, decreased HCO_3, elevated BUN, other values are normal; elevated Na^+ and BUN seen with dehydration

(3) Nutritional deficit: less than body requirements—seen with decreased HCO_3, but would have altered K^+

(4) Self-care deficit: feeding—no information to support this

68. The Answer is 3

A client is to receive 3,000 mL of 0.9% NaCl IV in 24 hours. The intravenous set delivers 15 drops per milliliter. The LPN/LVN would expect the flow rate to be how many drops of fluid per minute?

Reworded Question: What should the IV flow rate be?

Strategy: Use the formula and avoid making math errors.

Needed Info: Total volume × the drop factor divided by the total time in minutes

Category: Planning/Physiological Integrity/Pharmacological Therapies

(1) 21—inaccurate

(2) 28—inaccurate

(3) 31—CORRECT: (3,000 × 15) divided by (24 × 60)

(4) 42—inaccurate

69. The Answer is 4

The LPN/LVN cares for a client diagnosed with asthma. The physician orders neostigmine (Prostigmin) IM. Which of the following actions by the LPN/LVN is *MOST* appropriate?

Reworded Question: Can Prostigmin be administered to a client with asthma?

Strategy: "*MOST* appropriate" indicates that discrimination is required to answer the question.

Needed Info: Prostigmin: parasympathomimetic used to treat myasthenia gravis and as an antidote for nondepolarizing neuromuscular blocking agents; potentiates the action of morphine; side effects include nausea, vomiting, abdominal cramps, respiratory depression, bronchoconstriction, hypotension, and bradycardia; nursing considerations include monitor vital signs frequently, have atropine injection available, take with milk.

Category: Evaluation/Physiological Integrity/Reduction of Risk Potential

(1) Administer the medication—causes bronchoconstriction; notify physician

(2) Check the blood pressure and pulse—data collection; Prostigmin causes hypotension and bradycardia; important to monitor vital signs, but priority is to notify the RN or physician

(3) Ask the pharmacy if the medication can be given orally—medication used cautiously for clients with asthma

(4) Notify the physician—CORRECT: cholinergics can cause bronchoconstriction in asthmatic clients; may precipitate an acute asthmatic attack

70. The Answer is 4

The LPN/LVN cares for a client with a history of Addison's disease who has received steroid therapy for several years. The LPN/LVN would expect the client to exhibit which of the following changes in appearance?

Reworded Question: What changes are seen in a client after taking steroids long-term?

Strategy: All the options in an answer choice must be correct for the option to be right.

Needed Info: Meds: cortisone and hydrocortisone usually given in divided doses: 2/3 in morning and 1/3 in late afternoon with food to decrease GI irritation. Teach to report S/S of excessive drug therapy (rapid weight gain, round face, fluid retention).

Category: Data Collection/Physiological Integrity/ Physiological Adaptation

(1) Buffalo hump, girdle-obesity, gaunt facial appearance—hump and girdle-obesity true; gaunt face seen with lack of steroids

(2) Tanning of the skin, discoloration of the mucous membranes, alopecia, weight loss—tanning and weight loss seen with lack of steroids; rest not seen

(3) Emaciation, nervousness, breast engorgement, hirsutism—nothing to do with steroids; hirsutism: excessive growth of hair

(4) Truncal obesity, purple striations on the skin, moon face—CORRECT: due to excess glucocorticoids

71. The Answer is 1

The LPN/LVN is caring for a client who is jaundiced due to pancreatic cancer. The LPN/LVN should give the *HIGHEST* priority to which of the following needs?

Reworded Question: What is the highest priority for a client with pancreatic cancer?

Strategy: Remember Maslow.

Needed Info: Medical treatment: high-calorie, bland, low-fat diet; small, frequent feedings; avoid alcohol; anticholinergics; antineoplastic chemotherapy

Category: Planning/Physiological Integrity/Reduction of Risk Potential

(1) Nutrition—CORRECT: profound weight loss and anorexia occur with pancreatic cancer

(2) Self-image—jaundiced clients are concerned about how they look, but physiological needs take priority

(3) Skin integrity—jaundice causes dry skin and pruritis; scratching can lead to skin breakdown

(4) Urinary elimination—urine is dark due to obstructive process; kidney function is not affected

72. The Answer is 1

An 8-year-old boy is seen in a clinic for treatment of attention deficit hyperactivity disorder (ADHD). Medication has been prescribed for the child, along with family counseling. The LPN/LVN reinforces the teaching plan about the medication and discusses parenting strategies with the parents. Which of the following statements by the parents indicates that further teaching is necessary?

Reworded Question: What information is wrong for a child with ADHD?

Strategy: Be careful! You are looking for incorrect info.

Needed Info: ADHD: developmentally inappropriate inattention, impulsivity, hyperactivity. Treatment: medication (Ritalin), family counseling, remedial eduction, environmental manipulation (decrease external stimuli), psychotherapy.

Category: Evaluation/Psychosocial Integrity

(1) "We will give the medication at night so it doesn't decrease his appetite."—CORRECT: incorrect info; stimulants (Ritalin) used; side effects: insomnia, palpitations, growth suppression, nervousness, decreased appetite; give 6 hours before bedtime

(2) "We will provide a regular routine for sleeping, eating, working, and playing."—true

(3) "We will establish firm but reasonable limits on his behavior."—true

(4) "We will reduce distractions and external stimuli to help him concentrate."—true

73. The Answer is 4

A teenage client is admitted to the hospital with anorexia nervosa. Which of the following statements by the client requires immediate follow-up by the LPN/LVN?

Reworded Question: Which problem has the highest priority for this client?

Strategy: Remember Maslow's hierarchy of needs.

Needed Info: Anorexia nervosa: a disorder characterized by restrictive eating resulting in emaciation, disturbance in body image, and an intense fear of being obese. Physical needs must be met first in order to keep the client in stable condition. A difficult area to maintain is that of appropriate hydration and fluid and electrolyte balance.

Category: Planning/Psychosocial Integrity

(1) "My gums were bleeding this morning."—vitamin deficiencies occur in anorectic clients, but is not the highest priority

(2) "I'm getting fatter every day."—body image disturbance is a perceptual problem with anorectics, but is not the highest priority; this is a psychosocial need

(3) "Nobody likes me because I'm so ugly."—chronic low self-esteem is a psychodynamic factor, but is not the highest priority; this is a psychosocial need

(4) "I'm feeling dizzy and weak today."—CORRECT: fluid volume deficit is client's highest priority; dehydration is common and could lead to irreversible renal damage and vital-sign alterations

74. The Answer is 4

A client is admitted to the hospital for treatment of *Pneumocystis carinii* pneumonia and Kaposi sarcoma. The client tells the LPN/LVN that he has been considering organ donation when he dies. Which of the following responses by the LPN/LVN is *BEST*?

Reworded Question: Can this client be an organ donor?

Strategy: Think about each answer choice.

Needed Info: Criteria for organ/tissue donation: no history of significant disease process in organ/tissue to be donated; no untreated sepsis; brain death of donor; no history of extracranial malignancy; relative hemodynamic stability; blood group compatibility; newborn donors must be full-term (more than 200 g); only absolute restriction to organ donation is documented case of HIV infection. Family members can give consent. Nurse can discuss organ donation with other death-related topics (funeral home to be used, autopsy request).

Category: Implementation/Physiological Integrity/Physiological Adaptation

(1) "What does your family think about your decision?"—client has the right to make the decision

(2) "You will help many people by donating your organs."—clients with documented HIV are prohibited from donating organs

(3) "Would you like to speak to the Organ Donor Representative?"—passing the responsibility

(4) "That is not possible based on your illness."—CORRECT: clients with documented HIV are prohibited from donating organs

---

75. The Answer is 3

The LPN/LVN is caring for a client 2 days after a pancreatectomy for cancer of the pancreas. The LPN/LVN notes that there is minimal drainage from the nasogastric (NG) tube. It is *MOST* important for the LPN/LVN to take which of the following actions?

Reworded Question: What is the best action when an NG tube is not draining?

Strategy: Determine whether it is appropriate to collect data or implement.

Needed Info: Insertion of Levin/Salem sump: Measure distance from tip of nose to earlobe, plus distance from earlobe to bottom of xyphoid process. Mark distance on tube with tape and lubricate end of tube. Insert tube through nose to stomach. Offer sips of water and advance tube gently; bend head forward. Observe for respiratory distress. Secure with hypoallergenic tape. Verify tube position initially and before feeding. Aspirate for gastric contents and check pH. Inject approx 15 mL of air into stomach

while listening over epigastric area (not always accurate).

Category: Data Collection/Physiological Integrity/Basic Care and Comfort

(1) Notify the physician—should collect data first

(2) Monitor vital signs q 15 minutes—does not address lack of drainage

(3) Check the tubing for kinks—CORRECT: collect data prior to implementing; maintain tubing in a dependent position

(4) Replace the NG tube—collect data before implementing

---

76. The Answer is 3

The LPN/LVN plans to administer furosemide (Lasix) 20 mg PO to a client diagnosed with renal failure. The client asks the LPN/LVN why he is receiving this medication. Which of the following responses by the LPN/LVN is *BEST*?

Reworded Question: Why is Lasix given to a client diagnosed with chronic renal disease?

Strategy: Think about the action of Lasix.

Needed Info: Chronic renal failure is progressive, irreversible kidney injury caused by hypertension, diabetes mellitus, lupus erythematosus, and chronic glomerulonephritis; symptoms include anemia, acidosis, azotemia, fluid retention, and urinary output alterations; nursing care includes monitoring potassium levels, daily weight, intake and output, diet teaching about regulating protein intake, fluid intake to balance fluid losses, and some restrictions of sodium and potassium.

Category: Implementation/Physiological Integrity/Reduction of Risk Potential

(1) "To increase the blood flow to your kidney."—Lasix is a loop diuretic that inhibits sodium and chloride reabsorption at the proximal and distal tubules and the ascending loop of Henle

(2) "To decrease your circulating blood volume."—Lasix used to treat fluid overload due to chronic renal failure

(3) "To increase excretion of sodium and water."—CORRECT: nursing considerations when

administering Lasix include monitoring blood pressure, measuring intake and output, monitoring potassium levels; don't give at hour of sleep

(4) "To decrease the workload on your heart."—correcting the fluid overload will decrease the workload on the heart, but the primary reason Lasix is given to clients diagnosed with renal failure is to augment the kidney's functioning

77.   The Answer is 1

The LPN/LVN is reinforcing discharge teaching for a client with Parkinson's disease. To maintain safety, the LPN/LVN should make which of the following suggestions to the family?

Reworded Question: What is a correct client teaching for Parkinson's disease?

Strategy: Determine the outcome of each answer choice.

Needed Info: Symptoms: tremors, akinesia, rigidity, weakness, motorized propulsive gait, slurred monotonous speech, dysphagia, drooling, mask-like expression. Nursing care: Encourage finger exercises. Administer Artane, Cogentin, L-dopa, Parlodel, Sinemet, Symmetrel. Teach client ambulation modification. Promote family understanding of the disease (intellect/sight/hearing not impaired, disease progressive but slow, doesn't lead to paralysis). Refer for speech therapy, potential stereotactic surgery.

Category: Implementation/Physiological Integrity/ Basic Care and Comfort

(1) Install a raised toilet seat—CORRECT: helps client to be independent; also slightly elevate the back leg of chairs

(2) Obtain a hospital bed—no indications that this is needed

(3) Instruct the client to hold his arms in a dependent position when ambulating—should swing arms to assist in balance when walking

(4) Perform an exercise program during the late afternoon—activities should be scheduled for late morning when energy level is highest and client won't be rushed

78.   The Answer is 3

The LPN/LVN is reinforcing discharge teaching for a client with chronic pancreatitis. Which of the following statements by the client indicates that further teaching is necessary?

Reworded Question: What is an incorrect statement about pancreatitis?

Strategy: This is a negative question; you are looking for incorrect information.

Needed Info: Plan/implementation: nothing by mouth (NPO), gastric decompression. Meds: antacids, analgesics, antibiotics, anticholinergics. Maintain fluid/electrolyte imbalance. Monitor for signs of infection. Cough and deep-breathe; semi-Fowler's position. Monitor for shock and hyperglycemia. Provide total parenteral nutrition (TPN). Treatment of exocrine insufficiency: meds containing amylase, lipase, trypsin to aid digestion. Long-term: avoid alcohol; low-fat, bland diet; small, frequent meals. Monitor S/S of diabetes mellitus.

Category: Evaluation/Physiological Integrity/ Reduction of Risk Potential

(1) "I do not have to restrict my physical activity."— no specific restrictions on activity

(2) "I should take pancrelipase (Viokase) before meals."—pancreatic enzyme replacement; take before or with meals

(3) "I will eat 3 meals per day."—CORRECT: small, frequent feedings are most beneficial

(4) "I am not allowed to drink any alcoholic beverages."—complete abstinence from alcohol required

79.   The Answer is 3

Following a laparoscopic cholecystectomy, the client complains of abdominal pain and bloating. Which of the following responses by the LPN/LVN is *BEST*?

Reworded Question: What is the best intervention for a client complaining of free air pain?

Strategy: "*BEST*" indicates there may be more than one response that appears correct.

Needed Info: Cholecystectomy: removal of gallbladder. T-tube inserted to ensure drainage of bile from common bile duct until edema diminishes. Check amount of drainage (usually 500–1,000 mL/day, decreases as fluid begins to drain into duodenum). Protect skin around incision from bile drainage irritation (use zinc oxide or water-soluble lubricant). Keep drainage bag at same level as gallbladder. Maintain client in semi-Fowler's position after T-tube is removed; observe dressing for bile; notify physician if there is significant drainage. Evaluate pain to check for other problems. Monitor for signs of K^+ and Na^+ loss; flattened or inverted T-waves on EKG; muscle weakness; abdominal distension; headache; apathy; nausea or vomiting; jaundice.

Category: Implementation/Physiological Integrity/Physiological Adaptation

(1) "Increase your intake of fresh fruits and vegetables."—no indication of constipation

(2) "I'll give you the prescribed pain medication."—less pain medication needed with laparoscopic procedure

(3) "Why don't you take a walk in the hallway?"—CORRECT: "free air" pain caused by CO_2; ambulation will increase absorption

(4) "You may need an indwelling catheter."—pain due to retention of CO_2

80. The Answer is 3

The nursing team consists of an RN, two nursing assistants, and an LPN/LVN. The LPN/LVN would expect to be assigned to which of the following clients?

Reworded Question: What is a correct client assignment for an LPN/LVN?

Strategy: Think about each answer.

Needed Info: LPN/LVNs care for stable clients with predictable outcomes. Nursing assistants perform standard, unchanging procedures.

Category: Implementation/Safe and Effective Care Environment/Coordinated Care .

(1) A client scheduled for an MRI—requires assessment and teaching; should be cared for by RN

(2) An unconscious client who requires a bed bath—bed bath for an unconscious client can be assigned to the nursing assistant

(3) A client with a fracture who is in balanced suspension traction—CORRECT: LPN/LVN must care for client; collect data on client airway, adequate respirations, and circulatory status

(4) A client with diabetes who needs help bathing—nursing assistant can assist with bath

81. The Answer is 125

The physician orders 1 liter of D5 1/2 NS to run over 8 hours. The drip factor stated on the IV tubing is 15 gtt/mL. How many milliliters should the LPN/LVN expect to be infused every hour?

Reworded Question: How much fluid needs to run in every hour to infuse 1,000 mL in 8 hours?

Strategy: Think about the question being asked. Note that there is unnecessary information provided.

Needed Info: One liter is equal to 1,000 milliliters. Dividing the total amount of fluids to infuse by the number of hours in which the infusion should be completed equals hourly fluid amounts.

Category: Planning/Physiological Integrity/Pharmacological Therapies

1 liter = 1,000 mL; 1,000 mL/8 hours = 125 mL/hour

The correct answer is 125.

82. The Answer is 1

A client has a vagotomy with antrectomy to treat a duodenal ulcer. Postoperatively, the client develops dumping syndrome. Which of the following statements by the client indicates to the LPN/LVN that further dietary teaching is necessary?

Reworded Question: What is contraindicated for the client with dumping syndrome?

Strategy: Be careful! You are looking for incorrect information.

Needed Info: Antrectomy: surgery to reduce acid-secreting portions of stomach. Delays or eliminates gastric phase of digestion. Dumping syndrome occurs in clients after a gastric resection. It occurs after eating and is related to the reduced capacity of the stomach. Undigested food is dumped into the jejunum resulting in distention, cramping, pain, diarrhea 15–30 minutes after eating. Subsides in 6–12 months. S/S 5–30 minutes after eating: vertigo, tachycardia, syncope, diarrhea, nausea. Treatment: sedatives, antispasmodics, high-protein, high-fat, low-carbohydrate, dry diet. Eat in semirecumbent position, lying down after eating.

Category: Evaluation/Physiological Integrity/ Reduction of Risk Potential

(1) "I should eat bread with each meal."—COR-RECT: incorrect info; should decrease intake of carbohydrates

(2) "I should eat smaller meals more frequently."—true; 5–6 small meals

(3) "I should lie down after eating."—true; delays gastric emptying time

(4) "I should avoid drinking fluids with my meals."—true; no fluids 1 hour before, with, or 2 hours after meal

83.   The Answer is 3

The LPN/LVN reinforces discharge teaching with a client with emphysema. Which of the following statements by the client indicates that teaching was successful?

Reworded Question: What is true about emphysema?

Strategy: Determine the outcome of each answer choice.

Needed Info: Emphysema: chronic progressive respiratory disease caused by destruction of alveolar walls. Complications: acute respiratory infections, cardiac failure or cor pulmonale, cardiac dysrhythmias. Symptoms: cough, dyspnea, wheezing, barrel chest, use of accessory muscles to breathe. Treatment: bronchodilators, corticosteroids, cromolyn sodium, oxygen, diaphragmatic and pursed-lip breathing maneuvers, energy conservation, diet therapy.

Category: Evaluation/Physiological Integrity/Physiological Adaptation

(1) "Cold weather will help my breathing problems."—will exacerbate breathing problems by causing bronchospasms

(2) "I should eat 3 balanced meals but limit my fluid intake."—need small, frequent feedings to increase caloric intake, limit shortness of breath (SOB) caused by eating; hydration will liquify secretions

(3) "My outside activity should be limited when pollution levels are high."—CORRECT: pollution will act as irritant by causing bronchospasms

(4) "An intensive exercise program is important in regaining my strength."—unable to tolerate intensive exercise; conditioning program to conserve and increase pulmonary ventilation

84.   The Answer is 3

A client has been taking aluminum hydroxide (Amphojel) daily for 3 weeks. The LPN/LVN should be alert for which of the following side effects?

Reworded Question: What is a side effect of Amphojel?

Strategy: Remember common side effects.

Needed Info: Aluminum hydroxide (Amphojel): antacid that reduces the total amount of acid in the GI tract and elevates the gastric pH level. May cause hypophosphatemia. Shake suspension well and give with milk or water.

Category: Data Collection/Physiological Integrity/ Pharmacological Therapies

(1) Nausea—not common

(2) Hypercalcemia—seen with calcium-containing antacids (Tums); normal Ca 8.5–10.5 mg/dL

(3) Constipation—CORRECT: may need laxatives or stool softeners

(4) Anorexia—not common

85.   The Answer is 3

The LPN/LVN hears a client calling for help. The LPN/LVN enters the room and finds an elderly client in bilateral wrist restraints with a cool, pale right hand with no palpable radial pulse. Which of the following would be the most appropriate action for the LPN/LVN to take *FIRST*?

Reworded Question: What is the priority response to this situation?

Strategy: Think ABCs and about the risk restraints pose to circulation.

Needed Info: Loss of circulation: loss of all or part of a limb can occur in as little as 15 minutes when blood flow is absent.

Category: Planning/Safe and Effective Care Environment/Safety and Infection Control

(1) Leave to find the client's nurse—this delays the immediate intervention required to protect the hand

(2) Massage the client's wrist and hand—does not address the cause of the impaired hand circulation, delays intervention

(3) Remove the right wrist restraint—CORRECT: provides the most immediate and effective way to help return circulation to the wrist and hand; the LPN/LVN can call for help and turn on the client's call light for further assistance and assessment

(4) Reposition the client to reduce pressure—does not address the cause of the impaired hand circulation, delays intervention

86.   The Answer is 4

The LPN/LVN is reinforcing discharge teaching for a client with a new colostomy. The LPN/LVN knows teaching was successful when the client chooses which of the following menu options?

Reworded Question: What is the appropriate diet for a client with a colostomy?

Strategy: Recall the type of diet required and then select the menu that is appropriate.

Needed Info: Diet: a low-residue diet for 4–6 weeks post-op, avoiding gas-forming, odor-producing, or excessively laxative/ constipating foods.

Category: Evaluation/Physiological Integrity/ Reduction of Risk Potential

(1) Sausage, sauerkraut, baked potato, and fresh fruit—sausage and sauerkraut are gas-producing and should be avoided with a new colostomy

(2) Cheese omelet with bran muffin and fresh pineapple—bran muffin and fresh fruit are high-fiber (residue)

(3) Pork chop, mashed potatoes, turnips, and salad—turnips are odor-causing and salad is high-residue

(4) Baked chicken, boiled potato, cooked carrots, and yogurt—CORRECT: provides balanced nutrition, high protein, low residue, low fat, and non-irritating foods

87.   The Answer is 4

A client is admitted to the unit to rule out acute renal failure. The LPN/LVN would be *MOST* concerned if the client made which of the following statements?

Reworded Question: What is a symptom of acute renal failure?

Strategy: "*MOST* concerned" indicates you are looking for a symptom of acute renal failure.

Needed Info: Symptoms of oliguric phase of acute renal failure: urinary output less than 400 mL/day; irritability, drowsiness, confusion, coma; restlessness, twitching, seizures; increased serum K^+, BUN, creatinine, Ca^+, Na^+, pH; anemia; pulmonary edema, CHF, hypertension. Symptoms of diuretic or recovery phase: urinary output of 4–5 L/day; increased serum BUN; Na^+ and K^+ loss in urine; increased mental and physical activity.

Category: Data Collection/Physiological Integrity/ Physiological Adaptation

(1) "My urine is often pink-tinged."—seen with urinary tract infections or trauma; hematuria not usually a symptom of acute renal failure

(2) "It is hard for me to start the flow of urine."—urinary hesitancy not usually seen with acute renal failure

(3) "It is quite painful for me to urinate."—dysuria seen with urinary tract infections, not with acute renal failure

(4) "I urinate in the morning and again before dinner."—CORRECT: symptoms of acute renal failure include decreased urinary output (anuria or ologuria), increased urinary output, hypotension, tachycardia, lethargy; normal output 1,200–1,500 mL/day or 50–63 mL/hr, normal voiding pattern 5–6 times/day and once at night

88. The Answer is 2

The LPN/LVN is implementing the protocol for teaching a new mother how to breastfeed her newborn. The LPN/LVN knows that teaching has been successful if the client makes which of the following statements?

Reworded Question: What indicates that a newborn is receiving adequate nutrition when breastfeeding?

Strategy: Think about each statement. Is it true?

Needed Info: Breastfeeding is recommended for first 6–12 months of life; human milk is considered ideal food. Colostrum is secreted at first; clear and colorless; contains protective antibodies; high in protein and minerals. Milk is secreted after 2–4 days; milky white appearance; contains more fat and lactose than colostrum.

Category: Evaluation/Health Promotion and Maintenance

(1) "My baby's weight should equal her birthweight in 5–7 days."—breastfeeding infants should surpass birthweight in 10–14 days

(2) "My baby should have at least 6–8 wet diapers per day."—CORRECT: indicates newborn is ingesting an adequate amount of nutrition; should have at least 2 bowel movements per day

(3) "My baby will sleep at least 6 hours between feedings."—newborns feed approximately every 2–3 hours during the day and every 4 hours at night

(4) "My baby will feed for about 10 minutes per feeding."—should feed for approx. 15–20 minutes per breast

89. The Answer is 2

A client is admitted to the telemetry unit for evaluation of complaints of chest pain. Eight hours after admission, the client goes into ventricular fibrillation. The physician defibrillates the client. The LPN/LVN understands that the purpose of defibrillation is to do which of the following?

Reworded Question: Why is a client defibrillated?

Strategy: Think about each answer choice.

Needed Info: Defibrillation: produces asystole of heart to provide opportunity for natural pacemaker (SA node) to resume as pacer of heart activity

Category: Implementation/Physiological Integrity/Physiological Adaptation

(1) Increase cardiac contractility and cardiac output—inaccurate

(2) Cause asystole so the normal pacemaker can recapture—CORRECT: allows SA node to resume as pacer of heart activity

(3) Reduce cardiac ischemia and acidosis—inaccurate

(4) Provide energy for depleted myocardial cells—inaccurate

90. The Answer is 3

The LPN/LVN is caring for a client who suddenly complains of chest pains. The LPN/LVN knows that which of the following symptoms would be *MOST* characteristic of an acute myocardial infarction?

Reworded Question: What type of pain is characteristic in a myocardial infarction (MI)?

Strategy: Think about the cause of each type of pain.

Needed Info: MI signs and symptoms: chest pain radiating to neck, jaw, shoulder, back, or left arm; unrelieved by nitroglycerine. Also fever, apprehension, dizziness, diaphoresis, palpitations, shortness of breath.

Category: Data Collection/Physiological Integrity/Physiological Adaptation

(1) Colic-like epigastric pain—indicates GI disorder

(2) Sharp, well-localized, unilateral chest pain—symptoms of pneumothorax

(3) Severe substernal pain radiating down the left arm—CORRECT: crushing; may radiate; unrelated to emotion or exercise

(4) Sharp, burning chest pain moving from place to place—anxiety state

91. The Answer is 1

The physician orders packing for a nonhealing open surgical wound. Which of the following is the *FIRST* action by the LPN/LVN?

Reworded Question: Which first step is important prior to packing a wound?

Strategy: Determine what you need to know about the wound and dressing. "*FIRST* step" indicates priority.

Needed Info: Must observe a wound in order to properly care for the wound and client. Observation allows nurse to determine what materials are needed, whether another person will be needed to provided assistance, and whether the client will require pain medication prior to the dressing change. Open wounds require sterile technique.

Category: Planning/Safe and Effective Care Environment/Safety and Infection Control

(1) Identify wound size, shape, and depth—CORRECT: it is necessary to observe the wound to adequately prepare for a dressing change and select appropriate dressing materials

(2) Observe for wound drainage or discharge—this is indeed necessary, but not the first step

(3) Plan to set up for clean technique—an open wound requires sterile, not clean, technique

(4) Select the proper dressing material—this is a safe and expected practice, but not the first step

92. The Answer is 2

A client returns to the clinic 2 weeks after discharge from the hospital. He is taking wafarin sodium (Coumadin) 2 mg PO daily. Which of the following statements by the client to the LPN/LVN indicates that further teaching is necessary?

Reworded Question: What is contraindicated for Coumadin?

Strategy: Think about what each statement means and how it relates to Coumadin.

Needed Info: Coumadin: anticoagulant. Side effects: hemorrhage, fever, rash. Prothrombin time (PT) used to monitor effectiveness; PT usually maintained at 1.5–2 times normal. Antidote: vitamin K (aquamephyton). Nursing responsibilities: check for bleeding gums, bruises, nosebleeds, petechiae, melena, tarry stools, hematuria. Use electric razor, soft toothbrush; provide green leafy vegetables (contain vitamin K).

Category: Evaluation/Physiological Integrity/Pharmacological Therapies

(1) "I have been taking an antihistamine before bed."—no contraindication

(2) "I take aspirin when I have a headache."—CORRECT: inhibits platelet aggregation; effect lasts 3–8 days

(3) "I use sunscreen when I go outside."—correct behavior

(4) "I take Mylanta if my stomach gets upset."—correct information

93. The Answer is 3

To enhance the percutaneous absorption of nitroglycerine ointment, it would be *MOST* important for the LPN/LVN to select a site that is which of the following?

Reworded Question: What is the best site for nitroglycerine ointment?

Strategy: Think about each site.

Needed Info: Nitroglycerine: used in treatment of angina pectoris to reduce ischemia and relieve pain by decreasing myocardial oxygen consumption; dilates veins and arteries. Side effects: throbbing headache, flushing, hypotension, tachycardia. Nursing responsibilities: teach appropriate administration, storage, expected pain relief, side effects. Ointment applied to skin; sites rotated to avoid skin irritation. Prolonged effect up to 24 hours.

Category: Implementation/Physiological Integrity/Pharmacological Therapies

(1) Muscular—not most important

(2) Near the heart—not most important

(3) Non-hairy—CORRECT: skin site free of hair will increase absorption; avoid distal part of extremities due to less-than-maximal absorption

(4) Over a bony prominence—most important is that the site be non-hairy

94. The Answer is 3

When assisting the RN in planning care for a postoperative client, which of the following should be the *FIRST* choice of the LPN/LVN to reduce the client's risk for pooled airway secretions and decreased chest wall expansion?

Reworded Question: What respiratory intervention is the easiest and most cost-effective to implement?

Strategy: Identify standards of care to prevent respiratory complications for all hospitalized clients.

Needed Info: Causes of respiratory complications in the hospital setting: decreased mobility or immobility of acutely ill clients. To prevent potential complications: frequently reposition clients from side to side, get clients out of bed to a chair, assist clients to ambulate. These actions are cost-effective, easy, and standard practice.

Category: Planning/Physiological Integrity/Basic Care and Comfort

(1) Chest percussion—not necessary for the majority of clients and requires staff and/or respiratory therapy intervention

(2) Incentive spirometry—not necessary for the majority of clients, adds cost to care and requires a piece of equipment issued to the client

(3) Position changes—CORRECT: can be encouraged and accomplished easily for all clients without any additional expense for equipment or staff

(4) Postural drainage—not necessary for the majority of clients and requires staff and/or respiratory therapy intervention

95.   The Answer is 2

Which of the following actions by the LPN/LVN would be *MOST* helpful in preventing injury to elderly clients in a healthcare facility?

Reworded Question: What is the most frequent cause of injury for the elderly in a healthcare facility?

Strategy: Think about the primary injury category for the elderly.

Needed Info: Statistically, falls are the most frequent cause of injury for the hospitalized or institutionalized elderly adult. Must protect clients/residents from falls.

Category: Planning/Safe and Effective Care Environment/Safety and Infection Control

(1) Closely monitor the temperature of hot oral fluids—necessary, but not the most frequent cause of injury

(2) Keep unnecessary furniture out of the way—CORRECT: falls are the most common cause of injury, and maintaining an uncluttered environment can help prevent falls

(3) Maintain the safe function of all electrical equipment—necessary, but not the most frequent cause of injury

(4) Use safety protection caps on all medications—necessary, but bottles of medication should not be accessible to clients/residents

96.   The Answer is 4

Which of the following statements by a client during a group therapy session requires immediate follow-up by the LPN/LVN?

Reworded Question: Which statement indicates the possibility of impending danger?

Strategy: Think about which statement would make you question the client's intentions.

Needed Info: In *Tarasoff v. The Regents of the University of California* (1976), the court established a duty to warn of threats of harm to others. Failure to warn, coupled with subsequent injury to the threatened person, exposes the mental health professional to civil damages for malpractice. Based on this and other rulings in many states, the mental health caregiver must take responsibility to warn society of potential danger.

Category: Implementation/Psychosocial Integrity

(1) "I know I'm a chronically compulsive liar, but I can't help it."—this statement is revealing, but does not indicate impending threat

(2) "I don't ever want to go home; I feel safer here."—this statement is a response to anxiety or fear, but does not indicate immediate danger

(3) "I don't really care if I ever see my girlfriend again."—this statement does not imply a threat or impending violence

(4) "I'll make sure that doctor is sorry for what he said."—CORRECT: under the Tarasoff Act, a threatened person, including health profession-

als, must be warned about threats or potential threats to personal safety

97. The Answer is 4

A client newly diagnosed with Alzheimer's disease is admitted to the unit. Which of the following actions by the LPN/LVN is *BEST*?

Reworded Question: What is appropriate care for a client with Alzheimer's disease?

Strategy: Determine whether to collect data or implement.

Needed Info: Alzheimer's disease (senile dementia): chronic, progressive, degenerative, resulting in cerebral atrophy. S/S: changes in memory, confusion, disorientation, change in personality; most common after age 65. Nursing responsibilities: reorient as needed; speak slowly; place clocks and calendars in room; place bed in low position with side rails up.

Category: Data Collection/Psychosocial Integrity

(1) Place the client in a private room away from the nurses' station—should be in a semi-private room near nurses' station; needs frequent assessment

(2) Ask the family to wait in the waiting room while the nurse admits the client—familiar people decrease confusion of unfamiliar environment

(3) Assign a different nurse daily to care for the client—consistency is important

(4) Ask the client to state today's date—CORRECT: data collection is the first step in planning care

98. The Answer is 3

A female client visits the clinic with complaints of right calf tenderness and pain. It would be *MOST* important for the LPN/LVN to ask which of the following questions?

Reworded Question: What is a predisposing factor to developing deep vein thrombosis (DVT)?

Strategy: Determine why you would ask each question.

Needed Info: Thrombophlebitis (phlebitis, phlebothrombosis, or DVT): clot formation in a vein secondary to inflammation of vein or partial vein

obstruction. Risk factors: history of varicose veins, hypercoagulation, cardiovascular disease, pregnancy, oral contraceptives, immobility, recent surgery, or injury.

Category: Data Collection/Physiological Integrity/Pharmacological Therapies

(1) "Do you exercise excessively?"—could cause shin splints

(2) "Have you had any fractures in the last year?"—not relevant to client's complaints

(3) "What type of birth control do you use?"—CORRECT: increased risk of DVT with oral contraceptives

(4) "Are you under a lot of stress?"—should be concerned about possibility of DVT

99. The Answer is 1

Which of the following should be the LPN/LVN's *FIRST* priority in providing care for a client who has terminal ovarian cancer and has been weakened by chemotherapy?

Reworded Question: What is the most important information needed regarding this client?

Strategy: Think about basic needs of every client. Remember Maslow's hierarchy of needs.

Needed Info: Maslow's hierarchy of basic human needs: biological/physiological needs must be met before higher-level needs of safety and security, love and belonging, self-esteem, and self-actualization. Untreated pain affects all other biological/physiological needs: oxygenation, food and fluid intake, elimination, ability to rest/sleep, comfort, and activity level.

Category: Planning/Physiological Integrity/Basic Care and Comfort

(1) Assess if the client is experiencing pain—CORRECT: pain assessment enables the LPN/LVN to plan for the management of the client's pain and subsequently provide care to meet physiological and psychological needs

(2) Determine if the client is hungry or thirsty—important physiological needs that are difficult to meet for a client in pain

(3) Explore the client's feelings about dying—important psychological safety and security need that is difficult to meet for a client in pain

(4) Observe the client's self-care abilities—important safety and security need that is difficult to meet for a client in pain

100. The Answer is 2

The LPN/LVN in the postpartum unit cares for a client who delivered her first child the previous day. The LPN/LVN notes multiple varicosities on the client's lower extremities. Which of the following actions should the LPN/LVN perform?

Reworded Question: What is the best way to prevent thrombophlebitis?

Strategy: Think about what causes thrombophlebitis.

Needed Info: High risk of developing thrombophlebitis during pregnancy and immediate postpartum period. Thrombophlebitis: inflammation of vein associated with formation of a thrombus or blood clot. Other risk factors: prolonged immobility, use of oral contraceptives, sepsis, smoking, dehydration, and CHF. S/S: pain in the calf, localized edema of one extremity, positive Homans' sign (pain in calf when foot is dorsiflexed). Treatment: bed rest and elevation of extremity, anticoagulant (heparin).

Category: Planning/Health Promotion and Maintenance

(1) Teach the client to rest in bed when the baby sleeps—not preventive; bed rest can cause thrombophlebitis

(2) Encourage early and frequent ambulation—CORRECT: facilitates emptying of blood vessels in lower extremities

(3) Apply warm soaks for 20 minutes every 4 hours—not a preventive measure but an intervention used to treat; must be ordered by physician; can be intermittent or continuous

(4) Perform passive range-of-motion (ROM) exercises 3 times daily—early ambulation more effective; passive ROM retains joint function, maintains circulation; passive exercises: no assistance from client

101. The Answer is 2

The LPN/LVN cares for a client with a fracture of the left femur. A cast is applied. The LPN/LVN knows that which of the following exercises would be *MOST* beneficial for this client?

Reworded Question: What exercise is best for a client in a cast?

Strategy: Picture the client as described. Imagine client performing each type of exercise. Also think about the key words "*MOST* beneficial."

Needed Info: Fracture: break in continuity of bone. Complications: hemorrhage (bone vascular), shock, fat embolism (long bones), sepsis, peripheral nerve damage, delayed union, nonunion. Treatment: reduction (closed or open), immobilization (cast, traction, splints, internal and external fixation). Cast allows early mobility. Nursing responsibilities: teach isometric exercises.

Category: Planning/Physiological Integrity/Reduction of Risk Potential

(1) Passive exercise of the affected limb—nurse moves extremity; unable to do

(2) Quadriceps setting of the affected limb—CORRECT: isometric exercise: contraction of muscle without movement of joint; maintains strength

(3) Active range-of-motion exercises of the unaffected limb—not best

(4) Passive exercise of the upper extremities—need strengthening, not passive exercises

102. The Answer is: See Explanation

In preparation for a dressing change, the LPN/LVN puts on sterile gloves. Where should the LPN/LVN initially grip the first sterile glove?

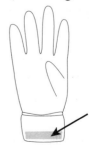

Reworded Question: What is the correct procedure for applying sterile gloves?

Strategy: Remember what part of the glove must remain sterile.

Needed Info: Absolutely necessary for the first glove of the pair to be donned in the proper fashion. Grasp the top end of the folded cuff without touching any part of the rest of the sterile glove to avoid contamination from nonsterile hands.

Category: Implementation/Safe and Effective Care Environment/Safety and Infection Control

103. The Answer is 2

A client is being discharged from the hospital following a right total hip arthroplasty. The LPN/LVN reinforces discharge teaching. Which of the following statements by the client would indicate that teaching was successful?

Reworded Question: What should a client do after a total hip arthroplasty?

Strategy: Determine which movements bring the right hip toward the median plane of the body (adduction).

Needed Info: Adduction: movement toward the median plane or midline of the body. Adduction precautions implemented to prevent hip dislocation: legs may not be crossed at knees or ankles, knees must be separated (most often with a special pillow). No hip flexion beyond 90 degrees.

Category: Planning/Physiological Integrity/Basic Care and Comfort

(1) "I can bend over to pick up something on the floor."—this describes flexion, not adduction, but is not allowed for total hip arthroplasty (THA) clients

(2) "I should not cross my ankles when sitting in a chair."—CORRECT: even though the client is only crossing her legs at the ankles, the leg is adducted

(3) "I need to lie on my stomach when sleeping in bed."—the prone position does not necessarily adduct the hip

(4) "I should spread my knees apart to put on my shoes."—this movement abducts the hip

104. The Answer is 725

The LPN/LVN cares for a client with continuous bladder irrigation. At 7 A.M., the LPN/LVN notes 4,200 mL of normal saline left in the irrigation bags. During the next shift (7 A.M. to 3 P.M.), the LPN/LVN hangs another 3,000 mL and empties a total of 5,625 mL from the urine drainage bag. At 3 P.M., there are 2,300 mL of irrigant left hanging. What is the actual urine output for the client from 7 A.M. to 3 P.M.?

Reworded Question: After subtracting the irrigant, what is the client's urinary output?

Strategy: Calculate irrigant used and subtract it from total fluid output to determine urinary output.

Needed Info: Accurate measurement of urinary output is critical. Subtract the irrigant used from the total fluid output to determine the urinary output.

Category: Implementation/Physiological Integrity/Basic Care and Comfort

The irrigant infused was 4,200 mL left at the beginning of the shift + 3,000 mL added − 2,300 mL remaining at the end of the shift = 4,900 mL infused as irrigant. Total output from the catheter bag was 5,625 mL − 4,900 mL of irrigant infused = 725 mL of urine as output.

The correct answer is 725.

105. The Answer is 1

The LPN/LVN observes activities on a medical/surgical unit. The LPN/LVN should intervene if which of the following is observed?

Reworded Question: What will cause the spread of infection?

Strategy: "Should intervene" indicates an incorrect action.

Needed Info: Standard precautions are used to prevent nosocomial infections; wash hands as soon as gloves are removed, between client contacts, between procedures or tasks with same client; gloves when touching blood, body fluids, or contaminated surfaces; masks, goggles, and gown if danger of splashes.

Category: Evaluation/Safe and Effective Care Environment/Safety and Infection Control

(1) A client's wife disposes of her husband's used tissue in the bedside container before opening the roommate's milk carton—CORRECT: contaminated hands cause cross-infections; instruct family about when handwashing is necessary and the correct procedure

(2) A nursing assistant removes her gloves and washes her hands for 15 seconds after emptying an indwelling urinary catheter—wash hands for at least 10 seconds after removing gloves after a procedure

(3) An LPN/LVN puts on a gown, gloves, mask, and goggles prior to inserting a nasogastric tube—appropriate technique; splashes may occur

(4) A visitor talks with a client diagnosed with methicillin-resistant *Staphylococcus aureus* (MRSA) wound infection while he eats his lunch—client in isolation may develop sense of loneliness; visiting with client during meals increases sensory stimulation

106. The Answer is 3

A client is admitted to the unit with complaints of nausea, vomiting, and abdominal pain. He is a type 1 diabetic (IDDM). Four days earlier, he reduced his insulin dose when flu symptoms prevented him from eating. The LPN/LVN observes the client and finds poor skin turgor, dry mucous membranes, and fruity breath odor. The LPN/LVN should be alert for which of the following problems?

Reworded Question: What do these symptoms indicate?

Strategy: Think about each answer choice.

Needed Info: Diabetes mellitus: disorder of carbohydrate metabolism: insufficient insulin to meet metabolic needs. Type 1 (juvenile): insulin dependent, prone to ketoacidosis. Type 2 (adult onset): controlled by diet and oral agents, non-ketosis prone. In keto-acidosis, the body becomes dehydrated from osmotic diuresis. The fruity breath odor develops from acetone, a component of ketone bodies. Rate and depth of respiration increase (Kussmaul) in attempt to blow off excess carbonic acid. Difference between ketoacidosis and HHNK—lack of ketonuria.

Category: Planning/Physiological Integrity/Reduction of Risk Potential

(1) Hypoglycemia—cause: too much insulin; blood sugar below 60 mg; S/S: tachycardia, perspiration, confusion, lethargy, lip numbness, anxiety, hunger

(2) Viral illness—not best answer

(3) Ketoacidosis—CORRECT: cause: insufficient insulin; S/S: polyuria, polydipsia, nausea and nauseating; dry mucous membranes, weight loss, abdominal pain, hypotension, shock, coma

(4) Hyperglycemic hyperosmolar nonketotic coma—(HHNK) extreme hyperglycemia (800–2,000 mg/dL) with absence of acidosis; some insulin production so don't mobilize fats for energy or form ketones; usually seen in type 2; cause: infections, stress, meds (steroids, thiazide diuretics), TPN; S/S: polyphagia, polyuria, polydipsia, glycosuria, dehydration, abdominal discomfort, hyperpyrexia, changes in level of consciousness (LOC), hypotension, shock; treatment: fluid replacement (2 L 0.45% NaCl over 2 hrs), K^+, Na^+, Cl^-, phosphates, insulin given IV

107. The Answer is 1

The LPN/LVN knows that it is *MOST* important for which of the following clients to receive his scheduled medication on time?

Reworded Question: Which medication, if given late, might cause harm to the client?

Strategy: Think about each answer.

Needed Info: Myasthenia gravis is deficiency of acetylcholine at myoneural junction; symptoms include muscular weakness produced by repeated movements that soon disappears following rest, diplopia, ptosis, impaired speech, and dysphagia.

Category: Planning/Physiological Integrity/Pharmacological Therapies

(1) A client diagnosed with myasthenia gravis receiving pyridostigmine bromide (Mestinon)—CORRECT: Mestinon is a cholinesterase inhibitor which increases acetylcholine concentration at the neuromuscular junction; early administration can precipitate a cholinergic crisis; late administration can precipitate myasthenic crisis

(2) A client diagnosed with bipolar disorder receiving lithium carbonate (Lithobid)—Lithobid is a mood stabilizer; targeted blood level = 1–1.5 mEq/L

(3) A client diagnosed with tuberculosis receiving isonicotinic acid hydrazide (INH)—INH is given in a single daily dose; side effects include hepatitis, peripheral neuritis, rash, and fever

(4) A client diagnosed with Parkinson's disease receiving levodopa (L-dopa)—L-dopa is thought to restore dopamine levels in extrapyramidal centers; sudden withdrawal can cause parkinsonian crisis; priority is to administer Mestinon

108. The Answer is 3

An 11-year-old boy is admitted to the hospital for evaluation for a kidney transplant. The LPN/LVN learns that the client received hemodialysis for 3 years due to renal failure. The LPN/LVN knows that his illness can interfere with this client's achievement of which of the following?

Reworded Question: What developmental stage is altered in a client due to this chronic disease?

Strategy: Picture the person described in the question. Think about his activities and interests. This helps eliminate incorrect answer choices. An 11-year-old is usually in grade school thinking about homework, or doing chores at home.

Needed Info: Eric Erikson developed a theory of the stages of personality development that progressed in predictable stages from birth to death. Other stages: autonomy versus shame and doubt (task of 1–3 yrs); initiative versus guilt (task of 3–6 yrs).

Category: Planning/Health Promotion and Maintenance

(1) Intimacy—young adult: 20–40 yrs; achieving sexual and loving relationship with another; alternative: isolation

(2) Trust—infancy; results from consistent care by a loving caretaker; teaches that basic needs will be met; alternative: mistrust

(3) Industry—CORRECT: 6–12 yrs; aspires to be the best; learns social skills, how to finish tasks; sensitive about school expectations; may be impaired due to absences from school, growth retardation, and emotional difficulties

(4) Identity—adolescence; peer groups important; used to define identity, establish body image, form new relationships; alternative: role diffusion

109. The Answer is 2, 3, 5, 6

The LPN/LVN notes that a 67-year-old client has an unsteady gait. The LPN/LVN should do which of the following? **Select all that apply.**

Reworded Question: What safety measures are appropriate for a client who is unsteady on his or her feet?

Strategy: Identify nonrestrictive safety measures.

Needed Info: Safety measures to help prevent falls include: rubber-soled (nonskid) shoes, removal of obstacles and clutter, a method of summoning the help of the nursing staff, assistance when out of bed, adequate lighting, safety bars and hand rails, and adaptive equipment including walkers and raised toilet seats as appropriate.

Category: Implementation/Safe and Effective Care Environment/Safety and Infection Control

(1) Apply a chest or vest restraint at night—restrictive and false imprisonment without a physician's orders

(2) Help the client put on nonskid shoes for walking—CORRECT: a choice that decreases fall risk without restricting the client

(3) Keep the call light within the client's reach—CORRECT: not restrictive and addresses the client's need to call for assistance when getting out of bed

(4) Lower the bed and raise all four side rails—lowering the bed is appropriate, but raising all the side rails only increases the height from which a client may fall while climbing over the side rails

(5) Provide adequate lighting—CORRECT: allows client to assess an unfamiliar hospital environment

(6) Remove obstacles and room clutter—CORRECT: provides clear access to room and bathroom

110. The Answer is 2

Haloperidol (Haldol) 5 mg tid is ordered for a client with schizophrenia. Two days later, the client complains of "tight jaws and a stiff neck." The LPN/LVN should recognize that these complaints are which of the following?

Reworded Question: Why does the client taking Haldol have these symptoms?

Strategy: Think about each answer choice.

Needed Info: Haldol is a med used in the treatment of psychotic disorders. High incidence of extrapyramidal reactions: pseudoparkinsonism (rigidity and tremors), akathisia (motor restlessness), dystonia (involuntary jerking, uncoordinated body movements), tardive dyskinesia (abnormal movements of lips, jaws, tongue). Schizophrenia: retreat from reality, flat affect, suspiciousness, hallucinations, delusions, loose associations, psychomotor retardation or hyperactivity, regression. Nursing responsibilities: maintain safety, meet physical needs, decrease sensory stimuli. Treatment: antipsychotic meds, individual therapy.

Category: Evaluation/Physiological Integrity/Pharmacological Therapies

(1) Common side effects of antipsychotic medications that will diminish over time—gets worse, untreated, life-threatening

(2) Early symptoms of extrapyramidal reactions to the medication—CORRECT: dystonic reaction, airway may become obstructed

(3) Psychosomatic complaints resulting from a delusional system—not accurate

(4) Permanent side effects of Haldol—reversible when treated with IV Benadryl

111. The Answer is 4

A client is receiving a continuous gastric tube feeding at 100 mL per hour. The LPN/LVN checks for feeding residual and finds 90 mL in the client's stomach. Which action should the LPN/LVN take?

Reworded Question: What are the standards and procedures for tube-feeding residuals?

Strategy: Think about electrolyte balance and gastric emptying.

Needed Info: Standard procedures for clients receiving continuous tube feedings: residuals and tube placement checked every 4 hours, position clients with head of bed elevated at least 30 degrees. To promote normal function: gastric residual volume with associated gastric enzymes and HCl acid should be returned to the stomach when residuals are under 150 mL, feeding should be stopped if the residual is over 50% of the volume fed over the last 1 hour.

Category: Physiological Integrity/Basic Care and Comfort/Analysis

(1) Discard the residual and continue the tube feeding—residuals under 150 mL should be returned to the stomach to maintain electrolyte balance; the feeding should be stopped because the residual is over 50% of the volume fed over 1 hour

(2) Discard the residual and stop the tube feeding—return the residual and stop the feeding

(3) Return the residual to the stomach and continue the tube feeding—return the residual and stop the feeding

(4) Return the residual to the stomach and stop the tube feeding—CORRECT: residuals less than 150 mL should be returned to the stomach to maintain electrolyte balance; the feeding should be stopped because the residual is over 50% of the volume fed over 1 hour

112. The Answer is 4

The LPN/LVN opens several sterile 4 × 4s on the client's over-bed table. The LPN/LVN knows that the sterile dressings will be contaminated if she does which of the following?

Reworded Question: What is incorrect sterile technique?

Strategy: List the basic principles of sterile technique.

Needed Info: To maintain sterility of sterile objects: may only touch other sterile objects, must remain in the LPN/LVN's view, must be above the LPN/LVN's waist, cannot be exposed to air for prolonged periods, must be located inside the 1-inch border of a sterile field or within the dressing packaging borders, sterile fluids must not contact a nonsterile object when fluids flow with gravity. The client's over-bed table is not sterile.

Category: Evaluation/Safe and Effective Care Environment/Safety and Infection Control

(1) Does not allow the dressings prolonged exposure to the air—a principle of sterile technique

(2) Keeps sterile 4 × 4s inside the border of the sterile packaging—a principle of sterile technique

(3) Positions the top of the table at or above waist level—a principle of sterile technique

(4) Pours sterile saline onto the opened sterile 4 × 4s on the table —CORRECT: capillary action and gravity lead to contamination of the sterile object because of contact between the nonsterile overbed table and the once-sterile fluid

113.   The Answer is 3

A client has adamantly refused all hygiene measures over the last 3 days. The LPN/LVN and the client are finally able to collaborate to achieve the hygiene goal of "self-administration of a complete bath once a day while in the hospital." To evaluate if this goal is met, the LPN/LVN should do which of the following?

Reworded Question: What is the most objective method to evaluate goal attainment of a psychomotor skill?

Strategy: Identify how you can best objectively determine if the client did bathe.

Needed Info: Goals and expected outcomes of nursing process provide the focus for the effectiveness of the planned nursing interventions. To validate that a goal has been met, measurable criteria are needed.

Category: Evaluation/Physiological Integrity/Basic Care and Comfort

(1) Ask the client if he has performed his daily bath—client confirmation of a bath is not measurable and may not always be reliable

(2) Bathe the client to be sure the hygiene goal is met—this does not support the goal of a self-administered bath

(3) Observe the client performing portions of his daily bath—CORRECT: direct observation pro-

vides the LPN/LVN with objective measurable data that the client has met the goal

(4) Remind the client to take his bath, providing the needed supplies—places all the responsibility on the client and does not actively create client compliance

114.   The Answer is: See Explanation

The LPN/LVN is caring for a client in labor. The MD palpates a firm, round form in the uterine fundus, small parts on the woman's right side, and a long, smooth, curved section on the left side. Based on these findings, where should the LPN/LVN anticipate auscultating the fetal heart?

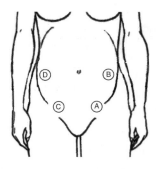

Reworded Question: If a fetus is left occiput anterior (LOA), where should the nurse listen for the fetal heart tone?

Strategy: Examine the diagram carefully. Know the woman's right from left.

Needed Info: Fetal reference point: Vertex presentation—dependent upon degree of flexion of fetal head on chest; full flexion/occiput (O), full extension chin (M), moderate extension (military) brow (B). Breech presentation—sacrum (S). Shoulder presentation—scapula (SC). Maternal pelvis is designated per her right/left and anterior/posterior. Position = relationship of fetal reference point to mother's pelvis; expressed as standard 3-letter abbreviation: left occiput anterior (LOA) (most common), left occiput posterior (LOP), right occiput anterior (ROA), right occiput posterior (ROP), left occiput transverse (LOT), right occiput transverse (ROT).

Category: Planning/Health Promotion and Maintenance

(1) A—CORRECT: point of maximum intensity for fetal heart with fetus in LOA position

(2) B—PMI location for fetus in LOP position

(3) C—PMI location for fetus in ROA position

(4) D—PMI location for fetus in ROP position

115. The Answer is 4

When completing data collection of an immobilized client, the LPN/LVN knows that he is most likely to observe edema in which of the following?

Reworded Question: Where does dependent edema occur in an immobile client? What position is the immobilized client usually in?

Strategy: Identify where dependent edema is likely to settle due to gravity in a client supine.

Needed Info: Immobile clients: most often horizontal in bed, gravity would cause fluid pooling at the most dependent place, namely, the sacrum. Mobile clients: fluids pool in dependent areas such as their feet and ankles.

Category: Data Collection/Physiological Integrity/Basic Care and Comfort

(1) Abdomen—not a likely place for dependent edema

(2) Feet and ankles—a primary place for edema in a client who is sitting up and/or out of bed walking

(3) Fingers and wrists—not a likely place to initially find dependent edema

(4) Sacrum—CORRECT: gravity causes dependent edema to develop at the sacrum in immobile clients

116. The Answer is 1

A client is preparing to take her 1-day-old infant home from the hospital. The LPN/LVN discusses the test for phenylketonuria (PKU) with the mother. The LPN/LVN's teaching should be based on an understanding that the test is *MOST* reliable in which of the following circumstances?

Reworded Question: When is the PKU test most reliable?

Strategy: Focus on the key words in the question. Think about what you know about the PKU test.

Needed Info: PKU: genetic disorder caused by a deficiency in liver enzyme phenylalanine hydroxylase. Body can't metabolize essential amino acid phenylalanine, allows phenyl acids to accumulate in the blood. If not recognized, resultant high levels of phenyl ketone in the brain cause mental retardation. Guthrie test: screening for PKU. Treatment: dietary restriction of foods containing phenylalanine. Blood levels of phenylalanine monitored to evaluate the effectiveness of the dietary restrictions.

Category: Implementation/Health Promotion and Maintenance

(1) After a source of protein has been ingested—CORRECT: recommended to be performed before newborns leave hospital; if initial blood sample is obtained within first 24 hours, recommended to be repeated at 3 weeks

(2) After the meconium has been excreted—no relationship; dark-green, tarry stool passed within first 48 hrs of birth

(3) After the danger of hyperbilirubinemia has passed—no relationship; excessive accumulation of bilirubin in blood; S/S: jaundice (yellow discoloration of skin); common finding in newborn; not cause for concern

(4) After the effects of delivery have subsided—no relationship

117. The Answer is 3

The LPN/LVN is caring for an Rh-negative mother who has delivered an Rh-positive child. The mother states, "The doctor told me about RhoGAM, but I'm still a little confused." Which of the following responses by the LPN/LVN is *MOST* appropriate?

Reworded Question: What is RhoGAM and why is it used?

Strategy: Remember what you know about RhoGAM.

Needed Info: RhoGAM: given to unsensitized Rh⁻ mother after delivery or abortion of an Rh⁺ infant or fetus to prevent development of sensitization. Rh⁻ mother produces antibodies in response to the Rh⁺ RBCs of fetus. If occurs during pregnancy, fetus is affected. If occurs during delivery, later pregnancies may be affected. An indirect Coombs' test is performed on the mother during pregnancy, and a direct Coombs' test is done on cord blood after delivery. If both are negative and the neonate is Rh⁺, the mother is given RhoGAM to prevent sensitization. RhoGAM is usually given to unsensitized mothers within 72 hrs of delivery, but may be effective when given 3–4 weeks after delivery. To be effective, RhoGAM must be given after the first delivery and repeated after each subsequent delivery. RhoGAM is ineffective against Rh⁺ antibodies that are already present in the maternal circulation. The administration of RhoGAM at 26–28 weeks' gestation is also recommended.

Category: Implementation/Health Promotion and Maintenance

(1) "RhoGAM is given to your child to prevent the development of antibodies."—not given to neonate

(2) "RhoGAM is given to your child to supply the necessary antibodies."—not given to neonate

(3) "RhoGAM is given to you to prevent the formation of antibodies."—CORRECT: prevents maternal circulation from developing antibodies

(4) "RhoGAM is given to you to encourage the production of antibodies."—not accurate; given to discourage antibody production

118. The Answer is 2

A woman is hospitalized with a diagnosis of bipolar disorder. While she is in the client activities room on the psychiatric unit, she flirts with male clients and disrupts unit activities. Which of the following approaches would be *MOST* appropriate for the LPN/LVN to take at this time?

Reworded Question: How should you deal with a client with bipolar disorder who is disruptive?

Strategy: Determine the outcome of each answer. Is it desirable?

Needed Info: Nursing responsibilities: accompany client to room when hyperactivity escalates, set limits, remain nonjudgmental.

Category: Planning/Psychosocial Integrity

(1) Set limits on the client's behavior and remind her of the rules—too confrontational

(2) Distract the client and escort her back to her room—CORRECT: clients are easily distracted; nonthreatening action

(3) Instruct the other clients to ignore this client's behavior—does not ensure safety

(4) Tell the client that she is behaving inappropriately and send her to her room—too confrontational; may agitate

119. The Answer is 1

A client is brought to the emergency room bleeding profusely from a stab wound in the left chest area. The client's vital signs are blood pressure 80/50, pulse 110, and respirations 28. The LPN/LVN should expect which of the following potential problems?

Reworded Question: What type of shock is described?

Strategy: Form a mental image of the person described.

Needed Info: Symptoms of hypovolemic shock: tachycardia, reduced output, irritability. Treatment: O₂, IV fluids to restore volume, adrenaline, Apresoline. Nursing responsibilities: check airway, vital signs, insert IV, check blood gases, CVP measurements, insert catheter, hourly I&O, position flat with legs elevated, keep warm.

Category: Planning/Physiological Integrity/Physiological Adaptation

(1) Hypovolemic shock—CORRECT: loss of circulating volume

(2) Cardiogenic shock—decrease in cardiac output; cause: cardiac dysfunction, MI, CHF

(3) Neurogenic shock—increase in vascular bed; cause: spinal anesthesia, spinal cord injury

(4) Septic shock—decreased cardiac output, hypotension; cause: gram+ or gram– bacteria

120. The Answer is 3

A client is admitted to the hospital for surgical repair of a detached retina in the right eye. In implementing the plan of care for this client postoperatively, the LPN/LVN should encourage the client to do which of the following?

Reworded Question: What should you do after surgery for a detached retina?

Strategy: Picture the client as described.

Needed Info: Detached retina: separation of retina from pigmented epithelium. S/S: curtain falling across field of vision, black spots, flashes of light, sudden onset. Treatment: surgical repair (photo-coagulation, electrodiathermy, cryosurgery, scleral buckling). Complications: infection, redetachment, increased intraocular pressure. Nursing responsibilities post-op: check eye patch for drainage, position with detached area dependent; no rapid eye movement (reading, sewing); no coughing, vomiting, sneezing.

Category: Planning/Physiological Integrity/Reduction of Risk Potential

(1) Perform self-care activities—activity restrictions depend on location and size of tear

(2) Maintain patches over both eyes—only affected eye covered

(3) Limit movement of both eyes—CORRECT: bed rest with eye patch or shield

(4) Refrain from excessive talking—no restriction

121. The Answer is 2

The LPN/LVN cares for a client receiving a balanced complete food by tube feeding. The LPN/LVN knows that the *MOST* common complication of a tube feeding is which of the following?

Reworded Question: What is a common complication of a tube feeding?

Strategy: Think about each answer choice. Focus on the words "*MOST* common" which means there may be more than one answer. And in this situation there is: #4 is a complication but is not common.

Needed Info: Tube feedings are used with clients unable to tolerate the oral route but with a functioning GI tract. May be given by intermittent or continuous infusion. Elevate head of bed 30–45 degrees. Give at room temp. Check for placement and residual before feeding or every 4–8 hrs (should be less than 50% of previous hour's intake). Replace residual to prevent fluid and electrolyte imbalances unless it appears abnormal (coffee ground–like material). Don't hang solution more than 6 hrs. Flush tubing with 20–30 mL water every 4 hrs. Change feeding set every 24 hrs. Balanced complete food product/supplement contains intact protein.

Category: Evaluation/Physiological Integrity/Basic Care and Comfort

(1) Edema—not frequently seen; if present physician change formula to contain less Na^+

(2) Diarrhea—CORRECT: intolerance to solution, rate; give slowly; other symptoms of intolerance: nausea and vomiting, aspiration, glycosuria, diaphoresis

(3) Hypokalemia—normal potassium 3.5–5.0 mEq/L; not commonly seen; common causes: diuretics, diarrhea, GI drainage

(4) Vomiting—can happen with rapid increase in rate; give feeding slowly

122. The Answer is 4

A 6-week-old infant is brought to the hospital for treatment of pyloric stenosis. The following nursing diagnosis is on the infant's care plan: "fluid volume deficit related to vomiting." The LPN/LVN would expect to see which of the following to support this diagnosis?

Reworded Question: What would indicate volume deficit?

Strategy: How does each answer relate to fluid volume deficit?.

Needed Info: Pyloric stenosis: obstruction of the sphincter between stomach and duodenum. Onset: within 2 months of birth. S/S: vomiting that becomes projectile. Treatment: surgery. Nursing responsibilities: small frequent feedings with glucose water or electrolyte solutions 4–6 hrs post-op. Small frequent feedings with formula 24 hrs post-op.

Category: Data Collection/Physiological Integrity/Physiological Adaptation

(1) The infant eagerly accepts feedings—may vomit after eating

(2) The infant vomited once since admission—don't assume will continue to vomit

(3) The infant's skin is warm and moist—normal; would be cool and dry with fluid volume deficit

(4) The infant's anterior fontanel is depressed—CORRECT: indicates dehydration

123. The Answer is 1

The LPN/LVN cares for a 4-year-old diagnosed with a fractured pelvis due to an auto accident. The LPN/LVN prepares the child for the application of a hip spica cast. It is *MOST* important for the LPN/LVN to take which of the following actions?

Reworded Question: How do you prepare a 4-year-old for the procedure?

Strategy: "*MOST* important" indicates that discrimination is required to answer the question.

Needed Info: Spica cast immobilizes the hip and knee. Preschool children (age 36 months to 6 years) fear injury, mutilation, and punishment; allow child to play with models of equipment; encourage expression of feelings.

Category: Planning/Health Promotion and Maintenance

(1) Obtain a doll with a hip spica cast in place—CORRECT: preschoolers need to see and play with dolls and equipment; explain procedure in simple terms and explain how it will affect the child

(2) Tell the child that the cast will feel cold when it is put on her skin—may feel a warm or burning sensation under cast while it dries due to chemical reaction between the plaster and the water

(3) Reassure the child that the cast application is painless—will be placed on special cast table that holds the child's body; turning to apply the cast may be painful

(4) Introduce the child to another child who has a hip spica cast—more important to allow child to play with doll with a hip spica cast; viewing the cast may be frightening

124. The Answer is 2

A woman comes to the clinic because she thinks she is pregnant. Tests are performed and the pregnancy is confirmed. The client's last menstrual period began on September 8 and lasted for 6 days. The LPN/LVN calculates that her expected date of confinement (EDC) is which of the following?

Reworded Question: How do you calculate the EDC?

Strategy: Perform the calculation required and check for math errors!

Needed Info: EDC or estimated date of delivery (EDD): calculated according to Nägele's rule (first day of the last normal menstrual period minus 3 months plus 7 days and 1 year). Assumes that every woman has a 28-day cycle and pregnancy occurred on 14th day. Most women deliver within a period extending from 7 days before to 7 days after the EDC.

Category: Implementation/Health Promotion and Maintenance

(1) May 15—too early

(2) June 15—CORRECT September 8 minus 3 months = June 8 plus 7 days plus one year = June 15 of next year

(3) June 21—EDC is calculated from first, not last day, of last normal menstrual period

(4) July 8—not accurate

125. The Answer is 3

A 2-month-old infant is brought to the pediatrician's office for a well-baby visit. During the examination, congenital subluxation of the left hip is suspected. The LPN/LVN would expect to see which of the following symptoms?

Reworded Question: What will you see with congenital hip dislocation?

Strategy: Form a mental image of the deformity.

Needed Info: Subluxation: most common type of congenital hip dislocation. Head of femur remains in contact with acetabulum but is partially displaced. Diagnosed in infant less than 4 weeks old S/S: unlevel gluteal folds, limited abduction of hip, shortened femur affected side, Ortolani's sign (click). Treatment: abduction splint, hip spica cast, Bryant's traction, open reduction.

Category: Data Collection/Health Promotion and Maintenance

(1) Lengthening of the limb on the affected side—inaccurate

(2) Deformities of the foot and ankle—inaccurate

(3) Asymmetry of the gluteal and thigh folds—CORRECT: restricted movement on affected side

(4) Plantar flexion of the foot—seen with clubfoot

126. The Answer is 4

After completing data collection, the LPN/LVN observes that a client is exhibiting early symptoms of a dystonic reaction related to the use of an antipsychotic medication. Which of the following actions by the LPN/LVN would be *MOST* appropriate?

Reworded Question: What is the first thing you do for a client with a dystonic reaction?

Strategy: Set priorities. Remember Maslow's hierarchy of needs.

Needed Info: Dystonic reaction: muscle tightness in throat, neck, tongue, mouth, eyes, neck, and back; difficulty talking and swallowing. Treatment: IM or IV Benadryl or Cogentin.

Category: Implementation/Psychosocial Integrity

(1) Reality test with the client and assure her that her physical symptoms are not real—real symptoms, not delusions

(2) Teach the client about common side effects of antipsychotic medications—physical needs highest priority

(3) Explain to the client that there is no treatment that will relieve these symptoms—Benadryl used IM or IV

(4) Notify the physician and obtain an order for IM Benadryl—CORRECT: emergency situation, can occlude airway

127. The Answer is 1

The LPN/LVN is preparing to perform mouth care for an unconscious client. Which of the following actions should the LPN/LVN take *FIRST*?

Reworded Question: Before initiating any care or procedure, what should the LPN/LVN do first to provide for client safety?

Strategy: Think ABCs when identifying first nursing action.

Needed Info: An unconscious client cannot protect himself from injury. Consider the ABCs. Sims' position: lying on left side with right knee and thigh drawn up to the chest. Gag reflex: prevents aspiration of secretions and food/fluid/objects.

Category: Data Collection/Physiological Integrity/Basic Care and Comfort

(1) Assess for the presence of a gag reflex—CORRECT: the LPN/LVN is responsible for determining if the client can clear his own airway or is at risk for occlusion or aspiration

(2) Place the client into Sims' position—an accurate position for mouth care for this client, but not the initial step

(3) Separate the teeth with a padded tongue blade—nothing should be used to separate the teeth; would likely lead to tooth damage

(4) Suction secretions from the oral cavity—an accurate procedural step that should occur after the client's gag reflex is determined

128. The Answer is 1

As a client nears death, the client's husband says, "I wish I could do something for her." Which of the following responses by the LPN/LVN is *MOST* appropriate?

Reworded Question: What is the most therapeutic communication for the husband?

Strategy: Think about the husband's need to help his wife.

Needed Info: End-of-life research: last of the senses of a dying person is believed to be hearing, reports of survivors support the reassurance they felt from the words of the caregivers present. Therapeutic communication: supports inclusion of significant others, supports "hope" or "usefulness" on the part of significant others.

Category: Evaluation/Psychosocial Integrity

(1) "It may be comforting to your wife if you talk to her calmly and clearly."—CORRECT: the client may actually hear her husband's communications; the husband is offered something to do that may be helpful to both the client and the spouse

(2) "Your wife does not know that you are here, but you can sit here with her."—the client may be aware that her husband is there, and it is nontherapeutic to exclude the husband from offering comfort

(3) "Unfortunately, there is little that you can do at this point."—it is nontherapeutic to exclude the husband from offering comfort

(4) "Why don't you take a break? It is just a matter of time now."—it is nontherapeutic to exclude the husband from offering comfort

129. The Answer is 4

The LPN/LVN provides care to clients in a long-term care facility. Four meal choices are available to the clients. The LPN/LVN should ensure that a client on a low-cholesterol diet receives which of the following meals?

Reworded Question: What should a client on a low-cholesterol diet eat?

Strategy: Remember which foods are part of a low-cholesterol diet.

Needed Info: Low-cholesterol diet should reduce total fat to 20–25% of total calories and reduce the ingestion of saturated fat. Carbohydrates (especially complex carbohydrates) should be 55–60% of calories. High-cholesterol foods: eggs, dairy products, meat, fish, shellfish, poultry.

Category: Implementation/Physiological Integrity/Basic Care and Comfort

(1) Egg custard and boiled liver—high amounts of cholesterol

(2) Fried chicken and potatoes—avoid fried foods

(3) Hamburger and french fries—avoid fried foods

(4) Grilled flounder and green beans—CORRECT: fish instead of meat; increase vegetables

130. The Answer is 465

The LPN/LVN removes a client's breakfast tray and notes that the client consumed 4 oz. of pudding, 4 oz. of gelatin, 6 ½ oz. of tea, and 5 oz. of apple juice. How many milliliters should the LPN/LVN record for the client's breakfast intake?

Reworded Question: Calculate the client's oral fluid intake in mL.

Strategy: Remember what is considered oral fluid intake.

Needed Info: Oral fluid intake: any liquid or food in more solid form that melts at room temperature.

Category: Data Collection/Physiological Integrity/Basic Care and Comfort

The calculation is 4 oz. gelatin + 6½ oz. of tea + 5 oz. of apple juice = 15½ oz. × 30 mL = 465 mL. Pudding does not melt at room temperature, so is not considered to be a liquid and therefore it is not included in the calculation.

The correct answer is 465.

131. The Answer is 2

The LPN/LVN cares for a client diagnosed with cholecystitis. The client says to the LPN/LVN, "I don't understand why my right shoulder hurts when the gallbladder is not by my shoulder!" Which of the following responses by the LPN/LVN is *BEST*?

Reworded Question: Why does the client's shoulder hurt?

Strategy: "*BEST*" indicates discrimination is required to answer the question.

Needed Info: Cholecystitis is inflammation of the gallbladder; indications include intolerance to fatty foods, indigestion, severe pain in right upper quadrant of abdomen radiating to back and right shoulder; leukocytosis, and diaphoresis.

Category: Implementation/Physiological Integrity/Physiological Adaptation

(1) "Sometimes small pieces of the gallstones break off and travel to other parts of the body."—gallstones do not become emboli

(2) "There is an invisible connection between the gallbladder and the right shoulder."—CORRECT: describes referred pain; when visceral branch of a pain receptor fiber is stimulated, vasodilation and pain may occur in a distant body area; right shoulder or scapula is the referred pain site for gallbladder

(3) "The gallbladder is on the right side of the body and so is that shoulder."—anatomically correct but is not the best explanation

(4) "Your shoulder became tense because you were guarding against the gallbladder pain."—possible; not the best explanation

132. The Answer is 4

A woman comes to the clinic at 32 weeks' gestation. A diagnosis of pregnancy-induced hypertension (PIH) is made. The LPN/LVN reinforces teaching performed by the RN. Which of the following statements by the client indicates that further teaching is required?

Reworded Question: What is not accurate about the care of a woman with PIH?

Strategy: This is a negative question. Look for incorrect information.

Needed Info: PIH, preeclampsia, toxemia: development of hypertension (increase 30 mmHg systolic or 15 mmHg diastolic) with proteinuria and/or edema (dependent or facial) after 20 weeks' gestation. Risk factors: parity (first-time mothers), age (younger than 20 or older than 35), geographic location (southern or western U.S.), multifetal gestation, hydatidiform mole, hypertension, and diabetes. Prevention: early prenatal care, identify high risk clients, recognize S/S early; bed rest lying on L side, daily weights. Treatment: urine checks for proteinuria; diet (increased protein and decreased Na^+). Can develop into eclampsia (convulsions or coma).

Category: Evaluation/Health Promotion and Maintenance

(1) "Lying in bed on my left side is likely to increase my urinary output."—true; bed rest promotes good perfusion of blood to uterus; decreases BP and promotes diuresis

(2) "If the bed rest works, I may lose a pound or two in the next few days."—true; causes diuresis; results in reduction of retained fluids; instruct to monitor weight daily and notify physician if notices abrupt increase even after resting in bed for 12 hrs

(3) "I should be sure to maintain a diet that has a good amount of protein."—true; replaces protein

lost in urine; increases plasma colloid osmotic pressure; avoid salty foods; avoid alcohol; drink 8 glasses of water daily; eat foods high in roughage

(4) "I will have to keep my room darkened and not watch much television."—CORRECT: incorrect info, not necessary; diversional activities helpful

133. The Answer is 4

The LPN/LVN collects data about a client's fluid balance. Which of the following findings *MOST* accurately indicates to the LPN/LVN that the client has retained fluid during the previous 24 hours?

Reworded Question: How can the LPN/LVN most accurately determine fluid retention?

Strategy: Look at the most conclusive means of determining fluid retention.

Needed Info: Means of evaluating fluid retention: recording fluid intake and output; determining areas of edema especially the sacrum, feet, and ankles; listening for wet lung sounds; and measuring short-term weight gain. Weight gain: most objective and accurate. Weight gain of 1 kilogram is equivalent to 1 liter of fluid.

Category: Data Collection/Physiological Integrity/Basic Care and Comfort

(1) Edema is found in both ankles—unable to consistently quantify this form of data

(2) Fluid intake is equal to fluid output—this is normal but does not account for insensible fluid loss through the skin and lungs

(3) Intake of fluid exceeds output by 200 mL—provides information, but does not eliminate the possibility of error recording all intake and output

(4) Weight gain of 4 pounds is noted—CORRECT: identifies fluid retention in a factual, accurate method and is unlikely to represent a gain of actual body substance (muscle or fat) in a 24-hour time frame

134. The Answer is 4

The LPN/LVN cares for a group of residents in a dependent-living facility. The LPN/LVN determines which of the following clients is *MOST* at risk to develop pneumonia?

Reworded Question: Who is most likely to develop pneumonia?

Strategy: Think about each answer.

Needed Info: Pneumonia is an inflammatory process that results in edema of lung tissues and extravasion of fluid into alveoli, causing hypoxia; symptoms include fever, leukocytosis, productive cough, dyspnea, and pleuritic pain.

Category: Evaluation/Health Promotion and Maintenance

(1) A 72-year-old female with left-sided hemiparesis after a cerebrovascular accident—advanced age is a risk factor, left-sided hemiparesis may affect inspiratory response

(2) A 76-year-old male with a history of hypertension and type 2 diabetes—age is a risk factor

(3) An 80-year-old female who walks 1 mile every day and has a history of depression—age is a risk factor

(4) An 87-year-old male who smokes and has a history of lung cancer—CORRECT: advanced age, smoking, underlying lung disease, malnutrition, and bedridden status are risk factors for development of pneumonia

135. The Answer is 2

The LPN/LVN is caring for a client diagnosed with bipolar disorder. Which of the following behaviors by the client indicates that a manic episode is subsiding?

Reworded Question: What indicates normalizing behavior?

Strategy: Think about the behaviors that indicate mania.

Needed Info: Manic clients may tease, talk, and joke excessively, usually cannot sit to eat and may need to carry fluids and food around in order to eat, often try to take a leadership position in an environment, and try to engage others.

Category: Data Collection/Psychosocial Integrity

(1) The client tells several jokes at a group meeting—reflects an elated mood and no real participation in the meeting; manic clients may tease, talk, and joke excessively

(2) The client sits and talks with other clients at mealtimes—CORRECT: manic clients have difficulty socializing because of flight of ideas and intrusiveness; usually cannot sit to eat and will carry fluids and food around

(3) The client begins to write a book about his life—manic clients often write voluminously; may help to express feelings, but does not reflect improvement, especially if thoughts are grandiose

(4) The client initiates an effort to start a radio station on the unit—manic clients often try to take a leadership position in an environment and try to recruit others

136. The Answer is 2

A mother brings her 4-year-old daughter to the pediatrician for treatment of chronic otitis media. The mother asks the LPN/LVN how she can prevent her child from getting ear infections so often. The LPN/LVN's response should be based on an understanding that the recurrence of otitis media can be decreased by which of the following?

Reworded Question: What will prevent the development of otitis media? What causes otitis media?

Strategy: Think about the causes of otitis media.

Needed Info: Otitis media: frequently follows respiratory infection; reduce occurrence by holding child upright for feedings, encourage gentle nose-blowing, teach modified Valsava maneuver (pinch nose, close lips and force air up through eustachian tubes), blow up balloons or chew gum, eliminate tobacco smoke or known allergens.

Category: Planning/Health Promotion and Maintenance

(1) Cover the child's ears while bathing—does not prevent otitis media

(2) Treat upper respiratory infections quickly—CORRECT: respiratory fluids are a medium for bacteria; antihistamines used

(3) Administer nose drops at bedtime—not preventative

(4) Isolate her child from other children—too extreme a measure

137. The Answer is 2

A man calls the Suicide Prevention Hotline and states that he is going to kill himself. Which of the following questions should the LPN/LVN ask *FIRST*?

Reworded Question: What is most important to know about a client who has threatened to kill himself?

Strategy: *"FIRST"* indicates priority.

Needed Info: Signs of suicide: symptoms of depression, client gives away possessions, gets finances in order, has a means, makes direct or indirect statements, leaves notes, increase in energy. Predisposing factors: male over age 50, teenagers between 15–19, poor social attachments, clients with previous attempts, clients with auditory hallucinations, overwhelming precipitating events (terminal disease, death or loss of loved one, failure at school, job).

Category: Data Collection/Psychosocial Integrity

(1) "What happened to cause you to want to end your life?"—does not determine immediate need for safety

(2) "How do you plan to kill yourself?"—CORRECT: lets you prioritize interventions to assure safety

(3) "When did you start to feel as though you wanted to die?"—does not determine immediate need for safety

(4) "Do you want me to prevent you from killing yourself?"—yes/no question, closed

138. The Answer is 2

Prior to the client undergoing a scheduled intravenous pyelogram (IVP), it would be *MOST* important for the LPN/LVN to ask which of the following questions?

Reworded Question: What do you need to know before an IVP?

Strategy: Think about each answer and how it relates to IVP.

Needed Info: IVP: radiopaque dye injected into the body and is filtered through the kidneys and excreted by the urinary tract. Visualizes kidneys, ureters, and bladder. Preparation: NPO midnight, cathartics evening before test. Injection of dye causes flushing of face, nausea, salty taste in mouth.

Category: Data Collection/Physiological Integrity/Reduction of Risk Potential

(1) "Do you have difficulty voiding?"—not most important

(2) "Do you have any allergies to shellfish or iodine?"—CORRECT: anaphylactic reaction; itching, hives, wheezing; treatment: antihistamines, O_2, CPR, epinephrine, vasopressor

(3) "Do you have a history of constipation?"—not essential info

(4) "Do you have frequent headaches?"—not most important

139. The Answer is 3

The LPN/LVN is assigned to a newly admitted elderly client in the hospital setting who states that she has no living relatives and only friends of her own age. One of the LPN/LVN's most immediate considerations for this client will be to help the RN implement which of the following?

Reworded Question: Given the information provided, what is a priority for this client?

Strategy: Look for the answer that addresses this client's individualized needs/situation.

Needed Info: Client lengths of stay are very short. Likely that this elderly client does not have anyone to assist with care or activities of daily living (ADLs) if needed upon discharge. Discharge planning: begins upon admission for all hospitalized clients. Concept map: a conceptual plan that integrates nursing care. Critical pathway: multidisciplinary plan for clinical interventions during hospitalization. Utilization group: classifies clients by disease or injury.

Category: Implementation/Safe and Effective Care Environment/Coordinated Care

(1) A concept map—a plan of care is necessary for every client

(2) A critical pathway—addresses only the acute-care stay

(3) A discharge plan—CORRECT: will provide for the appropriate support this client needs to return to the community or transfer to another level of care

(4) A utilization group—not an important consideration for this client

140. The Answer is 3

A woman delivers a 6 lb. 10 oz. baby girl. The mother observes the LPN/LVN in the delivery room place drops in her daughter's eyes. The mother asks the LPN/LVN why this was done. Which of the following responses by the LPN/LVN is *BEST*?

Reworded Question: Why are eyedrops placed in a newborn's eyes?

Strategy: "*BEST*" indicates that discrimination may be required to answer the question.

Needed Info: Prophylactic care of newborns includes administration of vitamin K to prevent hemorrhage; erythromycin and tetracycline are used for prophylactic eye care.

Category: Implementation/Health Promotion and Maintenance

(1) "The drops constrict your baby's pupils to prevent injury."—erythromycin or tetracycline do not cause myosis

(2) "The drops will remove mucus from your baby's eyes."—does not remove mucus from baby's eyes

(3) "The drops will prevent infections that might cause blindness."—CORRECT: precaution against opthalmia neonatorum (inflammation of the eyes due to gonorrheal or chlamydia infection)

(4) "The drops will prevent neonatal conjunctivitis."—conjunctivitis is inflammation of the conjunctiva

141. The Answer is 3

The LPN/LVN cares for a client admitted for a possible herniated intervertebral disk. Ibuprofen (Motrin), propoxyphene hydrochloride (Darvon), and cyclobenzaprine hydrochloride (Flexeril) are ordered PRN. Several hours after admission, the client complains of pain. Which of the following actions should the LPN/LVN take *FIRST*?

Reworded Question: What should you do first?

Strategy: Set priorities. Collect data before implementing.

Needed Info: Herniated disk: knifelike pain aggravated by sneezing, coughing, straining.

Category: Planning/Physiological Integrity/Pharmacological Therapies

(1) Administer ibuprofen (Motrin)—implementation; not first step

(2) Call the physician to determine which medication should be given—collect data before implementing

(3) Gather more information from the client about the complaint—CORRECT: collect data; first step in nursing process

(4) Allow the client some time to rest to see if the pain subsides—implementation; not first step

142. The Answer is 4

The LPN/LVN is completing a client's preoperative checklist prior to an early morning surgery. The nurse obtains the client's vital signs: temperature 97.4° F (36° C), radial pulse 84 strong and regular, respirations 16 and unlabored, and blood pressure 132/74. Which of the following actions should the LPN/LVN take *FIRST*?

Reworded Question: What should you do for a client with normal vital signs?

Strategy: Identify normal serum electrolyte values.

Needed Info: Normal electrolyte values (range may vary by laboratory): Na^+ (sodium) 135–145 mEq/L, K^+ (potassium) 3.6–5.4, Cl^- (chloride) 96–106 mEq/L, mEq/L = milliequivalents per liter.

Category: Data Collection/Physiological Integrity/ Reduction of Risk Potential

(1) Notify the physician of the client's vital signs—most physicians do not want to be notified about normal values

(2) Obtain orthostatic blood pressures lying and standing—there is no information to support this action

(3) Lower the side rails and place the bed in its lowest position—bed side rails should be raised, not lowered

(4) Record the data on the client's preoperative checklist—CORRECT: the vital signs are normal and should be recorded in the client's medical record

143. The Answer is 3

The LPN/LVN expects to see which of the following physiological changes in a client experiencing an episode of acute pain?

Reworded Question: What happens to the vital signs when a client is in pain?

Strategy: Think about the cause of each vital sign change. Is it consistent with pain?

Needed Info: Pain causes increased blood pressure and heart rate, which leads to increased blood flow to the brain and muscles; rapid irregular respirations lead to increased oxygen supply to brain and muscles; increased perspiration removes excessive body heat; increased pupillary diameter leads to increased eye accommodation to light.

Category: Data Collection/Physiological Integrity/Physiological Adaptation

(1) Decreased blood pressure—blood pressure increases to enhance alertness to threats

(2) Decreased heart rate—heart rate increases

(3) Decreased skin temperature—CORRECT: skin cools due to diaphoresis

(4) Decreased respirations—respirations increase

144. The Answer is 4

A client is transferred to an extended-care facility following a cerebrovascular accident (CVA). The client has right-sided paralysis and has been experiencing dysphagia. The LPN/LVN observes an aide preparing the client to eat lunch. Which of the following situations would require an intervention by the LPN/LVN?

Reworded Question: What option is wrong?

Strategy: This is a negative question. Determine if you are looking for a correct situation, or a problematic situation.

Needed Info: Dysphagia: difficulty swallowing. Provide support if necessary for the head, have the client sit upright, feed the client slowly in small amounts, place food on unaffected side of mouth. Maintain upright position for 30–45 minutes after eating. Good oral care after eating.

Category: Evaluation/Physiological Integrity/Reduction of Risk Potential

(1) The client is in bed in high Fowler's position—correct positioning, or may sit in chair

(2) The client's head and neck are positioned slightly forward—correct positioning; helps client chew and swallow

(3) The aide puts the food in the back of the client's mouth on the unaffected side—helps client handle food

(4) The aide waters down the pudding to help the client swallow—CORRECT: requires intervention, usually able to better handle soft or semi-soft foods; difficulty with liquids

145. The Answer is 2, 3, 4

During the LPN/LVN's morning data collection, a client's blood pressure is 146/92 with labored respirations of 24. There is red drainage on the client's IV dressing, and the client complains of pain in the left hip, depression, and hunger. The LPN/LVN identifies which of the following as subjective data? **Select all that apply.**

Reworded Question: What data have been reported by the client?

Strategy: Look for client-reported data.

Needed Info: Subjective data: client's perceptions. Objective data: information perceptible to the senses (sight, hearing, touch, smell, taste) or measurable data.

Category: Data Collection/Safe and Effective Care Environment/Coordinated Care

(1) Blood pressure—measurable objective data

(2) Depression—CORRECT: client-reported data

(3) Hip pain—CORRECT: client-reported data

(4) Hunger—CORRECT: client-reported data

(5) IV drainage—measurable objective data

(6) Respirations—measurable objective data

PART 3

NCLEX-PN®
EXAM RESOURCES

CHART OF CRITICAL THINKING PATHS

The chart on the reverse side of this page illustrates different paths you must choose from in order to correctly answer NCLEX-PN® exam test questions. The stepping stones stand for steps that you must follow in order to find the correct answer for that question type. Refer to Part 1, if necessary, to refresh your memory with respect to the various steps for each type of question. Tear out this page and use the chart to practice using this book's strategies when answering practice NCLEX-PN® exam-style questions.

Critical Thinking Paths to Correct Answers on the NCLEX-PN® Exam

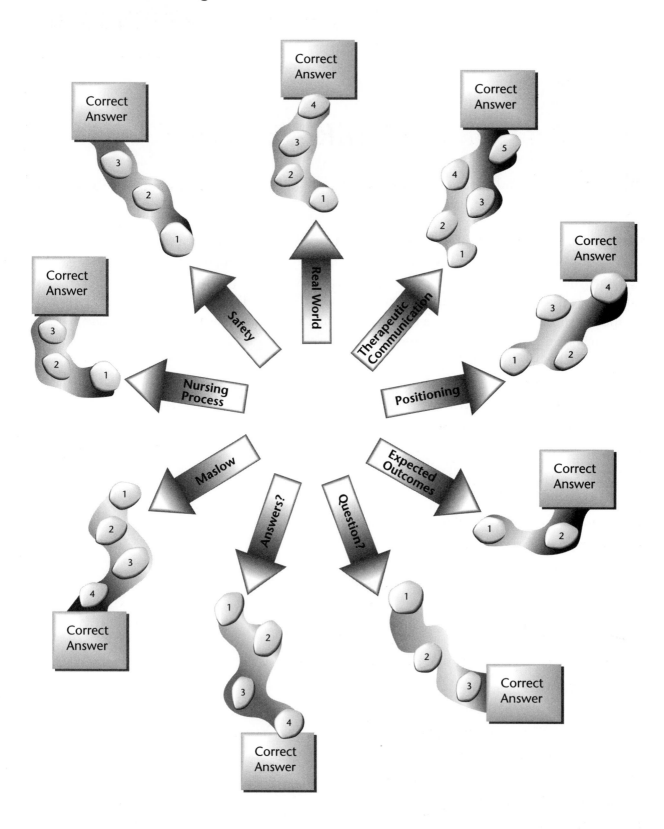

NURSING TERMINOLOGY

abduction – to move away from the midline

abraded – scraped

acetonuria – acetone in the urine

adduction – to move toward the midline

afebrile – without fever

albuminuria – albumin in the urine

ambulatory – walking

amenorrhea – absence of menstruation

amnesia – loss of or defective memory

ankyloses – stiff joint

anorexia – loss of appetite

anuria – total suppression of urination

apnea – short periods when breathing has ceased

arthritis – inflammation of joint

asphyxia – suffocation

atrophy – wasting

auscultation, auscultate – to listen for sounds

bradycardia – heart rate lower than 60 beats per minute

Cheyne-Stokes respirations – increasing dyspnea with periods of apnea

choluria – bile in the urine

clonic tremor – shaking with intervals of rest

conjunctivitis – inflammation of conjunctiva

coryza – watery drainage from nose

cyanotic – bluish in color due to poor oxygenation

defecation – bowel movement

dental caries – decay of the teeth

dentures – false teeth

diarrhea – excessive or frequent defecation

diplopia – double vision

distended – appears swollen

diuresis – large amount of urine voided

dorsal recumbent – lying on back, knees flexed and apart

dysmenorrhea – painful menstruation

dyspnea – difficulty breathing

dysrhythmia, arrhythmia – abnormal heartbeat

dysuria – painful urination

edematous – puffy, swollen

emaciated – thin, underweight

emetic – agent given to produce vomiting

enuresis – bed-wetting

epistaxis – nosebleed

eructation – belching

erythema – redness

eupnea – normal breathing

excoriation – raw surface

exophthalmos – abnormal protrusion of eyeball

extension – to straighten

fatigued – tired

feigned – pretended

fetid – foul

fixed – motionless

flaccid – soft, flabby

flatus, flatulence – gas in the digestive tract

flexion – bending

flushed – pink or hot

Fowler's position – semierect, knees flexed, head of bed elevated 45–60 degrees

gavage – forced feeding through a tube passed into the stomach

glossy – shiny

glycosuria – glucose in the urine

gustatory – dealing with taste

heliotherapy – using sunlight as a therapeutic agent

hematemesis – blood in vomitus

hematuria – blood in the urine

hemiplegia – paralysis of one side of the body

hemoglobinuria – hemoglobin in the urine

hemoptysis – spitting of blood

horizontal – flat

hydrotherapy – using water as a therapeutic agent

hyperpnea – rapid breathing

hypertonic – concentration greater than body fluids

hypotonic – concentration less than body fluids

infrequent – not often

insomnia – inability to sleep

instillation – pouring into a body cavity

intermittent – starting and stopping, not continuous

intradermal – within or through the skin

intramuscular – within or through the muscle

intraspinal – within or through the spinal canal

intravenous – within or through the vein

involuntary, incontinent – unable to control bladder or bowels

isotonic – having the same tonicity or concentration as body fluids

jackknife position – prone with hips over break in table and feet below level of head

jaundice – yellow color

knee-chest position – in face-down position resting on knees and chest

kyphosis – humpback, concavity of spine

labored – difficult, requires an effort

lacerated – torn, broken

lateral position – on the side, knees flexed

lithotomy position – on the back, buttocks near edge of table, knees well flexed and separated

lochia – drainage from the vagina after delivery

lordosis – sway-back, convexity of spine

manipulation, manipulate – to handle

menopause – cessation of menstruation

menorrhagia – profuse menstruation

metrorrhagia – variable amount of uterine bleeding occurring frequently but at irregular intervals

moist – wet

monoplegia – paralysis of one limb

mucopurulent – drainage containing mucus and pus

mydriasis – dilation of pupil

myopia – nearsightedness

myosis – contraction of pupil

nausea – desire to vomit

necrosis – death of tissue

nocturia – frequently voiding at night

obese – overweight

objective – able to document by other than observation

oliguria – scant urination, less than 400 mL per 24 hrs.

orthopnea – inability to breathe or difficulty breathing while lying down

palliative – offering temporary relief

pallor – white

palpation, palpate – to feel with hands or fingers

paraplegia – paralysis of legs

paroxysm – spasm or convulsive seizure

paroxysmal – coming in seizures

pediculi, pediculosis – lice

percussion, percuss – to strike

persistent – lasting over a long time

petechia – small rupture of blood vessels

photophobia – sensitive to light

photosensitivity – skin reaction caused by exposure to sunlight

pigmented – containing color

polyuria – increased amount of voiding

profuse, copious – large amount

projectile – ejected or projected some distance

pronation – turning downward

prone – on abdomen, face turned to one side

prophylactic – preventative

protruding – extending outward

pruritus – itching

ptosis – drooping eyelid

purulent – drainage containing pus

pyrexia – elevated temperature

pyuria – pus in the urine

radiating – spreading to distant areas

radiotherapy – using X-ray or radium as a therapeutic agent

rales, crackles – abnormal breath sounds

rapid – quickly

rotation – to move in circular pattern

sanguineous – bloody drainage

scanty – small amount

semi-Fowler's position – semi-erect, head of bed elevated 30–45 degrees

serous – drainage of lymphatic fluid

Sims' position – on left side, left arm behind back, left leg slightly flexed, right leg slightly flexed

sprain – wrenching of a joint

stertorous – snoring

stethoscope – instrument used for auscultation

strabismus – squinting

stuporous – partial unconsciousness

subcutaneous – under the skin

subjective – observed

sudden onset – started all at once

superficial – on the surface only

supination – turning upward

suppurating – discharging pus

syncope – fainting

syndrome – group of symptoms

tachycardia – fast heartbeat, greater than 100 beats per minute

tenacious – tough and sticky

thready – barely perceptible

tonic tremor – continuous shaking

Trendelenburg position – flat on back with pelvis higher than head, foot of bed elevated six inches

tympanic – filled with gas

urticaria – hives or wheals, eruption on skin or mucous membranes

vertigo – dizziness

vesicle – fluid-filled blister

visual acuity – sharpness of vision

void, micturate – to urinate or pass urine

COMMON MEDICAL ABBREVIATIONS

ABC – airway, breathing, circulation

abd. – abdomen

ABG – arterial blood gas

ABO – system of classifying blood groups

ac – before meals

ACE – angiotensin-converting enzyme

ACS – acute compartment syndrome

ACTH – adrenocorticotrophic hormone

ad lib – freely, as desired

ADH – antidiuretic hormone

ADL – activities of daily living

AFP – alpha-fetoprotein

AIDS – acquired immunodeficiency syndrome

AKA – above-the-knee amputation

ALL – acute lymphocytic leukemia

ALP – alkaline phosphatase

ALS – amyotrophic lateral sclerosis

ALT – alkaline phosphatase (formerly SGPT)

AMI – antibody-mediated immunity

AML – acute myelogenous leukemia

amt. – amount

ANA – antinuclear antibody

ANS – autonomic nervous system

AP – anteroposterior

A&P – anterior and posterior

APC – atrial premature contraction

aq. – water

ARDS – adult respiratory distress syndrome

ASD – atrial septal defect

ASHD – atherosclerotic heart disease

AST – aspartate aminotransferase (formerly SGOT)

ATP – adenosine triphosphate

AV – atrioventricular

BCG – Bacille Calmette-Guerin

bid – two times a day

BKA – below-the-knee amputation

BLS – basic life support

BMR – basal metabolic rate

BP – blood pressure

BPH – benign prostatic hypertrophy

bpm – beats per minute

BPR – bathroom privileges

BSA – body surface area

BUN – blood, urea, nitrogen

C – centigrade, Celsius

$\bar{\text{c}}$ – with

Ca – calcium

CA – cancer

CABG – coronary artery bypass graft

CAD – coronary artery disease

CAL – chronic airflow limitations

CAPD – continuous ambulatory peritoneal dialysis

caps – capsules

CBC – complete blood count

CC – chief complaint

cc – cubic centimeter

CCU – coronary care unit, critical care unit

CDC – Centers for Disease Control and Prevention

CHF – congestive heart failure

CK – creatine kinase

Cl – chloride

CLL – chronic lymphocytic leukemia

cm – centimeter

CMV – cytomegalovirus

CNS – central nervous system

CO – carbon monoxide, cardiac output

CO₂ – carbon dioxide

comp – compound

cont – continuous

COPD – chronic obstructive pulmonary disease

CP – cerebral palsy

CPAP – continuous positive airway pressure

CPK – creatine phosphokinase

CPR – cardiopulmonary resuscitation

CRP – C-reactive protein

C&S – culture and sensitivity

CSF – cerebrospinal fluid

CT – computerized tomography

CTD – connective tissue disease

CTS – carpal tunnel syndrome

cu – cubic

CVA – cerebrovascular accident or costovertebral angle

CVC – central venous catheter

CVP – central venous pressure

D&C – dilation and curettage

DC – discontinue

DCBE – double-contrast barium enema

DIC – disseminated intravascular coagulation

DIFF – differential blood count

dil. – dilute

DJD – degenerative joint disease

DKA – diabetic ketoacidosis

dL, dl – deciliter (100 mL)

DM – diabetes mellitus

DNA – deoxyribonucleic acid

DNR – do not resuscitate

DO – doctor of osteopathy

DOE – dyspnea on exertion

DPT – vaccine for diphtheria, pertussis, tetanus

Dr. – doctor

DRE – digital rectal exam

DVT – deep vein thrombosis

D/W – dextrose in water

Dx – diagnosis

ECF – extracellular fluid

ECG, EKG – electrocardiogram

ECT – electroconvulsive therapy

ED – emergency department

EEG – electroencephalogram

EMD – electromechanical dissociation

EMG – electromyography

ENT – ear, nose, and throat

ERCP – endoscopic retrograde cholangiopancreatography

ESR – erythrocyte sedimentation rate

ESRD – end-stage renal disease

ET – endotracheal tube

F – Fahrenheit

FBD – fibrocystic breast disease

FBS – fasting blood sugar

FDA – U.S. Food and Drug Administration

FFP – fresh frozen plasma

FHR – fetal heart rate

FHT – fetal heart tone

fl – fluid

FOBT – fecal occult blood test

4 × 4 – piece of gauze 4 inches by 4 inches; used for dressings

FSH – follicle-stimulating hormone

ft. – foot, feet (unit of measure)

FUO – fever of undetermined origin

g, gm – gram

GB – gallbladder

GCS – Glasgow coma scale

GFR – glomerular filtration rate

GH – growth hormone

GI – gastrointestinal

gr – grain

gtt – drops

GU – genitourinary

GYN – gynecological

h, hrs – hour, hours

(H) – hypodermically

Hb, Hgb – hemoglobin

HCG – human chorionic gonadotropin

HCO$_3$ – bicarbonate

Hct – hematocrit

HD – hemodialysis

HDL – high-density lipoprotein

Hg – mercury

Hgb – hemoglobin

HGH – human growth hormone

HHNK – hyperglycemia hyperosmolar nonketotic coma

HIV – human immunodeficiency virus

HLA – human leukocyte antigen

H$_2$O – water

HR – heart rate

HSV – herpes simplex virus

HTN – hypertension

Hx – history

Hz – hertz (cycles/second)

IAPB – intra-aortic balloon pump

IBBP – intermittent positive pressure breathing

IBS – irritable bowel syndrome

ICF – intracellular fluid

ICP – increased intracranial pressure

ICS – intercostal space

ICU – intensive care unit

I&D – incision and drainage

IDDM – insulin-dependent diabetes mellitus (type 1)

IgA – immunoglobulin A

IM – intramuscular

I&O – intake and output

IOP – increased intraocular pressure

IPG – impedance plethysmogram

IPPB – intermittent positive-pressure breathing

IUD – intrauterine device

IV – intravenous

IVC – intraventricular catheter

IVP – intravenous pyelogram or intravenous pyelography

JRA – juvenile rheumatoid arthritis

K⁺ – potassium

kcal – kilocalorie (food calorie)

kg – kilogram

KO, KVO – keep vein open

KS – Kaposi's sarcoma

KUB – kidneys, ureters, bladder

L, l – liter

lab – laboratory

lb. – pound

LBBB – left bundle branch block

LDH – lactate dehydrogenase

LDL – low-density lipoprotein

LE – lupus erythematosus

LH – luteinizing hormone

liq – liquid

LLQ – left lower quadrant

LOC – level of consciousness

LP – lumbar puncture

LPN, LVN – licensed practical nurse; licensed vocational nurse

Lt, lt – left

LTC – long-term care

LUQ – left upper quadrant

LV – left ventricle

m – minum, meter, micron

MAO – monoamine oxidase inhibitor

MAST – military antishock trousers

mcg – microgram

MCH – mean corpuscular hemoglobin

MCV – mean corpuscular volume

MD – muscular dystrophy, medical doctor

MDI – metered dose inhaler

mEq – milliequivalent

mg – milligram

Mg – magnesium

MG – myasthenia gravis

MI – myocardial infarction

mL, ml – milliliter

mm – millimeter

MMR – vaccine for measles, mumps, rubella

MRI – magnetic resonance imaging

MS – multiple sclerosis

N – nitrogen, normal (strength of solution)

NIDDM – non-insulin dependent diabetes mellitus (type 2)

Na⁺ – sodium

NaCl – sodium chloride

NANDA – North American Nursing Diagnosis Association

NG – nasogastric

NGT – nasogastric tube

NLN – National League for Nursing

noc – at night

NPO – nothing by mouth (nil per os)

NS – normal saline

NSAID – nonsteroidal anti-inflammatory drug

NSNA – National Student Nurses' Association

NST – non-stress test

O₂ – oxygen

OB-GYN – obstetrics and gynecology

OCT – oxytocin challenge test

OOB – out of bed

OPC – outpatient clinic

OR – operating room

o̅s – by mouth

OSHA – Occupational Safety and Health Administration

OTC – over-the-counter (drug that can be obtained without a prescription)

oz. – ounce

p̄ – with

P – pulse, pressure, phosphorus

PA Chest – posterior-anterior chest x-ray

PAC – premature atrial complexes

PaCO$_2$ – partial pressure of carbon dioxide in arterial blood

PaO$_2$ – partial pressure of oxygen in arterial blood

PAD – peripheral artery disease

Pap – Papanicolaou smear

pc – after meals

PCA – patient-controlled analgesia

pCO$_2$ – partial pressure of carbon dioxide

PCP – *Pneumocystis carinii* pneumonia

PD – peritoneal dialysis

PE – pulmonary embolism

PEEP – positive end-expiratory pressure

PERRLA – pupils equal, round, react to light and accommodation

PET – postural emission tomography

PFT – pulmonary function test

pH – hydrogen ion concentration

PICC – peripherally inserted central catheter

PID – pelvic inflammatory disease

PKD – polycystic disease

PKU – phenylketonuria

PMS – premenstrual syndrome

PND – paroxysmal nocturnal dyspnea

PO, po – by mouth

pO$_2$ – partial pressure of oxygen

PPD – positive purified protein derivative (of tuberculin)

PPE – personal protective equipment

PPN – partial parenteral nutrition

PRN, prn – as needed, whenever necessary

pro time – prothrombin time

PSA – prostate-specific antigen

psi – pounds per square inch

PSP – phenol-sulfonphthalein

PT – physical therapy, prothrombin time

PTCA – percutaneous transluminal coronary angioplasty

PTH – parathyroid hormone

PTSD – post-traumatic stress disorder

PTT – partial thromboplastin time

PUD – peptic ulcer disease

PVC – premature ventricular contraction

q – every

QA – quality assurance

qh – every hour

q 2 h – every two hours

q 4 h – every four hours

qid – four times a day

qs – quantity sufficient

R – rectal temperature, respirations, roentgen

RA – rheumatoid arthritis

RAI – radioactive iodine

RAIU – radioactive iodine uptake

RAS – reticular activating system

RBBB – right bundle branch block

RBC – red blood cell or red blood count

RCA – right coronary artery

RDA – recommended dietary allowance

resp – respirations

RF – rheumatic fever, rheumatoid factor

Rh – antigen on blood cell indicated by + or –

RIND – reversible ischemic neurologic deficit

RLQ – right lower quadrant

RN – registered nurse

RNA – ribonucleic acid

R/O, r/o – rule out, to exclude

ROM – range of motion (of joint)

Rt, rt – right

RUQ – right upper quadrant

Rx – prescription

$\bar{s}$ – without

S., Sig. – (Signa) to write on label

SA – sinoatrial node

SaO$_2$ – systemic arterial oxygen saturation (%)

sat sol – saturated solution

SBE – subacute bacterial endocarditis

SDA – same-day admission

SDS – same-day surgery

S/E – side effects

sed rate – sedimentation rate

SGOT – serum glutamic-oxaloacetic transaminase (see AST)

SGPT – serum glutamic-pyruvic transaminase (see ALT)

SI – International System of Units

SIADH – syndrome of inappropriate antidiuretic hormone

SIDS – sudden infant death syndrome

SL – sublingual

SLE – systemic lupus erythematosus

SMBG – self-monitoring blood glucose

SMR – submucous resection

SOB – shortness of breath

sol – solution

sp gr – specific gravity

spec. – specimen

$\overline{ss}$ – one half

SS – soapsuds

S/S, s/s – signs and symptoms

SSKI – saturated solution of potassium iodide

stat – immediately

STD – sexually transmitted disease

subcut , SubQ – subcutaneous

sx – symptoms

Syr. – syrup

T – temperature, thoracic (followed by the number designating specific thoracic vertebra)

T&A – tonsillectomy and adenoidectomy

tabs – tablets

TB – tuberculosis

T&C – type and crossmatch

TED – antiembolitic stockings

temp – temperature

TENS – transcutaneous electrical nerve stimulation

TIA – transient ischemic attack

TIBC – total iron binding capacity

tid – three times a day

tinct, tr. – tincture

TLC – total lymphocyte count

TMJ – temporomandibular joint

TPA, t-pa – tissue plasminogen activator

TPN – total parenteral nutrition

TPR – temperature, pulse, respiration

TQM – total quality management

TSE – testicular self-examination

TSH – thyroid-stimulating hormone

tsp. – teaspoon

TSS – toxic shock syndrome

TURP – transurethral prostatectomy

UA – urinalysis

um – unit of measurement

ung – ointment

URI – upper respiratory tract infection

UTI – urinary tract infection

VAD – venous access device

VDRL – Venereal Disease Research Laboratory (test for syphilis)

VF, Vfib – ventricular fibrillation

VPC – ventricular premature complexes

VS, vs – vital signs

VSD – ventricular septal defect

VT – ventricular tachycardia

WBC – white blood cell or white blood count

WHO – World Health Organization

WNL – within normal limits

wt – weight

X PO – 10 grains per orem

STATE LICENSING REQUIREMENTS

Note: State licensing requirements may have changed after this book was published. Contact your state board of nursing for the latest information.

ALABAMA

Board of Nursing
RSA Plaza, Suite 250
770 Washington Avenue
Montgomery, AL 36104
Mailing address:
P.O. Box 303900
Montgomery, AL 36130-3900
Phone: (334) 242-4060
Fax: (334) 242-4360
Website: *www.abn.alabama.gov*

Temporary Permit: 90 days; $50

Licensure Fee/By Examination: $85

Licensure Fee/By Endorsement: $85, plus $3.50 transaction fee

NCLEX-PN® Test Fee: $200

Reexamination Limitations: Must wait 45 days; $85

License Renewal: December 31, every odd year; $78.50 if renew by November 30; $203.50 if renew between December 1–December 31.

CEU Requirements: 24 contact hours per biennial renewal period. Nurses licensed by examination are required to have 4 contact hours of board-provided continuing education for the first renewal (included in the total number of hours to be earned). MED-CEU contact hours are no longer accepted.

ALASKA

Board of Nursing
Dept. of Community and Economic Development
Division of Occupational Licensing
550 W. 7th Avenue, Suite 1500
Anchorage, AK 99501
Phone: (907) 269-8161
Fax: (907) 261-8196
Website: *www.dced.state.ak.us/occl/pnur.htm*

Temporary Permit: Six months; $50

Licensure Fee/By Examination: $175 permanent license fee; $50 application fee, plus $59 fingerprint fee

Licensure Fee/By Endorsement: $175 permanent license fee; $50 application fee, plus $59 fingerprint fee

NCLEX-PN® Test Fee: $200

Reexamination Limitations: Must wait 45 days

License Renewal: September 30, every even year; $175

CEU Requirements: Method 1: Two of the three required for renewal: (1) 30 contact hours of CE, (2) 30 hours of uncompensated professional nursing activities, (3) 320 hours of employment as a registered nurse. Method 2: Completed a board-approved nursing refresher course. Method 3: Attained a degree or certificate in nursing, beyond the requirements of the original license, by successfully completing at least two required courses. Method 4: Successfully completed the National Council Licensing Examination.

ARIZONA

Board of Nursing
4747 N. 7th Street, Suite 200
Phoenix, AZ 85014
Phone: (602) 771-7800
Fax: (602) 771-7888
Website: *www.azbn.gov*

Temporary Permit: Six months, must have passed NCLEX exam; $50

Licensure Fee/By Examination: $300, plus $50 fingerprint fee

Licensure Fee/By Endorsement: $150, plus $50 fingerprint fee

NCLEX-PN® Test Fee: $200

Reexamination Limitations: Every 45 days; $100

License Renewal: April 1, every 4 years; $160, plus $2 convenience fee if renewed online

CEU Requirements: None

ARKANSAS

State Board of Nursing
University Tower Building
1123 South University, Suite 800
Little Rock, AR 72204-1619
Phone: (501) 686-2700
Fax: (501) 686-2714
Website: *www.arsbn.arkansas.gov*

Temporary Permit: Up to 6 months; $25

Licensure Fee/By Examination: $75, plus $41.25 for criminal background check

Licensure Fee/By Endorsement: $100, plus $41.25 for criminal background check

NCLEX-PN® Test Fee: $200

Reexamination Limitations: Must wait 45 days; $75

License Renewal: Birthday, every 2 years; $65

CEU Requirements: One of the following: (1) 15 contact hours of appropriately accredited practice-focused activities, (2) hold a current nationally recognized certification/recertification, or (3) completed a minimum of one college credit hour course in nursing with a grade of C or better during licensure period. Reinstatement from inactive status/late renewals of less than 5 years requires 20 contact hours of appropriately accredited activities. For each renewal, advanced practice nurses with prescriptive authority must complete an additional 5 contact hours of pharmacotherapeutics related to their specialty certification.

CALIFORNIA

California Board of Vocational Nursing and
  Psychiatric Technicians
2535 Capitol Oaks Drive, Suite 205
Sacramento, CA 95833
Phone: (916) 263-7800
Fax: (916) 263-7859
Website: *www.bvnpt.ca.gov*

Temporary Permit: Interim license for 6 months pending results of first exam; 6 months if by endorsement; $40

Licensure Fee/By Examination: $150, plus $51 fingerprint fee

Licensure Fee/By Endorsement: $75, plus $51 fingerprint fee

NCLEX-PN® Test Fee: $200

Reexamination Limitations: Must wait 45 days; $150

License Renewal: Every 2 years; $155

CEU Requirements: 30 contact hours every 2 years, does not apply to the first license renewal following initial issuance of license

COLORADO

Department of Regulatory Agencies
Board of Nursing
1560 Broadway, Suite 1370
Denver, CO 80202
Phone: (303) 894-2430
Fax: (303) 894-2821
Website: *www.dora.state.co.us/nursing*

Temporary Permit: Four months only by endorsement. Fee is included in application fee.

Licensure Fee/By Examination: $88 initial exam

Licensure Fee/By Endorsement: $43

NCLEX-PN® Test Fee: $200

Reexamination Limitations: Must wait 45 days; $75

License Renewal: August 31, every 2 years; $65

CEU Requirements: None

CONNECTICUT

Department of Public Health
LPN Licensure
410 Capitol Avenue
MS# 13PHO
P.O. Box 340308
Hartford, CT 06134-0308
Phone: (860) 509-7603
Fax: (860) 509-7553
Website: *www.state.ct.us/dph*

Temporary Permit: 90 days from completion of nursing program. Temporary permit also available for endorsement applicants, valid for 120 days, nonrenewable; must hold valid license in another state. Fee is included in application fee.

Licensure Fee/By Examination: $150

Licensure Fee/By Endorsement: $150

NCLEX-PN® Test Fee: $200

Reexamination Limitations: Must wait 45 days, no more than four times in 1 year

License Renewal: Last day of birth month, every year; $60

CEU Requirements: None

DELAWARE

Division of Professional Regulation
Board of Nursing
861 Silver Lake Boulevard
Cannon Building, Suite 203
Dover, DE 19904-2467
Phone: (302) 774-4500
Fax: (302) 739-2711
Website: *http://dpr.delaware.gov/boards/nursing*

Temporary Permit: 90 days by endorsement or 90 days from graduation date, pending results of first exam; $35

Licensure Fee/By Examination: $110

Licensure Fee/By Endorsement: $110

NCLEX-PN® Test Fee: $200

Reexamination Limitations: Must wait 45 days; can retake for up to 2 years; $20

License Renewal: February 28, even years; notified of amount of renewal fee at time of renewal

CEU Requirements: 24 contact hours every 2 years. Nurses licensed by exam are exempt from CE requirements for the first renewal after initial licensure. Minimum practice requirement of 1,000 hours in 5 years or 400 hours in 2 years.

DISTRICT OF COLUMBIA

Department of Health
Health Professional Licensing Administration
Board of Nursing
717 14th Street, NW, Suite 600
Washington, DC 20005
Phone: (877) 672-2174
Fax: (202) 727-8471
Website: *http://hpla.doh.dc.gov/hpla*

Temporary Permit: Supervised letters of practice, 90 days, $33

Licensure Fee/By Examination: $187

Licensure Fee/By Endorsement: $230

NCLEX-PN® Test Fee: $200

Reexamination Limitations: Must wait 45 days; $85

License Renewal: June 30, odd-numbered years; $145

CEU Requirements: 18 contact hours of CE in the licensee's current area of practice every 2 years.

Florida

Board of Nursing
4052 Bald Cypress Way, BIN C02
Tallahassee, FL 32399
Phone: (850) 245-4125
Fax: (850) 245-4172
Website: *www.doh.state.fl.us/mqa*

Temporary Permit: 90 days pending results of first exam; 60 days if by endorsement. Fee is included in licensure fee.

Licensure Fee/By Examination: $204 initial exam

Licensure Fee/By Endorsement: $223

NCLEX-PN® Test Fee: $200

Reexamination Limitations: Must wait 45 days; remedial training program is required after three attempts; $119

License Renewal: July 31, every odd year; $65

CEU Requirements: 24 contact hours every 2 years. One hour per month. Two hours in the prevention of medical errors; 1 hour in HIV prior to first renewal, (one time only); and 2 hours in domestic violence (every 3rd renewal, in addition to required 24 hours of general CE) by a provider approved by the state of Florida; proof of training in latter two prior to licensure. Nurses licensed by examination during the current renewal period are exempt from additional CE requirements for the first renewal period only.

Georgia

Board of Licensed Practical Nursing
237 Coliseum Drive
Macon, GA 31217-3858
Phone: (478) 207-2440
Fax: (478) 207-1354
Website: *www.sos.state.ga.us/plb/lpn*

Temporary Permit: None

Licensure Fee/By Examination: $40

Licensure Fee/By Endorsement: $75

NCLEX-PN® Test Fee: $200, plus $12 when registering by telephone

Reexamination Limitations: Every 91 days, 3 years maximum; $40

License Renewal: March 31, every odd year; $60

CEU Requirements: None

Hawaii

PVLD/DCCA
Attn: Board of Nursing
P.O. Box 3469
Honolulu, HI 96801
Phone: (808) 586-3000
Fax: (808) 586-2689
Website: *http://hawaii.gov/dcca/pvl/boards/nursing*

Temporary Permit: By endorsement with employment verification; pending verification of license from originating state

Licensure Fee/By Examination: $40

Licensure Fee/By Endorsement: $135 or $180, depending on the year license is issued. Noted on application information sheet.

NCLEX-PN® Test Fee: $200

Reexamination Limitations: Must wait 45 days

License Renewal: June 30, every odd year (deadline May 31); contact board for renewal fee

CEU Requirements: None

Idaho

Board of Nursing
280 North 8th Street, Suite 210
P.O. Box 83720
Boise, ID 83720-0061
Phone: (208) 334-3110
Fax: (208) 334-3262
Website: *http://ibn.idaho.gov*

Temporary Permit: 90 days if by endorsement, $25; 90 days Graduate Temporary License pending results of exam

Licensure Fee/By Examination: $105

Licensure Fee/By Endorsement: $140

NCLEX-PN® Test Fee: $200

Reexamination Limitations: Must wait 45 days

License Renewal: August 31, every even year; $90

CEU Requirements: None

ILLINOIS

Board of Nursing
James R. Thompson Center
100 West Randolph Street, Suite 9-300
Chicago, IL 60601
Phone: (312) 814-4500
Fax: (312) 814-3145
Website: *www.idfpr.com/dpr/WHO/nurs.asp*

Temporary Permit: Three-month approval letter by examination; 6 months by endorsement; $25

Licensure Fee/By Examination: $91

Licensure Fee/By Endorsement: $50

NCLEX-PN® Test Fee: $200

Reexamination Limitations: Must wait 45 days, can retake for 3 years from first writing to board

License Renewal: May 31, every odd year; $30

CEU Requirements: As of June 1, 2010, 20 hours of CE between June 1, 2010 and May 31, 2012

INDIANA

State Board of Nursing
Professional Licensing Agency
402 West Washington Street, Room W072
Indianapolis, IN 46204
Phone: (317) 234-2043
Fax: (317) 233-4236
Website: *www.in.gov/pla/nursing.htm*

Temporary Permit: 90 days if by endorsement; $10

Licensure Fee/By Examination: $50

Licensure Fee/By Endorsement: $50

NCLEX-PN® Test Fee: $200

Reexamination Limitations: Must wait 45 days

License Renewal: October 31, every even year; $50

CEU Requirements: None

IOWA

Board of Nursing
Riverpoint Business Park
400 SW 8th Street, Suite B
Des Moines, IA 50309-4685
Phone: (515) 281-3255
Fax: (515) 281-4825
Website: *http://nursing.iowa.gov*

Temporary Permit: 30 days if by endorsement. Fee is included in application fee.

Licensure Fee/By Examination: $143

Licensure Fee/By Endorsement: $169

NCLEX-PN® Test Fee: $200

Reexamination Limitations: Must wait 45 days; $93

License Renewal: 30 days prior to the 15th of month of birth, every 3 years; $99

CEU Requirements: 36 contact hours or 3.6 CEUs every 3 years

KANSAS

State Board of Nursing
Landon State Office Building
900 SW Jackson, Suite 1051
Topeka, KS 66612-1230
Phone: (785) 296-4929
Fax: (785) 296-3929
Website: *www.ksbn.org*

Temporary Permit: 120 days only by endorsement. Fee is included in application fee.

Licensure Fee/By Examination: $50

Licensure Fee/By Endorsement: $50

NCLEX-PN® Test Fee: $200

Reexamination Limitations: Must wait 45 days, can retake unlimited number of times; if applicant doesn't pass within 2 years, the applicant must provide an approved study plan.

License Renewal: Last day of birth month every odd year if you were born in an odd year, every even year if you were born in an even year; $60

CEU Requirements: 30 contact hours every 2 years

KENTUCKY

Board of Nursing
312 Whittington Parkway, Suite 300
Louisville, KY 40222-5172
Phone: (502) 429-3300, (800) 305-2042
Fax: (502) 429-3311
Website: *www.kbn.ky.gov*

Temporary Permit: No temporary work permits are issued to new graduates. Six months by endorsement. Fee included in application fee.

Licensure Fee/By Examination: $110, plus $15 for criminal background report

Licensure Fee/By Endorsement: $150, plus $19.25 fingerprint fee

NCLEX-PN® Test Fee: $200

Reexamination Limitations: Must wait 46 days

License Renewal: September 15–October 31, annually; $50 if online; paper renewal requires application request form and a $40 additional fee

CEU Requirements: 14 contact hours every year; 2 hours of mandatory AIDS CE approved by the Kentucky Cabinet for Health Services once every 10 years. A one-time, 3-hour domestic violence requirement must be completed within 3 years of the date of initial licensing.

LOUISIANA

State Board of Practical Nurse Examiners
3421 N. Causeway Boulevard, Suite 505
Metairie, LA 70002
Phone: (504) 838-5791
Fax: (504) 838-5279
Website: *www.lsbpne.com*

Temporary Permit: Pending results of first exam. Fee is included in application fee. Permit becomes void when exam results received. If by endorsement, 90 days: $50

Licensure Fee/By Examination: $100, plus $18 for criminal background check

Licensure Fee/By Endorsement: $100, plus $18 for criminal background check

NCLEX-PN® Test Fee: $200

Reexamination Limitations: Must wait 45 days, can retake up to four times

License Renewal: January 31, every year; $80

CEU Requirements: None

MAINE

Board of Nursing
161 Capitol Street
#158 State House Station (mailing address)
Augusta, ME 04333
Phone: (207) 287-1133
Fax: (207) 287-1149
Website: *www.maine.gov/boardofnursing*

Temporary Permit: 90 days. Fee is included in application fee. Only by endorsement.

Licensure Fee/By Examination: $50

Licensure Fee/By Endorsement: $50

NCLEX-PN® Test Fee: $200

Reexamination Limitations: Must wait 45 days

License Renewal: Birthday, every 2 years; $50

CEU Requirements: None

MARYLAND

Board of Nursing
4140 Patterson Avenue
Baltimore, MD 21215-2254
Phone: (410) 585-1900
Fax: (410) 358-3530
Website: *www.mbon.org/main.php*

Temporary Permit: 90 days by endorsement, not renewable; must submit separate application with $40

Licensure Fee/By Examination: $100

Licensure Fee/By Endorsement: $100

NCLEX-PN® Test Fee: $200

Reexamination Limitations: Must wait 45 days; $100

License Renewal: Prior to 28th day of month of birth, every year; $55

CEU Requirements: None

MASSACHUSETTS

Board of Registration in Nursing
239 Causeway Street, 2nd Floor
Boston, MA 02114
Phone: (617) 973-0800
Fax: (617) 973-0894
Website: *www.mass.gov/dpl/boards/rn*

Temporary Permit: Not granted

Licensure Fee/By Examination: $230

Licensure Fee/By Endorsement: $275

NCLEX-PN® Test Fee: $200

Reexamination Limitations: Must wait 45 days; $80

License Renewal: Birthday, every odd year; $120

CEU Requirements: 15 contact hours every 2 years

MICHIGAN

Bureau of Health Professions
Michigan Department of Community Health
Board of Nursing
Ottawa Towers North
611 West Ottawa, 1st Floor
Lansing, MI 48933
Phone: (517) 335-0918
Fax: (517) 373-2179
Website: *www.michigan.gov/healthlicense*

Temporary Permit: Not available

Licensure Fee/By Examination: $54, plus $62.75 fingerprinting fee

Licensure Fee/By Endorsement: $54, plus $62.75 fingerprinting fee

NCLEX-PN® Test Fee: $200

Reexamination Limitations: Must wait 45 days, up to six attempts within 3 years. Must pass within 1 year or three attempts or review course. After six failures, must attend education program.

License Renewal: March 31, every 2 years; $60

CEU Requirements: 25 credits every 2 years; at least 1 hour in pain and symptom management

MINNESOTA

Board of Nursing
2829 University Avenue, SE #200
Minneapolis, MN 55414-3253
Phone: (612) 617-2270
Fax: (612) 617-2190
Website: *www.nursingboard.state.mn.us*

Temporary Permit: 60 days, license by exam; $60. One year if by endorsement, no fee.

Licensure Fee/By Examination: $105, plus $10.50 eLicensing surcharge

Licensure Fee/By Endorsement: $105, plus $10.50 eLicensing surcharge

NCLEX-PN® Test Fee: $200

Reexamination Limitations: Must wait 45 days. Must retake within 1 year or application becomes null; $60.

License Renewal: Birth month, every 2 years; $93.50

CEU Requirements: 12 contact hours every 2 years

MISSISSIPPI

Board of Nursing
1080 River Oaks Drive, Suite A100
Flowood, MS 39232
Phone: (601) 987-4188
Fax: (601) 364-2352
Website: *www.msbn.state.ms.us/*

Temporary Permit: 90 days by endorsement; $25

Licensure Fee/By Examination: $60

Licensure Fee/By Endorsement: $60

NCLEX-PN® Test Fee: $200

Reexamination Limitations: Must wait 46 days; maximum of eight times per year, $60

License Renewal: October 1–December 31, every odd year; $100

CEU Requirements: None

MISSOURI

Board of Nursing
3605 Missouri Boulevard
P.O. Box 656
Jefferson City, MO 65102-0656
Phone: (573) 751-0681
Fax: (573) 751-0075
Website: *www.pr.mo.gov/nursing.asp*

Temporary Permit: Six months. Fee is included in application fee. Only by endorsement.

Licensure Fee/By Examination: $41 initial exam

Licensure Fee/By Endorsement: $51

NCLEX-PN® Test Fee: $200

Reexamination Limitations: Must wait 45 days; $40

License Renewal: May 31, every even year; $52

CEU Requirements: None

MONTANA

Department of Labor and Industry
Board of Nursing
301 South Park, Suite 401
P.O. Box 200513
Helena, MT 59620-0513
Phone: (406) 841-2345
Fax: (406) 841-2305
Website: *www.nurse.mt.gov*

Temporary Permit: 90 days by exam only; $25

Licensure Fee/By Examination: $100

Licensure Fee/By Endorsement: $200

NCLEX-PN® Test Fee: $200

Reexamination Limitations: Must wait 45 days, can retake up to five times in 3 years. After failing twice, must present a plan of study to the board before next retake. If applicant doesn't pass within 3 years, must take Nursing Program before sixth retake.

License Renewal: December 31, every even year; $100

CEU Requirements: None

NEBRASKA

Board of Nursing
301 Centennial Mall South, 3rd Floor
P.O. Box 94986
Lincoln, NE 68509-4986
Phone: (402) 471-4376
Fax: (402) 471-1066
Website: *www.hhs.state.ne.us/crl/nursing/ nursingindex.htm*

Temporary Permit: 60 days if by endorsement. Fee is included in licensing fee.

Licensure Fee/By Examination: $123

Licensure Fee/By Endorsement: $123

NCLEX-PN® Test Fee: $200

Reexamination Limitations: Must wait 45 days

License Renewal: October 31, every odd year; $123.

CEU Requirements: 20 contact hours within the last renewal period, 10 hours of which must be peer reviewed and approved.

NEVADA

Board of Nursing
5011 Meadowood Mall Way, Suite 300
Reno, NV 89502
Phone: (775) 687-7700
Fax: (775) 687-7707
Website: *www.nursingboard.state.nv.us*

Temporary License: Three months, not renewable. Fee is included in application fee.

Licensure Fee/By Examination: $90, plus $51.25 fingerprint card fee

Licensure Fee/By Endorsement: $95, plus $51.25 fingerprint card fee

NCLEX-PN® Test Fee: $200

Reexamination Limitations: Must wait 45 days, can retake up to three times, then only with remediation.

License Renewal: Birthday, every 2 years; $100

CEU Requirements: 30 contact hours every 2 years at renewal. One-time requirement of 4 hours on bioterrorism. New grads may be exempt from CE requirements for their first renewal period.

NEW HAMPSHIRE

Board of Nursing
21 South Fruit Street, Suite 16
Concord, NH 03301
Phone: (603) 271-2323
Fax: (603) 271-6605
Website: *www.state.nh.us/nursing*

Temporary Permit: Six months or until results of first exam are received and license is issued; $20

Licensure Fee/By Examination: $120, plus $55.25 for Criminal Record Release Authorization

Licensure Fee/By Endorsement: $120, plus $55.25 for Criminal Record Release Authorization

NCLEX-PN® Test Fee: $200

Reexamination Limitations: Must wait 45 days

License Renewal: Birthday, every 2 years; $100

CEU Requirements: 30 contact hours every 2 years

NEW JERSEY

Board of Nursing
P.O. Box 45010
124 Halsey Street, 6th Floor
Newark, NJ 07101
Phone: (973) 504-6430
Fax: (973) 648-3481
Website: *www.njconsumeraffairs.gov/nursing/*

Temporary Permit: Not available

Licensure Fee/By Examination: $200, plus $25.30 for criminal history background check

Licensure Fee/By Endorsement: $200, plus $66.30 fingerprinting fee and $25.30 for criminal history background check

NCLEX-PN® Test Fee: $200

Reexamination Limitations: Must wait 45 days; only with remediation after three attempts

License Renewal: May 31, every 2 years; $120

CEU Requirements: 30 contact hours every 2 years

NEW MEXICO

Board of Nursing
6301 Indian School Road NE, Suite 710
Albuquerque, NM 87110
Phone: (505) 841-8340
Fax: (505) 841-8347
Website: *www.bon.state.nm.us*

Temporary Permit: 24 weeks from graduation if application process is completed within 12 weeks of graduation. Fee is included in application fee; must have NM employment verified. Six months if by endorsement, fee is $50.

Licensure Fee/By Examination: $110 initial exam, plus $44 for criminal background check

Licensure Fee/By Endorsement: $110, plus $44 for criminal background check

NCLEX-PN® Test Fee: $200

Reexamination Limitations: Must wait 45 days; $60; can retake up to three times; thereafter, must take a refresher course first.

License Renewal: Every 2 years from date of issue; $93

CEU Requirements: 30 contact hours every 2 years

NEW YORK

Board of Nursing
NYS Education Department
Office of the Professions
Division of Professional Licensing Services, Nurse Unit
89 Washington Avenue
2nd Floor West Wing
Albany, NY 12234-1000
Phone: (518) 474-3817, ext. 280
Fax: (518) 474-3398
Website: *www.op.nysed.gov/prof/nurse*

Temporary Permit: Must have completed all other requirements for licensure except the licensing examination. Valid for 1 year from date of issue or until 10 days after the applicant is notified of failure on the licensing examination, whichever occurs first. Graduates of New York state nursing programs may be employed without permit for 90 days immediately following graduation; $35.

Licensure Fee/By Examination: $143 (includes first license and 3-year registration)

Licensure Fee/By Endorsement: $143

NCLEX-PN® Test Fee: $200

Reexamination Limitations: Must wait 45 days

License Renewal: Every 3 years; $65

CEU Requirements: 3 contact hours on infection control every 4 years

NORTH CAROLINA

Board of Nursing
4516 Lake Boone Trail
Raleigh, NC 27602
Phone: (919) 782-3211
Fax: (919) 781-9461
Website: *www.ncbon.com*

Temporary Permit: None for new graduates. By endorsement: 6 months or until the endorsement is approved, whichever occurs first; not renewable. Fee is included in application fee.

Licensure Fee/By Examination: $70; $38 criminal background check

Licensure Fee/By Endorsement: $150 plus $38 fingerprint fee; initial application fee, $100

NCLEX-PN® Test Fee: $200

Reexamination Limitations: Must wait 45 days; $65

License Renewal: Month of birth, every 2 years; $92

CEU Requirements: Various options to fulfill continuing competency requirement, including 30 contact hours of CE

NORTH DAKOTA

Board of Nursing
919 South 7th Street, Suite 504
Bismarck, ND 58504-5881
Phone: (701) 328-9777
Fax: (701) 328-9785
Website: *www.ndbon.org*

Temporary Permit: By endorsement: 90 days; fee is included in endorsement fee. By exam: 90 days after the date of issue or upon notification of exam results, whichever occurs first.

Licensure Fee/By Examination: $110, plus $20 for criminal history record check

Licensure Fee/By Endorsement: $110, plus $20 for criminal history record check

NCLEX-PN® Test Fee: $200

Reexamination Limitations: Must wait 45 days, can retake up to five times in 3 years; $110

License Renewal: December 31 of the year you receive your initial license; after initial licensure, every 2 years; $90

CEU Requirements: 12 contact hours required in the 2 years leading up to renewal. If first renewal by exam, CE is not required. If first renewal by endorsement, 6 contact hours are required by date of first renewal.

OHIO

Board of Nursing
17 South High Street, Suite 400
Columbus, OH 43215-7410
Phone: (614) 466-3947
Fax: (614) 466-0388
Website: *www.nursing.ohio.gov*

Temporary Permit: 180 days if by endorsement, not renewable. Fee is included in endorsement application fee. Written verification required.

Licensure Fee/By Examination: $75

Licensure Fee/By Endorsement: $75

NCLEX-PN® Test Fee: $200

Reexamination Limitations: Must wait 45 days; $75

License Renewal: June 30, every even year; $65

CEU Requirements: 24 hours in a 2-year period, except in the case of first renewal after licensure by examination. One of 24 hours must pertain to Ohio law.

OKLAHOMA

Board of Nursing
2915 North Classen Boulevard, Suite 524
Oklahoma City, OK 73106
Phone: (405) 962-1800
Fax: (405) 962-1821
Website: *www.ok.gov/nursing*

Temporary Permit: 90 days if by endorsement; $10

Licensure Fee/By Examination: $85

Licensure Fee/By Endorsement: $85

NCLEX-PN® Test Fee: $200

Reexamination Limitations: Must wait 45 days; can retake for 2 years; $85

License Renewal: Last day of birth month, every 2 years; $75

CEU Requirements: None

OREGON

Board of Nursing
17938 SW Upper Boones Ferry Road
Portland, OR 97224
Phone: (971) 673-0685
Fax: (971) 673-0684
Website: *www.osbn.state.or.us*

Temporary Permit: None

Licensure Fee/By Examination: $160, plus $52 for criminal background check

Licensure Fee/By Endorsement: $195, plus $52 for criminal background check

NCLEX-PN® Test Fee: $200

Reexamination Limitations: Must wait 45 days, can retake for up to 3 years from the date of graduation; $25

License Renewal: By midnight the night before birthdate, every odd year if you were born in an odd year, every even year if you were born in an even year; $130

CEU Requirements: One-time requirement of 7 hours of pain management-related CE. One hour must be a course provided by the Oregon Pain Management Commission.

PENNSYLVANIA

Board of Nursing
P.O. Box 2649
Harrisburg, PA 17105-2649
Phone: (717) 783-7142
Fax: (717) 783-0822
Website: *www.dos.state.pa.us/bpoa*

Temporary Permit: One year maximum; examination results preempt permit, $35

Licensure Fee/By Examination: $35 if educated in PA; $100 if educated out of state

Licensure Fee/By Endorsement: $100

NCLEX-PN® Test Fee: $200

Reexamination Limitations: Must wait 45 days, $30

License Renewal: June 30 every even year; $60

CEU Requirements: None

RHODE ISLAND

Board of Nurse Registration and Nursing
  Education
105 Cannon Building
Three Capitol Hill
Providence, RI 02908
Phone: (401) 222-5700
Fax: (401) 222-3352
Website: *www.health.ri.gov/hsr/professions/
  nurses.php*

Temporary Permit: Pending results of first exam but no longer than 90 days after graduation; 90 days if by endorsement. Not renewable. No fee.

Licensure Fee/By Examination: $90

Licensure Fee/By Endorsement: $90

NCLEX-PN® Test Fee: $200

Reexamination Limitations: Must wait 45 days; $130

License Renewal: Before February 15, every 2 years; $90

CEU Requirements: 10 contact hours in preceding 2 years

South Carolina

Board of Nursing
P.O. Box 12367
Columbia, SC 29211-2367
Phone: (803) 896-4550
Fax: (803) 896-4525
Website: *www.llr.state.sc.us/pol/nursing*

Temporary Permit: 90 days by endorsement only; $10

Licensure Fee/By Examination: $77

Licensure Fee/By Endorsement: $114; with permit $124

NCLEX-PN® Test Fee: $200

Reexamination Limitations: Must wait 45 days, can retake up to four times in 1 year, then must remediate; $45

License Renewal: By April 30 every 2 years; $64

CEU Requirements: One of the following, every 2 years: (1) 30 CE contact hours, (2) maintenance of certification or recertification by a national certifying body, (3) completion of an academic program of study in nursing or a related field, or (4) verification of competency and number of hours practiced as evidenced by employer certification

South Dakota

Board of Nursing
4305 S. Louise Avenue, Suite 201
Sioux Falls, SD 57106-3115
Phone: (605) 362-2760
Fax: (605) 362-2768
Website: *www.doh.sd.gov/boards/nursing/*

Temporary Permit: 90 days from graduation pending results of first exam; 90 days if by endorsement; $25

Licensure Fee/By Examination: $100, plus $43.25 for criminal background check

Licensure Fee/By Endorsement: $100, plus $43.25 for criminal background check

NCLEX-PN® Test Fee: $200

Reexamination Limitations: Must wait 45 days, can retake a maximum of four times per year in 3 years, then must requalify; $100

License Renewal: Birthday, every 2 years; $90

CEU Requirements: None

Tennessee

Board of Nursing
Heritage Place, MetroCenter
227 French Landing, Suite 300
Nashville, TN 37243
Phone: (615) 532-5166
Fax: (615) 741-7899
Website: *http://health.state.tn.us/Boards/Nursing*

Temporary Permit: Six months if by endorsement; $25

Licensure Fee/By Examination: $90

Licensure Fee/By Endorsement: $115

NCLEX-PN® Test Fee: $200

Reexamination Limitations: Must wait 45 days, can retake for up to 3 years, then only with remediation; $100

License Renewal: Last day of month of birth, every 2 years; $65

CEU Requirements: Continued practice requirement over a 5-year period

Texas

Board of Nursing
333 Guadalupe, Suite 3-460
Austin, TX 78701
Phone: (512) 305-7400
Fax: (512) 305-7401
Website: *www.bon.state.tx.us*

Temporary Permit: 120 days by endorsement, 6-month permits issued for completing a refresher course; no extensions; $25

Licensure Fee/By Examination: $139

Licensure Fee/By Endorsement: $200

NCLEX-PN® Test Fee: $200

Reexamination Limitations: Must wait 45 days; unlimited testing within 4 years of eligibility; $139 retake fee

License Renewal: Every even year for those born in even years, every odd year for those born in odd years (initial licensure period ranges from 6 months to 29 months depending on birth year); $55

CEU Requirements: 20 contact hours (two CEUs) or achievement of an approved national nursing certification, every 2 years. Nurses licensed by exam or by endorsement are exempt from CE requirements for the first renewal after initial licensure.

UTAH

Board of Nursing
Heber M. Wells Building, 4th Floor
160 East 300 South
Salt Lake City, UT 84111
Phone: (801) 530-6628
Fax: (801) 530-6511
Website: *www.dopl.utah.gov/licensing/nursing.html*

Temporary Permit: Four months; $50

Licensure Fee/By Examination: $100

Licensure Fee/By Endorsement: $100

NCLEX-PN® Test Fee: $200

Reexamination Limitations: Must wait 45 days

License Renewal: January 31, every even year; $58

CEU Requirements: Must have practiced not less than 400 hours during 2 years preceding application for renewal, or have completed 30 contact hours, or have practiced not less than 200 hours and completed 15 contact hours during 2 years preceding application for renewal.

VERMONT

Board of Nursing
Office of Professional Regulation
National Life Building North Fl.2
Montpelier, Vermont 05620-3402
Phone: (802) 828-2396
Fax: (802) 828-2484
Website: *www.vtprofessionals.org/opr1/nurses*

Temporary Permit: 90 days pending results of exam, 90 days if by endorsement; $25

Licensure Fee/By Examination: $90

Licensure Fee/By Endorsement: $150

NCLEX-PN® Test Fee: $200

Reexamination Limitations: Must wait 45 days; various review requirements if fail between 2–4 times; if fail 5 times, must contact Board of Nursing Office; $30

License Renewal: January 1 every even year; $95

CEU Requirements: Minimum practice requirement of 960 hours in 5 years or 400 hours in 2 years

VIRGINIA

Board of Nursing
Department of Health Professions
Perimeter Center
9960 Mayland Drive, Suite 300
Richmond, Virginia 23233
Phone: (804) 367-4515
Fax: (804) 527-4455
Website: *www.dhp.virginia.gov/nursing*

Temporary Permit: 90 days pending results of exam; 30 days by endorsement, which may be extended at the discretion of the board

Licensure Fee/By Examination: $130

Licensure Fee/By Endorsement: $130

NCLEX-PN® Test Fee: $200

Reexamination Limitations: Must wait 45 days; $25

License Renewal: Last day of month of birth, every even year for those born in even years, every odd year for those born in odd years; $95

CEU Requirements: None

WASHINGTON

Nursing Care Quality Assurance Commission
310 Israel Road SE
P.O. Box 47864
Olympia, WA 98504-7864
Phone: (360) 236-4700
Fax: (360) 236-4738
Website: *www.doh.wa.gov/hsqa/Professions/Nursing*

Temporary Permit: None

Licensure Fee/By Examination: $92

Licensure Fee/By Endorsement: $92

NCLEX-PN® Test Fee: $200

Reexamination Limitations: Must wait 45 days

License Renewal: Birthday, every year; $96

CEU Requirements: Not mandatory

WEST VIRGINIA

Board of Examiners for Registered Professional
 Nurses
101 Dee Drive
Charleston, WV 25311-1620
Phone: (304) 558-3596
Fax: (304) 558-3666
Website: *www.lpnboard.state.wv.us*

Temporary Permit: 90 days pending results of first exam; 90 days if by endorsement; $10

Licensure Fee/By Examination: $75

Licensure Fee/By Endorsement: $50

NCLEX-PN® Test Fee: $200

Reexamination Limitations: Must wait 45 days; additional requirements are needed after two attempts; $75

License Renewal: Between March 1 and June 30, every even year; $25

CEU Requirements: 24 contact hours of CE and 400 hours of practice in each 2-year reporting period.

WISCONSIN

Department of Regulation and Licensing
1400 East Washington Avenue
Madison, WI 53703
Mailing Address: P.O. Box 8935
Madison, WI 53708-8935
Phone: (608) 266-2112
Fax: (608) 261-7083
Website:
 http://drl.wi.gov/profession.asp?profid=22&locid=0

Temporary Permit: 90 days pending results of exam; 90 days if by endorsement; $10

Licensure Fee/By Examination: $90

Licensure Fee/By Endorsement: $82

NCLEX-PN® Test Fee: $200

Reexamination Limitations: Must wait 45 days; $15

License Renewal: April 30 every odd year; $82

CEU Requirements: None

WYOMING

Board of Nursing
1810 Pioneer Avenue
Cheyenne, WY 82001
Phone: (307) 777-7601
Fax: (307) 777-3519
Website: *http://nursing-online.state.wy.us*

Temporary Permit: 90 days by endorsement or by exam. Fee is included in application fee. Temporary permit is not renewable.

Licensure Fee/By Examination: $195

Licensure Fee/By Endorsement: $195

NCLEX-PN® Test Fee: $200

Reexamination Limitations: Must wait 45 days, can retake a maximum of 10 times within 5 years of graduation; $195

License Renewal: December 31, every even year; $110

CEU Requirements: 20 contact hours in last year or combination of nursing practice and contact hours, or minimum practice requirement of 1,600 hours in 5 years or 500 hours in 2 years.

PEARSON PROFESSIONAL CENTERS OFFERING NCLEX-PN® EXAMINATIONS

The following is a listing of some NCLEX-PN® examination sites. More sites may be available in your area. For more information, please visit the website of the National Council of State Boards of Nursing at *ncsbn.org*.

U.S. EXAMINATION SITES

Alabama

2 Chase Corporate Drive, Suite 20
Birmingham, AL 35244

401 Lee Street NE, Suite 602
Decatur, AL 35602

Carmel Plaza
2623 Montgomery Hwy., Suite 4
Dothan, AL 36303

Executive Center One
900 Western America Circle, Suite 212
Mobile, AL 36609

400 East Blvd., Suite 103
Montgomery, AL 36117

Alaska

Denali Towers North Building
2550 Denali Street, Suite 511
Anchorage, AK 99503

American Samoa

Pago Plaza
PO Box AC, Suite 222
Pago Pago, AS 96799

Arizona

555 W. Iron Avenue, Suite 102
Mesa, AZ 85210

2501 West Dunlap Avenue, Suite 260
Phoenix, AZ 85021

Merrill Lynch Building
5210 East Williams Circle, Suite 722
Tucson, AZ 85711

Arkansas

1401 S. Waldron Road, Suite 208
Fort Smith, AR 72903

Conway Building
10816 Executive Center Drive, Suite 209
Little Rock, AR 72211

Landmark Building
210 North State Line Avenue, Suite B100
Texarkana, AR 71854

California

Anaheim Corporate Plaza
2190 Towne Centre Place, Suite 300
Anaheim, CA 92806

7555 N. Palm Avenue, Suite 205
Fresno, CA 93711

South Bay Centre
1515 West 190th Street, Suite 405
Gardena, CA 90248

1551 McCarthy Blvd., Suite 108
Milpitas, CA 95035

Transpacific Center
1000 Broadway, Suite 470
Oakland, CA 94607

Centrelake Plaza
3401 Centrelake Drive, Suite 675
Ontario, CA 91761

Union Bank Building
70 S. Lake Avenue, Suite 840
Pasadena, CA 91101

2190 Larkspur Lane, Suite 400
Redding, CA 96002

3010 Lava Ridge Court, Suite 170
Roseville, CA 95661

8950 Cal Center Drive, Suite 215
Sacramento, CA 95826

Sunroad Financial Plaza
11770 Bernardo Plaza Court, Suite 463
San Diego, CA 92128

9619 Chesapeake Drive, Suite 208
San Diego, CA 92123

140 East Via Verde, Suite 110
San Dimas, CA 91773

201 Filbert Street, Suite 200
San Francisco, CA 94133

Gill Office Building
1010 South Broadway, Suite F
Santa Maria, CA 93454

Westlake Corporate Centre
875 Westlake Blvd., Suite 106
WestLake Village, CA 91361

Colorado

The Triad
5660 Greenwood Plaza Blvd., Suite 510
Greenwood Village, CO 80111

University Center Professional Building
41 Montebello Road, Suite 312
Pueblo, CO 81001

Lake Arbor Plaza
9101 Harlan Street, Suite 320
Westminster, CO 80030

Connecticut

Merritt on the River - North Tower
20 Glover Avenue, Suite 19
Norwalk, CT 06850

35 Thorpe Avenue, Suite 105
Wallingford, CT 06492

Putnam Park
100 Great Meadow Road, Suite 404
Wethersfield, CT 06109

Delaware

The Kays Building
1012 College Road, Suite 104
Dover, DE 19904

111 Continental Drive, Suite 109
Newark, DE 19713

District of Columbia

1615 L Street NW, Suite 410
Washington, DC 20036

Florida

Premier Point South
237 South Westmonte Drive, Suite 245
Altamonte Springs, FL 32714

1191 East Newport Center Drive, Suite PHA
3rd Floor, Penthouse A
Deerfield Beach, FL 33442

Union Street Station
201 SE 2nd Avenue, Suite 208
Gainesville, FL 32601

Spring Lake Business Center
Building 3
8659 Baypine Road, Suite 305
Jacksonville, FL 32256

8615–8617 South Dixie Highway
Miami, FL 33143

1707 Orlando Central Parkway, Suite 300
Orlando, FL 32809

Royal Palm at Southpoint
1000 South Pine Island Road, Suite 260
Plantation, FL 33324

M & I Bank Building
1777 Tamiami Trail, Suite 508
Port Charlotte, FL 33948

Baypoint Commerce Center
877 Executive Center Drive, Suite 350
St. Petersburg, FL 33702

2286–2 Wednesday Street
Tallahassee, FL 32308

Sabal Business Center 5
3922 Coconut Palm Drive, Suite 101
Tampa, FL 33619

Georgia

2410 Westgate Blvd., Suite 102
Albany, GA 31707

1117 Perimeter Center West, Suite 311 East
Atlanta, GA 30338

The Entrusted Building
3420 Norman Berry Road, Suite 275
Atlanta, GA 30354

Augusta Riverfront Center
One 10th Street, Suite 640
Augusta, GA 30901

Riverside Corporate Center
4885 Riverside Drive, Suite 101
Macon, GA 31210

Georgetown Center
785 King George Blvd., Suite C
Savannah, GA 31419

Guam

267 South Marine Drive, 2nd Floor, Suite 2E
Tamuning, GU 96913

Hawaii

Airport Center Building
3049 Ualena Street, Suite 406
Honolulu, HI 96819

Idaho

Spectrum View Business Center
1951 South Saturn Way, Suite 200
Boise, ID 83709

Illinois

200 West Adams Street, Suite 1105
Chicago, IL 60606

103 Airway Drive, Suite 1
Marion, IL 62959

Norwoods Professional Building
4507 N. Sterling Avenue, Suite 302
Peoria, IL 61615

Gateway Executive Park
1827 Walden Office Square, Suite 540
Schaumburg, IL 60173

3000 Professional Drive, Lower Level, Suite C
Springfield, IL 62703

Indiana

Bank of Evansville Building
4424 Vogel Road, Suite 402
Evansville, IN 47715

Dupont Office Center Building 2
9921 Dupont Circle Drive West, Suite 140
Fort Wayne, IN 46825

2629 Waterfront Parkway East Drive, Suite 100
Indianapolis, IN 46214

Pyramids at College Park
3500 DePauw Blvd., Bldg. 2, 8th Floor, Suite 2080
Indianapolis, IN 46268

Chase Building
8585 Broadway, Suite 745
Merrillville, IN 46410

630 Wabash Avenue, Suite 221
Terre Haute, IN 47807

Iowa

Wells Fargo Building
327 2nd Street, Suite 370
Coralville, IA 52241

Northwest Bank & Trust Company
100 East Kimberly Road, Suite 401
Davenport, IA 52806

4300 South Lakeport, Suite 204
Sioux City, IA 51106

Colony Park Office Building
3737 Woodland Avenue, Third Floor, Suite 340
West Des Moines, IA 50266

Kansas

Hadley Center
205 E. 7th Street, Suite 237
Hays, KS 67601

Gage Center Office Suites
4125 SW Gage Center Drive, Suite 201
Topeka, KS 66604

Equity Financial Center
7701 E. Kellogg, 7th Floor, Suite 750
Wichita, KS 67207

Kentucky

Alumni Office Park
2317 Alumni Park Plaza, Suite B-130
Lexington, KY 40517

1941 Bishop Lane, Suite 713
Louisville, KY 40218

Louisiana

Corporate Atrium Building
5555 Hilton Avenue, Suite 430
Baton Rouge, LA 70808

2800 Veterans Blvd., Suite 256
Metairie, LA 70002

Pierremont Office Park
920 Pierremont Road, Suite 212
Shreveport, LA 71106

Maine

10 Ridgewood Drive, Suite 2
Bangor, ME 04401

201 Main Street, Suite 4A
Westbrook, ME 04092

Maryland

3108 Lord Baltimore Drive, Suite 103
Baltimore, MD 21244

Bethesda Towers
4350 East West Highway, Suite 525
Bethesda, MD 20814

9891 Broken Land Parkway, Suite 108
Columbia, MD 21046

1315 Mount Herman Road, Suite B
Salisbury, MD 21804

Massachusetts

Park Square
31 St. James Avenue, Suite 725
Boston, MA 02116

295 Devonshire Street, 2nd Floor
Boston, MA 02110

Monarch Place
1414 Main Street, Suite 1110
Springfield, MA 01144

Reservoir Place
1601 Trapelo Road, Suite 203
Waltham, MA 02451

255 Park Avenue, 6th Floor, Suite 604
Worcester, MA 01609

Michigan

Burlington Office Center I
325 E. Eisenhower Parkway, Suite 3A
Ann Arbor, MI 48108

Waters Building
161 Ottawa NW, Suite 307
Grand Rapids, MI 49503

3390 Pine Tree Road, Suite 101
Lansing, MI 48911

Rublein Building
290 Rublein Street, Suite B
Marquette, MI 49855

Travelers Tower I
26555 Evergreen Road, Suite 850
Southfield, MI 48076

City Center Building
888 W. Big Beaver Road, Suite 490
Troy, MI 48084

Minnesota

5601 Green Valley Drive, Suite 150
Bloomington, MN 55437

Triad Building
7101 Northland Circle, Suite 102
Brooklyn Park, MN 55428

Washington Drive Executive Center
3459 Washington Drive, Suite 107
Eagan, MN 55122

North Shore Bank Place
4815 West Arrowhead Road, Suite 100
Hermantown, MN 55811

Greenview Office Building
1544 Greenview Drive SW, Suite 200
Rochester, MN 55902

Mississippi

1755 Lelia Drive, Suite 404
Jackson, MI 39211
Woodlands Office Park

431 W. Main Street, Suite 340
Tupelo, MS 38801

Missouri

Buttonwood Building
3610 Buttonwood Drive, Suite 102A
Columbia, MO 65201

Ward Parkway Corporate Centre
9200 Ward Parkway, Suite 101
Kansas City, MO 64114

Blue Ridge Tower
4240 Blue Ridge Blvd., Suite 705
Kansas City, MO 64133

2833 (A) East Battlefield, Suite 106
Springfield, MO 65804

Center Forty Building
1600 S. Brentwood Blvd., Suite 120
St. Louis, MO 63144

10805 Sunset Office Drive, Suite 402
St. Louis, MO 63127

Montana

Transwestern 1 Building
404 North 31st Street, Suite 230
Billings, MT 59101

Arcade Building
111 N. Last Chance Gulch, Suite 4K
Helena, MT 59601

Nebraska

44 Corporate Place Office Park
300 North 44th Street, Suite 104
Lincoln, NE 68503

Nebraskaland Bank Building
121 N. Dewey, Suite 212
North Platte, NE 69101

Omni Corporate Park
10832 Old Mill Road, Suite 4
Omaha, NE 68154

Nevada

Tower Building
101 Convention Center Drive, Suite 330
Las Vegas, NV 89109

Corporate Point
5250 S. Virginia, Suite 301
Reno, NV 89502

New Hampshire

Capital Plaza
2 Capital Plaza, 3rd Floor
Concord, NH 03301

New Jersey

1125 Atlantic Avenue, Suite 107
Atlantic City, NJ 08401

1099 Wall Street West, Suite 104
Lyndhurst, NJ 07071

100 Village Blvd., Suite 201
Princeton, NJ 08540

1543 State Route 27, Lower Level–Basement
Somerset, NJ 08873

New Mexico

Bank of Albuquerque Building
2500 Louisiana Blvd. NE, Suite LL–1B
Albuquerque, NM 87110

New York

1365 Washington Avenue, Suite 107
Albany, NY 12206

45 Main Street, Suite 706
Brooklyn, NY 11201

6700 Kirkville Road, Suite 204
East Syracuse, NY 13057

421–423 East Main Street, Suite 100
Endicott, NY 13760

2950 Express Drive South, Suite 145
Islandia, NY 11722

100 William Street, Suite 1200
New York, NY 10038

500 Fifth Avenue, Suite 3120
New York, NY 10110

9734 64th Road
Rego Park, NY 11374

The Design Center
3445 Winton Place, Suite 238
Rochester, NY 14623

Gardens Office I
1110 South Avenue, Suite 400
Staten Island, NY 10314

122 Business Park Drive, Suite 4
Utica, NY 13502

18564 US Route 11, Suite 7
Watertown, NY 13601

Cross West Office Center
399 Knollwood Road, Suite 218
White Plains, NY 10603

Centerpointe Corporate Park
325 Essjay Road, Suite 104
Williamsville, NY 14221

North Carolina

One Town Square
One Town Square Blvd., Suite 350
Asheville, NC 28803

4601 Charlotte Park Drive, Suite 340
Charlotte, NC 28217

1105 Corporate Drive, Suite B
Greenville, NC 27858

8024 Glenwood Avenue, Suite 106
Raleigh, NC 27612

Market Street Central
2709 Market Street, Suite 206
Wilmington, NC 28405

Stratford Oaks
514 S. Stratford Road, Knollwood Level
Winston-Salem, NC 27104

North Dakota

Kirkwood Office Tower
919 S. 7th Street, Suite 400
Bismarck, ND 58504

1150 Prairie Parkway, Suite 103
West Fargo, ND 58078

Northern Mariana Islands

Del Sol Building
Suite 102, P.O. Box 505140
Saipan 96950

Ohio

Springside Center
231 Springside Drive, Suite 125
Akron, OH 44333

3201 Enterprise Parkway, Suite 10, Basement
Beachwood, OH 44122

11300 Cornell Park Drive, Suite 140
Cincinnati, OH 45242

355 E. Campus View Blvd., Suite 140
Columbus, OH 43235

Imperial Plaza Office Building
1129 Miamisburg-Centerville Road, Suite 203
Dayton, OH 45449

OffiCenter 2
700 Taylor Road, Suite 180
Gahanna, OH 43230

Metro Woods Building
1789 Indian Wood Circle, Suite 120
Maumee, OH 43537

2001 Crocker Road, Suite 350
Westlake, OH 44145

Oklahoma

5100 N. Brookline, Suite 282
Oklahoma City, OK 73112

7136 South Yale
Executive Center I, Suite 418
Tulsa, OK 74136

Oregon

Park Plaza West, Building 3
10700 SW Beaverton Hillsdale Hwy, Suite 595
Beaverton, OR 97005

3560 Excel Drive, Suite 105
Medford, OR 97504

The VA Outpatient Clinic Building
1660 Oak Street SE, Suite 250
Salem, OR 97301

Pennsylvania

Commerce Corporate Center II
5100 W. Tilghman Street, Suite B-30
Allentown, PA 18104

Edgewood Plaza Place
3123 West 12th Street, Suite D
Erie, PA 16505

801 East Park Drive, Suite 101
Harrisburg, PA 17111

Pennsylvania Business Campus
110 Gibraltar Road, Suite 227
Horsham, PA 19044

205 Granite Run Drive, Suite 130
Lancaster, PA 17601

1800 John F Kennedy (JFK) Blvd., 10th Floor,
 Suite 1001
Philadelphia, PA 19103

Digital Place Office Complex
1500 Ardmore Blvd., Suite 401
Pittsburgh, PA 15221

2 Penn Center Blvd.
Penn Center Blvd. & Campbell's Run Road
Building 2, Suite 109
Pittsburgh, PA 15276

Stadium Office Park
330 Montage Mountain Road, Suite 102
Scranton, PA 18507

Valley Forge Office Center
530 E. Swedesford Road, Suite 109
Wayne, PA 19087

Puerto Rico

Plaza Scotiabank
273 Ponce de Leon Avenue, Suite 501
San Juan, PR 00917

Rhode Island

301 Metro Center Blvd., Suite 103
Warwick, RI 02886

South Carolina

Westpark Center II Building
107 Westpark Blvd., Suite 170
Columbia, SC 29210

Halton Commons Office Park
301 Halton Road, Suite D1
Greenville, SC 29606

Rivergate Center II
4975 LaCrosse Road, Suite 255
North Charleston, SC 29406

South Dakota

VanBuskirk Office Building
5101 South Nevada Avenue, Suite 130
Sioux Falls, SD 57108

Tennessee

Franklin Building
5726 Marlin Road, Suite 310
Chattanooga, TN 37411

Sun Trust Bank Building
207 Mockingbird Lane, Suite 401
Johnson City, TN 37604

Keystone Center
135 Fox Road, Suite C
Knoxville, TN 37922

6060 Poplar Avenue, Suite LL01
Memphis, TN 38119

Riverview Building
545 Mainstream Drive, Suite 410
Nashville, TN 37228

Texas

500 Chestnut Street, Suite 856
Abilene, TX 79602

1616 S. Kentucky, Suite C305
Amarillo, TX 79102

South Park One
1701 Directors Blvd., Suite 350
Austin, TX 78744

BBVA Compass Building
301 Congress Avenue, Suite 565
Austin, Texas 78701

Prosperity Bank Building
6800 West Loop S., Suite 405
Bellaire, TX 77401

Corona South Building
4646 Corona Drive, Suite 175
Corpus Christi, TX 78411

12801 North Central Expressway, Suite 820
Dallas, TX 75243

4110 Rio Bravo Drive, Suite 222
El Paso, TX 79902

14425 Torrey Chase Blvd., Suite 240
Houston, TX 77014

8876 Gulf Freeway Building
8876 Gulf Freeway, Suite 220
Houston, TX 77017

500 Grapevine Highway, Suite 401
Hurst, TX 76054

Wells Fargo Center
1500 Broadway Street, Suite 1113
Lubbock, TX 79401

Building 4
3300 North A Street, Suite 228
Midland, TX 79705

Stonewater Tower West
6100 Bandera Road, Suite 407
San Antonio, TX 78238

10000 San Pedro, Suite 175
San Antonio, TX 78216

One America Center
909 East Southeast Loop 323, Suite 625
Tyler, TX 75701

Wells Fargo Bank Building
1105 Wooded Acres Drive, Suite 406
Waco, TX 76710

Utah

Draper Technology Center
11734 Election Road, Suite 180
Draper, UT 84020

Business Depot Ogden
1150 South Depot Drive, Suite 130
Ogden, UT 84404

Vermont

30 Kimball, Suite 202
South Burlington, VT 05403

Virginia

Graves Mill Office Park
424 Graves Mill Road, Suite 200-A
Lynchburg, VA 24502

825 Diligence Drive, Suite 120
Newport News, VA 23606

3900 Westerre Parkway, Suite 202
Richmond, VA 23233

Northpark Business Center
6701 Peters Creek Road, Suite 108
Roanoke, VA 24019

8391 Old Courthouse Road, Suite 201
Vienna, VA 22182

Virgin Islands

Nisky Center, Suite 730 East Wing
St. Thomas, VI 00802

Washington

Oaksdale Center
1300 SW 7th Street, Suite 113
Renton, WA 98055

10700 Meridian Avenue North, Suite 407
Seattle, WA 98133

Mullan Centre
1410 N. Mullan Road, Suite 203
Spokane Valley, WA 99206

1701 Creekside Loop, Suite 110
Yakima, WA 98902

West Virginia

BB&T Square
300 Summers Street, Suite 430
Charleston, WV 25301

The Jackson & Kelly Building
150 Clay Street, Suite 420
Morgantown, WV 26505

Wisconsin

Bishops Woods Centre
13555 Bishops Court, Suite L10
Brookfield, WI 53005

3610 Oakwood Mall Drive, Suite 102
Eau Claire, WI 54701

Johnson Bank Building
7500 Green Bay Road, Suite 311
Kenosha, WI 53142

Prairie Trail Office Suites II
8517 Excelsior Drive, Suite 202
Madison, WI 53717

Wyoming

Aspen Creek
800 Werner Court, Suite 310
Casper, WY 82601

INTERNATIONAL EXAMINATION SITES

Australia

Level 6 , 287 Elizabeth Street
Sydney, New South Wales 2000

Canada

Commerce Court Building
4190 Lougheed Hwy, Suite 103
Burnaby, British Columbia V5C 6A8
Canada

21 St. Clair Avenue East, Suite 501
Toronto, Ontario M4T 1L9
Canada

7705 17th Avenue
Montreal, Quebec H2A 2S4
Canada

Hong Kong

Grand Millenium Plaza
Room 503, 5th Floor
181 Queen's Road, Central
Hong Kong

India

Pochampalli House, 1-10-72/A/2, 3rd Floor
S P Road, Begumpet,
Hyderabad, Andhra Pradesh 500016
India

Yousuf Sarai Community Centre
4th Floor, Building 18, Ramnath House
New Delhi, Delhi 110049
India

Trade Center, 3rd Floor, # 45
Dickenson Road
Bangalore, Karnataka 560042
India

Building 9, 1st Floor
Solitaire Corporate Park, 167 Andheri
J B Nagar Link Rd., Chakala, Andheri (East)
Mumbai, Maharashtra 400093
India

6th Floor, Nelson Chambers, E Block,
115, Nelson Manickam Road,
Aminijikarai,
Chennai, Tamil Nadu 600 029
India

Japan

12F Osaka Dai-Ichi Seimei Bldg,
1-8-17 Umeda
Kita-ku
Osaka-shi, Osaka 530-0001
Japan

4th Floor, Kojimachi Shimura Building
4-1-5, Kojimachi,
Chiyoda-ku, Tokyo 102-0083
Japan

Mexico

Industrial Atoto
Atlacomulco 500, 4th Floor
Naucalpan, Estado de Mexico 53519
Mexico City, Distrito Federal
Mexico

Philippines

Trident Tower, 27th Floor
312 Senator Gil Puyat Avenue,
Makati City,
Manila 1227
Philippines

Taiwan

12F-3, No 163
Sec. 1 Keelung Road,
Union Century Building
Taipei
Taiwan

United Kingdom

190 High Holborn
London WC1V 7BH
United Kingdom

INTERNET RESOURCES

INTERNET PORTALS

Because Web addresses tend to change, and listings on the Internet are frequently added or deleted, it is necessary to verify and update these listings periodically. The websites listed below provide annotated, searchable databases, including direct hyperlinks, to sites of interest. These websites also contain additional resources not mentioned in this book:

- American Nurses Association *nursingworld.org*
- Cybernurse *cybernurse.com*
- Google *directory.google.com/Top/Health/Nursing*
- Medi-Smart Resource Directory *medi-smart.com*
- Lippincott's Nursing Center *nursingcenter.com*
- Ultimate Nurse *ultimatenurse.com*
- Welch Web Subject Guides *welch.jhu.edu/internet/nursing.html* This is the Johns Hopkins University site for nurses and includes links to MEDLINE and CINAHL, in addition to many other useful sites.

CLINICAL NURSING RESOURCES

Internet Portals

Use the following websites to select the clinical resources most useful to you. A sampling of what they have to offer appears below:

- The National Library of Medicine Gateway to the U.S. National Library of Medicine and National Institutes of Health
  http://gateway.nlm.nih.gov/gw/Cmd?Overview.x
- Nursing Spectrum/NurseWeek *nurse.com*

Additional Websites

- Auscultation Assistant (hear actual heart and breath sounds) *wilkes.med.ucla.edu/intro.html*

- Cumulative Index to Nursing and Allied Health Literature (CINAHL) *ebscohost.com/cinahl/*

- 2010 Edition Delmar Nurse's Drug Handbook Online Database *nursespdr.com*

- Online Journal of Issues in Nursing *nursingworld.org/ojin*

- PDA cortex listservs *pdacortex.com/listserv.htm* Listservs, newsgroups, and electronic newsletters, including listserv communities with a nursing-specific link for those using personal digital assistants (PDAs).

- PubMed *ncbi.nlm.nih.gov/pubmed*

HEALTHCARE ASSOCIATIONS AND GOVERNMENT ORGANIZATIONS

- American Academy of Pediatrics *aap.org*
- American Diabetic Association *diabetes.org*
- American Heart Association *americanheart.org/HEARTORG/*
- American Hospital Association *aha.org*
- American Medical Association *ama-assn.org*
- American Psychiatric Association *psych.org*
- American Psychological Association *apa.org*
- American Public Health Association *apha.org*
- American Red Cross *redcross.org*
- Centers for Disease Control and Prevention (CDC) *cdc.gov*
- Health Insurance Portability and Accountability Act *cms.gov/HIPAAGenInfo/01_Overview.asp*
- The Joint Commission *jointcommission.org*
- Mayo Clinic *mayoclinic.com*
- National Institutes of Health *nih.gov*
- Office of Advancement of Telehealth *hrsa.gov/telehealth*
- To check the status of pending or passed legislation *nursingworld.org/MainMenuCategories/ANAPoliticalPower.aspx*
- U.S. Department of Health and Human Services *healthfinder.gov*
- U.S. Department of Labor Bureau of Labor Statistics Occupational Outlook Handbook (published annually) *stats.bls.gov/oco/ocos102.htm*
- U.S. Food and Drug Administration *fda.gov*
- World Health Organization *who.int*

ANCC Magnet Status Health Organizations

Healthcare organizations granted Magnet status have characteristics and outcomes that are positive for clients, nurses, and employers. In these organizations, client satisfaction is high, with shorter lengths of stay; nursing satisfaction is high, with nurses reporting more control over their nursing practice; employers report lower burnout rates and an enhanced ability to attract and retain nurses. To find out if a hospital in your area is a magnet facility, visit: *www.nursecredentialing.org/Magnet/FindaMagnetFacility.aspx*

CAREER MANAGEMENT

Employment

- Monster.com *monster.com*
- Nursing Jobs at Nurse.com *nurse.com/Jobs*
- The New York Times *jobmarket.nytimes.com/pages/jobs*

Resumes and Cover Letters

- Career Journal *jobstar.org*
- Kaplan Career Center *kaptest.com*
- Monster.com *career-advice.monster.com/*

Interview Assistance

- Monster.com *career-advice.monster.com/*

Job Fairs

- *http://jobsearch.about.com/od/jobfairs/a/jobfairtips.htm*

SELF-CARE AND STRESS MANAGEMENT RESOURCES

These additional websites are specific to stress management and contain long lists of hyperlinks:

- Caring for the Nurse *care-nurse.com*
- Holistic-Online.com *holistic-online.com/stress/stress_home.htm*
- Rx for Sanity *rxforsanity.com*
- Stress Management and Nursing Burnout Prevention *medi-smart.com/nursing-articles/tips-for-first-year-nurses/stress-management-and-nursing-burnout*
- Stress Virtual Library *vl-site.org/stress/index.html*

INDEX

Note: "f" following page number indicates figure.

nursing assistants, 89
nursing communication, U.S.-style, 132–134
nursing interventions, types of, 15
nursing practice, in United States, 131–132
nursing process, 14–16
    data collection, 14
    evaluation, 17–16
    implementation, 15–16
    planning, 14–15
    strategy for priority questions, 73–77
nursing school exam questions
    compared to NCLEX-PN® questions, 21–24
    example of, 21
nursing terminology, 235–239

O

ordered response question *see* drag-and-drop
    question/ordered response question
outcomes, expected, 15, 47–49

P

Pearson Professional Centers, offering NCLEX-
    PN® exam, 267–276
pharmacological therapies, 12
    example of questions on, 12
    nursing actions included within, 12
    overview of subcategory, 12
    percentage of questions on, 12
physician, notifying, as answer choice, 63–64
physiological adaptation, 13
    example of questions on, 13
    overview of subcategory, 13
    percentage of questions on exam, 13
physiological integrity, overview of category, 11–13
planning
    as part of nursing process, 14–15
    example of questions on, 15
    steps in, 15
positioning questions, strategies, 93–98
positioning, critical path diagram, 93*f*
positions
    dorsal recumbent, 98
    elevation of extremity, 98
    essential to know, 98

feet and legs elevated, 98
    Fowler's, 98
    knee-chest, 98
    lithotomy, 98
    modified Trendelenburg, 98
    prone, 98
    side lateral, 98
    Sims', 98
    supine (flat), 98
    Trendelenburg, 98
practice test, 149–172
practice test answer key, 175
practice test answers and explanations, 177–229
practice test scores, understanding, 173
priority questions
    Maslow strategy, 69–73
    nursing process (data collection vs. implement)
        strategy, 73–77
    strategies for, 67–83
prone position, 98
psychosocial integrity, 10–11
    example of questions on, 11
    nursing actions included within, 10–11
    overview of category, 10–11
    percentage of questions on, 10

Q

R

real-world nursing, vs. NCLEX-PN® exam, 55–65
real-world strategy, critical path diagram, 56*f*
recall/recognition, level of question in nursing test,
    21
reduction of risk potential, 12–13
    example of questions on, 13
    nursing actions included within, 12
    overview of subcategory, 12–13
    percentage of questions on, 12
reflecting, using as therapeutic response, 99
registered nurse (RN), 85–92
    scope of practice/roles, 88
    coordination with LPNs/LVNs, 88
registration process, NCLEX-PN®, 112–113
rescheduling, NCLEX-PN® exam, 115–116

knowledge-based, example 21
levels in nursing tests, illustration of, 21*f*
multiple-choice, 36–54
on communication, 99–103
on coordination of care, 7–8, 85–92
on positioning, 93–98
on priority, 68–83
rewording, 39–41
sample U.S.-style communication, 135–143
select all that apply, 29, 30–31, 118,119
test taker
becoming better, 25–27
successful, characteristics of, 25
unsuccessful, characteristics of, 25–26
therapeutic communications, 99–101
therapeutic responses, examples of, 99
TOEFL®, 130
Kaplan programs for, 145–146
TOEIC® test program, 131
Trendelenburg position, 98
TSE®, 130
TWE®, 130

U

UAP *see* unlicensed assistive personnel
understanding/comprehension, level of question, 21*f*, 22
United States, nursing practice in, 131–132
United States, style of nursing communication, 132–134
unlicensed assistive personnel (UAP), 85, 88, 89, 92

V

visas, work, 131
visualization, as mental preparation technique, 109–110
vocabulary, and international nurses, 144

W

"why", in communication question answer choices, 100
work visas, 131